Historical Atlas of

DERMATOLOGY AND
DERMATOLOGISTS

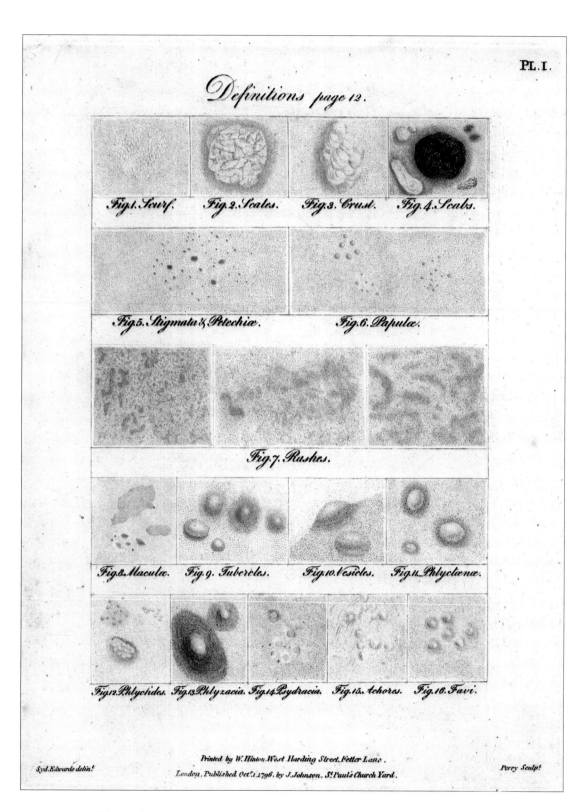

Plate 1 from Robert Willan's "On cutaneous diseases," London, 1808.

Historical Atlas of DERMATOLOGY AND DERMATOLOGISTS

John Thorne Crissey, M.D.

Clinical Professor of Medicine (Dermatology), Keck School of Medicine,
University of Southern California, Los Angeles, California
Attending Dermatologist, Los Angeles County-University of Southern California
Medical Center, Los Angeles, California

Lawrence Charles Parish, M.D.

Clinical Professor of Dermatology and Cutaneous Biology, and Director of
the Jefferson Center for International Dermatology, Jefferson Medical College,
Thomas Jefferson University, Philadelphia, Pennsylvania

and

Karl Holubar, M.D., F.R.C.P.

Professor of Dermatology and of the History of Medicine, Institute for the
History of Medicine, University of Vienna, Vienna, Austria

The Parthenon Publishing Group
International Publishers in Medicine, Science & Technology

A CRC PRESS COMPANY
BOCA RATON   LONDON   NEW YORK   WASHINGTON, D.C.

**Library of Congress
Cataloging-in-Publication Data**
Data available on request

**British Library Cataloguing
in Publication Data**
Crissey, John Thorne
  Historical atlas of dermatology and dermatologists
  1. Dermatologists 2. Dermatology - History
  I. Title II. Parish, Lawrence Charles III. Holubar, Karl
  616.5'00922

  ISBN 1-84214-100-7

Published in the USA by
The Parthenon Publishing Group
345 Park Avenue South
10th Floor
New York, NY 10010, USA

Published in the UK and Europe by
The Parthenon Publishing Group
23–25 Blades Court, Deodar Road
London SW15 2NU, UK

Copyright © 2002 The Parthenon Publishing Group

Printed and bound by Bookcraft (Bath) Ltd.,
Midsomer Norton, UK

CONTENTS

PREFACE

This is an atlas; the pictures are the thing. Most of them came from our own private libraries; all three of us have been compulsive collectors for many years. Others were generously contributed by donors from all over the Western World, and a significant number were extracted from the magnificent resources of the University of Vienna Institute for the History of Medicine. Many have never been published before.

Space constraints effectively defeated any attempt at completeness, especially in sections dealing with the heavily populated dermatologic landscape of more recent times. We have tried to select individuals representative of each era, workers who dealt seriously with the dermatologic concerns of the day, or who through their opinions or behavior project the color and ambience of the period in which they lived. We have also included typical examples of the books, journals, instruments, and devices that made up the annals and paraphernalia of the specialty as it evolved. The texts accompanying each image represent attempts at *molto in parvo* exposition, summing up the nature, significance, or purpose of the image. The entire work is arranged as a sort of illustrated time line, moving from early to late.

We wish to thank Drs. Vincent Afsahi, Joaquin Calap Calatayud, Stella Fatovic-Ferencic, Thomas Fitzpatrick, Roy Forsey, Irwin Freedberg, Arnold Gurevitch, Robert Jackson, Stephen Kurtin, Willard Marmelzat, Thomas Rea, Albrecht Scholz, Gerard Tilles, Daniel Wallach, Wolfgang Weyers, Joseph Witkowski, David T. Woodley, and John Yarborough for their help in supplying pictures, tracking down elusive bits and sources of information, or checking for errors. The comments, suggestions, and personal experiences of these individuals also provided valuable information on the proper route to follow to get from here to there.

The library of the late Dr. Max Wolf and his wife Margareta has been most helpful in the preparation of this work.

John Thorne Crissey, M.D.

Lawrence Charles Parish, M.D.

Karl Holubar, M.D., F.R.C.P.

August, 2001

INTRODUCTION

Protodermatology. From the Egypt of the Pharaohs to the Renaissance, literature, both lay and medical, is dotted with isolated descriptions of skin, hair and nail problems. This atlas begins with several examples. The earliest known attempt to consider these problems as a group is to be found in a section of the general medical treatise "De Medicina" of the Roman writer Celsus. A few of the entities he described two thousand years ago are recognizable even now – alopecia areata, furunculosis, and kerion, for example. Most are not.

In the "De Morbis Cutaneis," of Mercurialis, the first book devoted entirely to the subject, we find a more focused attempt to name and classify skin diseases. The work, which appeared in 1572, is a transcription of a set of lectures designed for medical students, and from it one suspects there may have been more to 16th century dermatology than meets the eye. It is difficult to believe that these lectures, with their profusion of disease names and treatment recommendations, could have been delivered, accepted, and committed to print if Mercurialis were unable in some way to demonstrate in the clinic or at the bedside the proper diagnostic category in which to place the eruptions observed. Unfortunately, the baroque terminology, inadequate disease descriptions, and constant immersion of the text in Galenical fancies reduce our understanding of the majority of the conditions considered to the level of speculation.

The fascinating works of Daniel Turner, Anne-Charles Lorry, and Josef Von Plenck – the "protodermatologists" of 18th century – also suffer from descriptive imprecision and Galenical overkill. In his "Doctrina de Morbis Cutaneis" (1778) Plenck, for example, lists 114 diseases or affections of skin, hair, and nails, most described in two or three sentences. Included are 8 types of herpes (not one of which is vesicular), 6 varieties of aphthae, 10 erythemas, and 7 kinds of scabies. Number 7 in the scabies list, he believed, might be associated with worms or mites.

Whatever the limitations of these earlier writers, by the end of the 18th century there existed a limited but substantial clinical database of skin diseases, adequately described or striking enough in appearance to constitute a recognizable part of the everyday experience of physicians and the general public alike. Vitiligo, scrofuloderma, elephantiasis, smallpox, measles, erysipelas, warts, favus, cutaneous horns, and furunculosis are typical representatives of this group. For the great mass of eruptions, however, chaos prevailed. The various forms of "eczema," the majority of the papulo-squamous eruptions, the vesiculo-bullous diseases, the ringworms, the syphilids, and the manifestations of scabies, for example, were lumped together or subdivided arbitrarily in the medical works of the time. These conditions were considered loosely under a variety of names, herpes, dartres, tetters, lichens, impetigines, and the like, none of which was satisfactorily defined. Despite these deficiencies, the texts of the time contain little in the way of complaints, apologies, or expressions of disappointment over the woeful state of the arts in dermatologic matters. They sail along instead under the apparent assumption that the readers would already be familiar with many of the conditions named, and properly instructed by the author with respect to the rest.

Complaints began in earnest at the end of the eighteenth century and the beginning of the nineteenth, and the number one complainer was the Yorkshire Englishman, Robert Willan. A highly educated physician and scholar, Willan reviewed the entire dermatologic literature with a critical eye, credited the "Ancients" with some success in describing those dermatologic conditions so striking in appearance they could hardly be missed, and took his contemporaries and immediate predecessors severely to task for their shortcomings in handling the subject. They misinterpreted the writings of the Ancients, he charged, and formulated patently artificial arrangements in which they crowded everything into 2 or 3 categories or multiplied endlessly the number of skin diseases by applying new names to different stages or minor variations in the same condition. Some, he continued, generated fuzzy speculations on pathogenesis and cause as well, and constructed equally fuzzy classification schemes in accordance with these speculations. The proper characterization of the individual entities caught up in this tangle was one of the major achievements of the dermatology of the nineteenth century, and it was greatly facilitated by

the meticulous work of the English master.

An Era of Disease Description and Classification (1776–1850). Robert Willan did more than complain. Working in general medicine at the Public Dispensary in London, he became interested in skin diseases. As early as 1784 he began to sketch and make notes on the eruptions he encountered. His interest intensified, and for the first time a physician with access to significant numbers of cutaneous problems actually scrutinized the lesions with the express purpose of recording every variation in configuration, color, and arrangement. When he had accumulated a large amount of morphologic information of this sort and correlated it at the same time with other signs and symptoms, he defined and named a large set of skin diseases, some new and some old, and looked for a way to classify them in an appropriate manner. He found it in the work of Josef Von Plenck who, a generation earlier, had classified his rag tag collection of skin problems according to the type of lesion that predominated – vesicles, pustules, and the like. Willan adopted Plenck's idea, reduced the categories from 14 to 9, and presented his findings in a masterwork entitled "On cutaneous diseases, Part 1," which appeared in sections from 1798 to 1808. The clarity of the disease presentations in the book and the usefulness of diagnostic tools provided by the lesion definitions brought a measure of order to the field of skin diseases where previously chaos had reigned. The value of the work was further enhanced by the inclusion of 33 hand colored copper plate engravings depicting the diseases described. Plate 1 in the collection illustrates Willan's conception of what we now call the essential or elementary lesions. It is reproduced as the frontispiece to this atlas, and because of the power and utility of the idea it represents, could well be considered the most important dermatologic illustration ever published.

Willan died before he could finish Part 2 of "On cutaneous diseases." His friend and pupil, Thomas Bateman, completed the work and published the whole as "A practical synopsis of cutaneous diseases according to the arrangement of Dr. Willan." (1813). Four years later, Bateman gathered together all of Willan's plates and added a few of his own, including the first picture of molluscum contagiosum, which disease he himself had been the first to describe. He published the collection as "Delineations of cutaneous disease." These three works – the Willan text and the Bateman synopsis and atlas – subsequently altered completely the way physicians of the time found their way step by step to a proper dermatologic diagnosis. Examine the eruption carefully, they were instructed; identify the essential lesions; consult a Willanist text for the diseases that produce such lesions, and immediately your differential diagnostic list will be reduced to manageable size. The method, much modified of course, is still in use today. The successful inauguration of the concept in "On cutaneous diseases" has earned Willan the title "the Father of Modern Dermatology." It is a title well deserved.

Across the channel, the brilliant, flamboyant Frenchman, Baron Jean Louis Alibert, approached the same problems in quite another way. Originally intended for the Church, Alibert was freed up by the French Revolution. He turned to medicine, and shortly after graduation in 1799, was placed in charge of l'Hôpital Saint Louis in Paris. The post was not the most desirable. In contrast to its later preeminence in dermatology, St. Louis was at the time a suburban repository for rejects from the more centrally located hospitals of Paris, including large numbers of cutaneous disasters. Alibert saw in this "uncharted ocean of disease" (his own phrase) a route to fame and fortune, and he took full advantage of his opportunity. By 1806 he had seen and catalogued enough cutaneous pathology to publish a gigantic and beautifully illustrated work on skin diseases, and the teaching clinic he founded had become so popular it had to be moved outdoors to accommodate the crowds of physicians who came from all over the world to attend. Alibert's own description of his clinic dwells on the kindness of the nuns who brought the patients to the stage to be demonstrated, and the wonderful results obtained in healing the sick and instructing the physicians who attended. A hyper-romantic painting of the clinic in progress hangs now in the city hall in Alibert's hometown, Villefranche de Rouergue. In it the master is caught and preserved forever in a saviour-like pose, surrounded by admiring assistants and by patients who look like siblings of Lazarus.

The conduct of the clinic was not in fact so decorous as Alibert and his artist would have us believe. Three days a week Alibert arrived in his magnificent equipage and took his place on the stage. Dressed in satin knee britches and Napoleonic hat he strode back and forth vigorously exchanging quips with the patients. His speech, exceptionally fluent, bubbled with simile and metaphor. A syphilitic prostitute became "a priestess of Venus wounded by a perfidious dart of love." Patients were placed on display with the names of their disorders in letters two inches high inked on placards placed across their chests. Paintings of diseases were hung from the trees, and bold theatrics were employed to get the message across. To impress the spectators with the amount of scale in exfoliative dermatitis, for example, Alibert suddenly dumped a boxful, fresh from the wards, on the occupants of the front row seats. It was a hit show, and it ran for years.

Alibert was assisted at Saint Louis by Laurent Biett, a Swiss dermatologist who trained with the Baron and resided permanently in Paris. The two men were great friends. As sharp and shrewd an observer as any physician of the era, Biett was a rising star in his own right. His clinics at Saint Louis, although less theatrical than those of his teacher, were well attended and much admired. When the Bourbons returned to power in France, Alibert was appointed to the post of personal physician to King Louis XVIII and was continually preoccupied with the royal health from 1814 until the death of the king in 1824. On returning to his dermatologic teaching, Alibert made an unpleasant discovery. Biett, whom he had left in charge, had been to England, had brought back the Willan system, and had installed it at St. Louis. Alibert himself had classified and named skin diseases on the basis of a whole series of shared signs and symptoms. He was appalled at what he considered the superficiality of Willan's morphologic approach, and deeply wounded at Biett's perceived betrayal. He wrapped himself in mystery, surrounded himself with scholars, and announced that a thorough refutation of the whole Willan business would be forthcoming. Tension mounted when Biett announced that a rebuttal would follow shortly. It was the warm, romantic, Catholic, French extrovert against the cool, scientific, protestant Swiss introvert. The day was cold when Alibert chose to make his stand, but the clinic was crowded, and Alibert gave the speech of his life, unveiling at the climax, and to tumultuous applause, two huge paintings of his new system – his tree of dermatoses – trunk, branches, twigs representing interrelationships of the various diseases as he saw them. His triumph was short lived. A few days later, before the very same audience, Biett calmy uprooted the newly planted tree, and clearly demonstrated the superiority of the Willan system. This confrontation was merely the first in the long struggle in dermatology to come to terms with the question of the relationship of the skin to the total corpus. There were to be further confrontations in the future.

Alibert is remembered now, not for his impractical classification system, nor even for the many diseases he was the first to describe – mycosis fungoides, keloids, cutaneous leismaniasis, and more. His fame rests properly on his organization of the first great dermatologic training center and on his dynamic approach to teaching. The zest, the élan and éclat he brought to the subject focused the attention of the medical world on the diseases of the skin to an unprecedented degree. The potent combination of Alibertian spirit and the eminently practical approach of Robert Willan served as a source of inspiration to a talented group of young physicians in the next generation, who embraced the study of the skin and its problems with enthusiasm, and dermatology as a specialty came into its own.

Willan, Bateman, Alibert, and selected plates from their atlases, are all on display in the pages of our own atlas, along with Biett and the famous tree of dermatoses.

Thanks largely to the fame of Alibert and the presence of l'Hôpital Saint Louis, Paris was clearly the number one dermatolgic center in the early decades of the nineteenth century. It was the home of a hard working, contentious, observant cadre of men known as the French Willanists. They were influenced in varying degrees by the teachings of Biett. Included in the group were Pierre-François-Olive Rayer, Pierre-Louis-Alphée Cazenave, Camille Gibert, and Alphonse Devergie. All are noted in the pages of this atlas. These men busied themselves with the refinement of Willan's list of essential lesions. They picked through the English master's roster of skin diseases as well, confirming the valid, rejecting the spurious, renaming many, and adding new discoveries of their own. By the time their stars began to fade at the halfway mark of the century, they had assembled a solid collection of cutaneous diseases that corresponded to reality far better than any that had gone before.

The development of a dermatologic language and the meticulous characterization and description of all the eruptions in terms that everyone could understand – those were the goals of Willan and his Willanist successors. These individuals saw the delineation and separation of clinical patterns for diagnostic purposes as the very first order of business, a task that had to be completed before any further progress could be made. Camille Gibert went to the heart of the matter in the following sentences, which date from 1839. His purpose in writing them was to chastise Pierre Baumès of Lyon, who had classified skin diseases on the basis of a set of causes invisible to everyone else:

Doubtless the considerations of cause and of nature are of the highest importance for the practitioner; doubtless M. Baumès has given proofs of his clinical experience and philosophy by endeavoring to place them prominently forward, but let us beware of forgetting that we must first learn how to recognize the evil before we can undertake its cure.

The dermatologists of this period were not oblivious to questions of pathogenesis and cause. They simply did not have the tools to investigate these matters in any significant way. It should be noted, however, that as the result of the skill with which they and their clinical successors practiced their arts, those who later came into possession of the proper tools had the inestimable advantage of being able to work with reasonably homogeneous groups of patients with diseases genuinely *sui generis.*

Mainstream European dermatology in the latter half of the 19th century. Ferdinand von Hebra and his students Moriz Kaposi, Isidor Neumann, Heinrich Auspitz, and Phillip Joseph Pick at the University of Vienna Medical School, comprised without question the most talented and inventive dermatologic team at the middle and three quarter marks of the nineteenth century. All these individuals are on display in the pages that follow. Together they made quantum leaps in clinical descriptive precision and tied clinically observed morphology in with the new discoveries in pathology – first gross, later microscopic. Hebra himself laid the groundwork for experimental dermatology in a series of experiments in which he painted croton oil and other irritants on normal skin to produce "artificial eczema" – his term for primary irritation contact dermatitis. The members of the Vienna school also welcomed enthusiastically the new discoveries in mycology, and later bacteriology, and applied them successfully to the study of skin diseases. From the 1850s to the onset of World War I, these men, the clinics they conducted, and the forums they sponsored, attracted students in great numbers from every part of the globe.

British dermatology followed a different path. Erasmus Wilson and William Tilbury Fox were the dominant figures in the middle decades of the century. Fox died young; Wilson lived a long and productive life. He wrote the era's most successful textbook in English and published an enormously popular work for the general public on the care of the skin that did a great deal to acquaint the man and woman in the street with the fact that skin specialists existed and were available for consultation. He also published the first journal in English devoted to dermatology, was the first to describe a number of skin diseases, including lichen planus, and annoyed his colleagues by his propensity for loudly sounding his personal trumpet.

The stubborn opposition of the nineteenth century British medical establishment to specialization, along with the failure to establish training centers comparable to l'Hôpital St. Louis and the Viennese Allgemeines Krankenhaus, delayed the development of British dermatology beyond clinical concerns. Nevertheless, the continuous development of stubbornly independent,

practical dermatologists who were subject neither to the pressures of institutional pecking rows nor to rigid systems of thought imposed from higher up, resulted in a great many refreshing observations on skin diseases that had escaped notice of the anointed at the grand institutions on the Continent. Members of the late century group known as "the big five" are representative of the type. The most prominent among them was Henry Radcliffe-Crocker, but he shared the limelight with Henry Grundy Brooke, Thomas Colcott Fox, John James Pringle, and Malcolm Morris. Joining them in many endeavors was the extraordinarily gifted and versatile sometime dermatologist, Jonathan Hutchinson. All these individuals grace the pages of our atlas.

Dermatology in mid-nineteenth century France followed a path uniquely its own. Ernest Bazin and Alfred Hardy had been installed as the dominant dermatologists at l'Hôpital St. Louis. True students of Alibert, and trained as internists, they decried the morphologic approach of the French Willanists, which they considered a pernicious disregard of the obvious relationship of skin lesions to disturbances in the organism as a whole. To these men there were few if any "skin diseases;" all lesions were manifestations of diatheses or constitutional diseases. With respect to two of their favorites, syphilis and the tuberculous diathesis, they were on reasonably firm ground, but the rest of their creations – arthritism, herpetism, and the like – had no basis in reality. Their outspoken rejection of the morphologic approach generated an equally intense reaction on the part of the French Willanists and resulted in a notorious series of heated quarrels in print. Alphonse Devergie, chief spokesman for the Willanists, charged that the work of Bazin and Hardy "introduced prejudice into science, diverted students from the studies necessary to prepare them for practice, substituted dreams and figments of the imagination for good sound observation, and hypothesized the hypothetical to the point where all of the past has been destroyed and nothing new established in its place." The fur flew. These debates were not merely examples of quarrelsome French professors at each other's throats; they were in fact salutary dialectics essential to a more flexible and sensible conception of the relation of outer skin to inner self.

Ernest Besnier, successor to Bazin at l'Hôpital St. Louis, swept away the diathetic turgidity later in the century and elevated French dermatology once more to parity with the specialty as it existed in Germany and Austria. He was amply assisted in this task by an outstanding group of inventive, industrious colleagues that included Émile Vidal, Charles Lailler, Adrien Doyon, Jean-LouisBrocq, Jean Darier, and Raymond Sabouraud, all of whom appear later in this atlas.

In the late decades of the nineteenth century and the early years of the twentieth, German dermatologists came to the fore, particularly the dynamic collection of individuals associated with centers in Breslau, Berlin, and Hamburg. Many appear in the pages of this atlas.

Albert Neisser, chairman of the department of dermatology at Breslau, demonstrated his talent for investigative work early in his career; in 1879, at the age of 24, he identified the gonococcus as the cause of gonorrhea. He devoted most of his professional life to intensive research on every aspect of syphilis, which disease was the scourge of Europe at the time. He was the co-author with August Wassermann of the 1906 classic report on the complement fixation test for the disease. Neisser's laboratory became a Mecca for research minded dermatologists from everywhere. Thirty-four of his trainees later became directors of university skin clinics and dermatological departments of large teaching hospitals.

The dermatology of nineteenth century *fin de siècle* Berlin, with its mixture of university-based and private or "polyclinic" facilities staffed by adventurous dermatologists willing to step over the then accepted boundaries of the specialty, has a distinctly modern flavor. On the traditional side, the university clinic of Edmund Lesser was the site of the momentous 1905 demonstration by Fritz Schaudinn and Erich Hoffmann that a spirochete is the cause of syphilis. Less conventional were the activities of that restless experimenter, Heinrich Koebner, who founded the city's first true polyclinic, a private outpatient facility that was something new for Germany, although Auspitz had opened a similar facility earlier in Vienna. More freewheeling, even radical, were the Berlin dermatologists Edmund Saalfeld and Ernst Kromayer, pioneers in the development of cosmetic dermatologic surgical procedures. Kromayer in particular defied convention to the maximum, combining an ostentatious and luxurious life style with the revolutionary politics of the hard German Left.

Paul Gerson Unna, pupil of Hebra and Auspitz, and Hyperion of the independent dermatologists, set up in a suburb of Hamburg the ultimate in private facilities. He called it the Dermatologikum, and within its walls conducted the sort of clinical, research, and teaching activities that would ordinarily be associated with the dermatology department of a university center. His true forte was histopathology, and young dermatologists everywhere who wished to master that art signed up for his famous course on the subject and spent rewarding and profitable time with the Hamburg master. Hundreds of papers emanated from Unna's pen, based on observations made in the wards and laboratories of the Dermatologikum – original disease descriptions, therapeutic innovations, new histologic stains and cellular discoveries, tips and practical hints for the dermatologist in practice, and much more. By the end of the nineteenth century, Unna was in all probability the best-known dermatologist in the world.

Pan-European amalgamation: 1866 to 1914. The diversity of the specialty as it was practiced in the leading European centers was a constant source of communication problems. Despite decades of devotion to descriptive precision and uniformity, loose ends and misunderstandings abounded. These problems were addressed and ameliorated considerably through the medium of three great textbooks published in the last half of the nineteenth century. The first was the five-volume New Sydenham Society translation of the Hebra-Kaposi treatise, which appeared in sections from 1866 to 1880. The opinions and marvelous contributions of the Vienna school were made abundantly clear to physicians in the English-speaking world by this work, confirming the observations of those dermatologists who had had the good fortune personally to observe Hebra and his students in action. The second

was Adrien Doyon's 1881 French translation of the Kaposi "Vorlesungen," thoroughly annotated by Ernest Besnier, through which the many differences in the dermatology of France and the German-speaking world were aired, confronted and, more often than not, resolved. The third was the 1896 English translation of Unna's exhaustively detailed "Histopathologie" that pulled together the observations of the Hamburg master and other microscopists and served as a reference standard for the confusing differences in terminology that hindered progress in this young and rapidly developing field. The influence of these books was complemented by decisions on the part of progressive journal editors to include material on observations made in foreign clinics and furnish summaries of their published reports in languages other than their own.

Dermatologic differences cannot, of course, be resolved through the printed page alone. Equally important are the personal meetings and the actual examination of patients made possible by international congresses convened at intervals in different countries. The first of these took place in Paris in 1889. Participants in these early sessions were able to size one another up, face-to-face, and judge the depth, weight and trustworthiness of colleagues whom they may previously have known only through the written word. They brought along and shared their photographs, wax and cardboard-paste moulages, cultures, slides, specimens, and newly designed instruments. Commercial exhibits appeared. Formal dinners, entertainments, and sightseeing expeditions were organized. Everyone came away better acquainted and better informed, and little by little the nationalistic differences that had often impeded the progress of European dermatology gave way to a more comfortable and enlightened uniformity.

And finally, at this the halfway point in our summary of dermatology, let it be recognized appreciatively that the specialty is a European invention, created from scratch by European physicians, with very little help from anyone else. A century of intense effort on their part resulted in an enormous catalogue of skin diseases beautifully and accurately described, great teaching centers, professional organizations, international meetings, and wonderfully productive research programs. Virtually every facet of the specialty as it has evolved through the twentieth century and into the twenty-first can be traced to European efforts in the nineteenth.

The Rise of American Dermatology. Dermatology in the United States began in the 1830s and 40s with two men who studied briefly in the skin clinics of Paris during the postgraduate tour of European medical facilities that was *de rigeur* at the time for those graduates of American medical schools who could afford it. Henry Daggett Bulkley was the first. A Yale graduate, he spent some time in the clinics of Biett and Gibert, set up a practice in New York, and discovered that despite the brevity of his exposure to dermatology, he knew more about the subject than any of his colleagues. In 1836, he established the Broome Street Infirmary for Diseases of the Skin and a year later delivered a series of lectures on dermatology, the first ever in North America. Noah Worcester, a Dartmouth graduate, studied in the Parisian clinics in

1841, later joined the faculty of the newly founded Medical School of Ohio in Cincinnati, and in 1845 wrote America's first dermatologic textbook, "Diseases of the Skin." It is a well-executed exposition of the French Willanist approach. Neither man exerted much influence on the future development of American dermatology. Bulkley lost interest and became one of New York's leading internists. Worcester died young, of tuberculosis.

United States dermatology as we know it began in the turbulent years that followed the Civil War, years that saw explosive growth in every aspect of American enterprise, industrial, scientific, medical, and more. Philadelphia, Boston, and New York took the lead, serving as home bases for a group of highly intelligent and immoderately ambitious dermatologic pioneers that included, for example, Louis Duhring, James Clark White, Henry Granger Piffard, and George Henry Fox. All were American medical school graduates who journeyed to Europe for post-graduate training in the 1870s and beyond. *Amerikanische Wandervögel,* Unna called them – American migratory birds – and their favorite roosting place was the Vienna clinic of Ferdinand Hebra and his students. There they struggled manfully to master the German language, studied hard, and returned home determined to establish an American version of the specialty on a par with their favorite European model. These individuals are well represented in our atlas. In the last two decades of the nineteenth century and the early years of the twentieth, they established university professorships and organized regional and national dermatologic societies. They wrote textbooks, recognized and described new skin diseases, and published specialty journals in which to record their discoveries. Training centers and programs multiplied, and American dermatology, thriving now and here to stay, came to resemble its Central European counterpart in every respect but one – basic dermatologic research. That deficiency came to be remedied as a direct result of momentous world events.

World War I (1914–18) largely put an end to the flights of the *Wandervögel,* although a few individuals of note – Marion Sulzberger for example – continued to make the trip in the 1920s. The home grown dermatologic infrastructure was by this time adequate to meet American needs. Post-war devastation, the humiliation of the losers, the Communist revolution, and the Great Depression combined to destabilize Europe, resulting in the rise of Fascism, which in its most virulent form settled in Germany when Adolf Hitler came to power in 1933. Hitler's horrendous anti-Jewish policies soon led to the displacement and degradation of Jews in every walk of life and culminated in the holocaust. All branches of German and Austrian medicine were severely affected, but none more than dermatology, which from the beginning had been a specialty open to and favored by Jewish physicians. 27% of the 2078 dermatologists in Germany in 1933 were Jewish. Proportions were even higher in Austria. Dozens of the luckier ones fled, most of them to the United States. Those who stayed disappeared, committed suicide or, as in the case of Abraham Buschke and Karl Herxheimer, were locked away in concentration camps and left to die.

Arriving in the United States, the German and Austrian refugees found American dermatology in the midst of an extensive program of modernization. The American Board of Dermatology was organized in 1932. The Society for Investigative Dermatology (SID) was founded in 1937, and the American Academy of Dermatology met for the first time in 1938. The SID in particular attracted the attention of the refugees, who brought with them the European tradition in which academic dermatologists were expected to combine clinical expertise with investigational effort. The perfect exemplar of this group is Rudolf Baer, who arrived in the United States from Germany (via Switzerland) in 1934, joined Marion Sulzberger in basic research on contact dermatitis, and embraced the SID enthusiastically. Following World War II, he joined the faculty of the New York Skin and Cancer Unit as a clinical investigator and spent the rest of his life working for a better balance between clinical and research activities in American dermatology. Variations on the Baer story can be found in the lives of many of the other new arrivals. The group is well represented in the pages of this atlas.

American hegemony; homogeneous dermatology: 1946 to the 1970s. The United States emerged from World War II in far better condition than any of its allies or enemies. Its physical plant was undamaged and its economy stronger than ever. Concerned that post-war devastation would play into the hands of the Soviet Union and result in the wholesale takeover of Western Europe by forces inimical to American interests, the United States instituted the European Recovery Program (the Marshall Plan, 1948–1952). Billions of dollars were injected into the economies of West Germany and sixteen other nations, hastening recovery in all phases of national life, including medicine. Along with the rest of the specialties, European dermatologic departments began to rebuild.

In the United States, large numbers of ambitious young physicians who had seen the value and benefits of specialization during their years in the military service, returned to civilian life and crowded into residency training programs. Dermatology was a favorite choice, and many of the new residents immediately fell under the spell of the Rudolf Baers and Stephen Rothmans, who preached and embodied the union of clinical know-how with investigative effort. Exciting American research reports generated by the maturing crop of new residents began to appear in the literature and caught the eye of the young European dermatologic trainees who were stimulated to examine first hand the sources of these reports and if possible join in the activities as well. A new wave of Wandervögel flights began, this time from east to west. When the visitors returned home, they spread the word and revised their facilities and programs along the American lines. The result was that dermatology in the Western World became more homogeneous than ever before. Post-war recovery in Japan lagged somewhat, but when it reached a critical mass, young Japanese dermatologists also headed for the United States to broaden their horizons; they returned home with American ideas and worked diligently to bring the Japanese version of the specialty up to speed.

The homogeneous era was characterized by an impressive series of therapeutic advances – topical and systemic corticosteroids, penicillin and other antibiotics, griseofulvin, methotrexate, calciferol, PABA and other effective sun screens, PUVA, benzoyl peroxide, and tretinoin, complemented as well by the widespread availability and use of liquid nitrogen, which prior to World War II had been difficult to obtain. Dermabrasion, the importation of the Mohs surgical technique into the realm of dermatology, hair transplantation, and the introduction of laser ablation also belong to this era. Many of these discoveries and activities are noted and celebrated in the pages that follow.

In 1969 the newly formed Joint Committee on Planning for Dermatology presented to the National Institutes of Health a report that recommended the establishment of a national biomedical communications network for the specialty. To this end, a task force formed by the American Academy of Dermatology (AAD) spent the next ten years assembling a variety of useful dermatologic databases and searching out the best way to make them available to dermatologists by electronic means. By 1986, the "Infonet" had been developed to connect users' personal computers to large computers maintained at the national headquarters of the AAD. It was the beginning of the computer age for dermatology. Since then, computers worldwide have entered into nearly every activity associated with the specialty – information storage and retrieval, preparation and presentation of teaching materials, travel arrangements, office record keeping and billing procedures, and much more. The impact has been profound. The marriage of computer and Internet has in fact become the most powerful force ever in diminishing regional differences in the practice of dermatology. The end is nowhere in sight.

This time period is also noteworthy for the increase in the participation of women in dermatology. Women have been active in the specialty in the Western World at least since 1907, but in small numbers until relatively recently. In the United States the increase began in earnest in the 1960s, *pari passu* with the increase in enrolment of women in medical schools. By 1993, women constituted 23% of American Academy of Dermatology membership and were represented in leadership positions in numbers commensurate with their age groups. In 1999 their numbers approached 30%; they continue to rise. The effect has been less unsettling than many of the old guard expected, and their presence has brought new concerns to the attention of the specialty, broadened its perspectives, and enhanced its appeal.

It should be noted that the homogeneity characteristic of the period was not absolute. The abandonment of venereology in the 1950s put American dermatology at odds with its European counterparts. The most conspicuous sign of this abandonment, the decision to drop the term syphilology from the specialty board certificate, was based on the conviction that the massive decline in the incidence of the disease following the introduction and widespread use of penicillin and other antibiotics would soon render the designation unnecessary. Unintended consequences resulted. When AIDS burst upon the scene in the 1970s, American dermatology, no longer identified with the world of sexually transmitted diseases, found itself at the periphery of the massive response effort mounted worldwide, despite the fact that cutaneous changes are an extremely important part of the catalogue of signs and symptoms.

Dermatologic transformation and fragmentation: 1970s to the present. Signs of strain and threats of fragmentation were already evident in the optimism and heady progress characteristic of dermatology in the years following World War II.

These disruptive trends differ from country to country; they are functions of the interaction of government, medicine, and the various economic systems in place. In the United States, it is becoming increasingly difficult to answer the simple questions: What is dermatology and what is a dermatologist? For better or worse, American trends in medicine, along with entertainment, cuisine, dress, and behavior, tend to seep into other cultures, whether the recipients of the seepage appreciate it or not. Dermatologists of other nations may therefore catch a glimpse of what the future holds for them by considering the American experience in recent years.

Economic strength combined with the successful union of the strong American clinical infrastructures and imported European research traditions that began in the 1930s and 40s has resulted in the past four decades in series of dermatologic investigational triumphs unprecedented in history. Pigment cell biology was clarified, and the unsuspected immunologic capabilities of the keratinocyte revealed. The elegantly complicated structure of the dermal-epidermal junction was worked out a step at a time, pinpointing the defects that allow it sometimes to fall apart. Cellular matrix constituents were shown to be complex and beautifully designed for their supportive function, but subject to disturbances which, thanks to research, are better understood now than ever before. The mediators of inflammation and the cells that produce them have been identified one by one, along with the unlikely chain of immunologic events that leads to the clinical manifestations of allergic contact dermatitis. The Langerhans cell has been rescued from structural and functional limbo and recognized for its key role in antigen presentation. Examples of these and other research triumphs are on display in the pages that follow.

These activities were not exclusively American, to be sure, but it cannot be denied that most of the investigations were initiated or conducted in the United States. Many of the research advances were facilitated by the incorporation of Ph.Ds into dermatologic faculty positions, and by the multiplication of dermatologists of a new breed, whose interests from the beginning lay in research, with the clinical aspects of their positions relegated to a place of lesser importance. A significant number of these dermatologists had earned both an M.D. and a basic science Ph.D degree.

Research dermatology is in a way a victim of its own success. Its activities have sometimes resulted in the alienation of clinical dermatologists who do not see the relevance to their daily problems of the abstruse basic science reports that appear in their journals. Clinicians are also put off at times by preferences shown to the stars of bench research in faculty appointments and departmental chairmanships, and in allocations of funds and space. Problems have been lessened to some extent by the recent shift in emphasis in dermatologic research away from investigations at the molecular level to considerations more applicable to the problems of pathogenesis and more readily appreciated by those in practice. Moreover, clinicians are intrigued by the new genomics, with its implied promise of gene therapies potentially effective in conditions they are at present completely powerless to control. They are also impressed by the advances in cutaneous pharmacology that have already paid off at the clinical level and augur well for the development of still more effective medications targeting specific biological defects discovered in bench research. Nevertheless, bench research investigators and their clinical colleagues continue to cultivate separate gardens and set agendas that clash.

Dermato-histopathology, essentially a nineteenth century invention, was brought to new heights in the twentieth, confirming the centrality of the biopsy to success in many diagnostic situations. It has also led to the identification of new cutaneous disease entities based more on observable cellular interactions than clinical findings. Typical examples are presented in the body of this work. The success and increasing complexity of the subject, along with perceived economic benefits and preservation of turf, led to sub-specialization and special certification in the United States. That in turn has had the unintended consequence of further separation of the dermatopathologist from mainstream dermatology, with a fall-off in mainstream interest and support to a point that some believe will result in the end of dermatopathology as a dermatologic discipline.

Pediatric dermatology sub-specialization, with its separate journals and meetings, and agitation for special certification, has created still another division that weakens the cement holding the specialty together. Geriatric sub-specialization is also gaining strength.

Problematic, too, is the surgical explosion of the last thirty years – hair transplants, scalp reductions, skin peels and resurfacing, laser procedures, sclerotherapy, tattooing, collagen and botulinum toxin injections, liposuction, soft tissue augmentation, and the like – driven by the all-powerful engine of economics, at least in North America. Continually expanded and refined, many dermatologic surgical procedures require special training and expensive equipment; they make increasing demands on departmental funds and on teaching time in the post-graduate curriculum that threaten to split the specialty into competing medical and surgical camps

These things are not going to go away. They have a life of their own, and those who try to turn back the clock will find themselves in the position of the formidable King Canute, who sat on an English beach a thousand years ago, commanded the incoming tide to stop, and ended up soaking wet. If dermatology is to survive in its present form, it will need leaders who can unite and extract the best from the divisive factions noted above and still remain devoted to the preservation of the 200 year-old core, the nidus around which all these other elements have crystallized. It is essential that those in positions of power emphasize and constantly renew the one thing that most impresses both the medical world and the public in general – the ability of dermatologists to identify eruptions accurately and therefore manage skin problems better than anyone else. That ability is the special chain that links together the diverse set of individuals whose pictures and accomplishments appear on the pages of this atlas.

EARLY OBSERVATIONS

Egyptian medicine, as presented in the Edwin Smith and Ebers papyri (ca. 1600 BC and 1550 BC) contains many references to skin diseases and the topical medications used to treat them. Unfortunately the diseases themselves are so sketchily described that other than such obvious entities as baldness, canities, and wrinkling, it is usually impossible to assign a modern name to the problems treated. Many, including both skin and hair disturbances, were attributed to *whdw* (pronounced ukhedu), the number one toxin in the Egyptian pathogenetic scheme. *Whdw* originates in the colon and in disease states makes its way into internal organs as well as the skin.

A large number of substances, many of them disgusting, were incorporated in Egyptian topical medications. Here, too, the nature of the plant derivatives utilized can often be identified only tentatively.

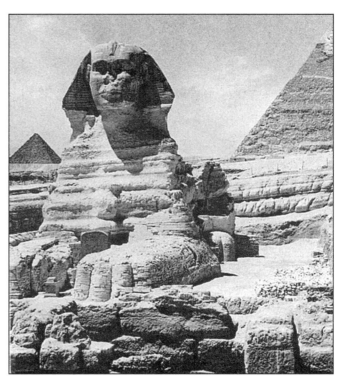

The Great Sphinx at Giza, Egypt. It is a portrait of King Khafre, 4th King of the 4th Dynasty (2550 B.C.E.).

To the right are the indications and instructions for the application of one of the earliest dermatological preparations ever recorded (ca. 1600 B.C.E.). The instructions are preceded by a detailed description of the proper method of compounding the ointment. "Let there be brought a large quantity of *hemayet*-fruit, about two khar," it begins. Hemayet was probably a form of fenugreek. The fruit was husked, winnowed, dried, soaked, boiled, washed, etc., and ended up as a mass or ointment with the consistency of clay. It was difficult to make, no doubt, but if it lived up to any of the promises recorded by that ancient scribe, certainly well worth the effort.

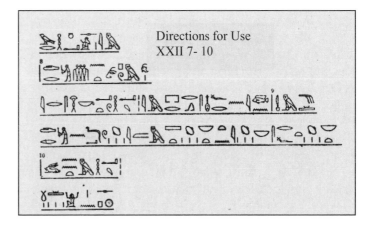

Translation: "Anoint a man therewith. It is a remover of wrinkles from the head. When the flesh is smeared therewith, it becomes a beautifier of the skin, a remover of blemishes, of all disfigurements, of all signs of age, of all weaknesses that are in the flesh. Found effective myriads of times." - The Edwin Smith Papyrus

XXXI Τῶν δ' ἐντόμων ὅσα σαρκοφάγα μὲν μή ἐστι, ζῇ
δὲ χυμοῖς σαρκὸς ζώσης, οἷον οἵ τε φθεῖρες καὶ αἱ
ψύλλαι καὶ κόρεις, ἐκ μὲν τῆς ὀχείας πάντα γεννᾷ
τὰς καλουμένας κονίδας, ἐκ δὲ τούτων ἕτερον οὐδὲν
25 γίγνεται πάλιν. αὐτῶν δὲ γίγνονται τούτων αἱ μὲν
ψύλλαι ἐξ ἐλαχίστης σηπεδόνος (ὅπου γὰρ ἂν κόπρος
ξηρὰ γένηται, ἐνταῦθα συνίστανται), οἱ¹ δὲ κόρεις
ἐκ τῆς ἰκμάδος τῆς ἀπὸ τῶν ζώων συνισταμένης
ἐκτός, οἱ δὲ φθεῖρες ἐκ τῶν σαρκῶν. γίγνονται δ'
ὅταν μέλλωσιν οἷον ἴονθοι μικροί, οὐκ ἔχοντες πύον·
30 τούτους ἐάν τις κεντήσῃ, ἐξέρχονται φθεῖρες. ἐνίοις
δὲ τοῦτο συμβαίνει τῶν ἀνθρώπων νόσημα, ὅταν
ὑγρασία πολλὴ ἐν τῷ σώματι ᾖ· καὶ διεφθάρησάν
τινες ἤδη τοῦτον τὸν τρόπον, ὥσπερ Ἀλκμᾶνά τέ
φασι τὸν ποιητὴν καὶ Φερεκύδην τὸν Σύριον. καὶ
ἐν νόσοις δέ τισι γίγνεται πλῆθος φθειρῶν.

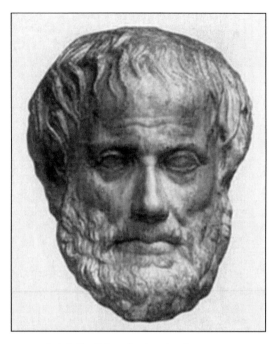

Above: extract from Aristotle's *Historia Animalium*,
Book V, Section XXXI.

Aristotle, Macedonian teacher,
philosopher, scientist. (384-322 B.C.E.).

Below: Translation of the extract.

We go on now to insects which though not carnivorous live on the juices of living flesh - insects such as lice, fleas, and bugs. All these as the result of copulation generate what are called nits, and from these nothing further is produced. The slightest quantity of putrefying matter gives rise to fleas (they are found taking shape where there is any dry excrement); bugs are produced out of the moisture from living animals as it congeals outside them; lice are produced out of flesh. When lice are going to be produced, as it were small eruptions form, but without any purulent matter in them; and if these are pricked, lice emerge. Some people get this disease when there is a great deal of moisture in the body ; some indeed have been killed by it, as Alkman the poet is said to have been, and Pherekydes the Syrian. Further, in certain diseases large numbers of lice appear.

Aristotle is routinely cited as the first to describe lice in any recognizable form. To a degree the citation is accurate. Shown to the left is everything he had to say on the subject, both in his own language and in translation. The paragraph does not present the sage of Macedonia at his best. That lice and fleas suck the juices of living flesh, and nits arise from copulation are valid observations - but the statement that nits produce nothing and bugs emerge mysteriously from congealment of body moisture helped to perpetuate the grand error of spontaneous generation that impeded progress in the understanding of biology for another 2000 years. Lice, of course, do not emerge from pricked skin lesions either. To Ferdinand Hebra, that portion of Aristotle's account constitutes in fact the first description of scabietic lesions and recovery of the scabies mite.

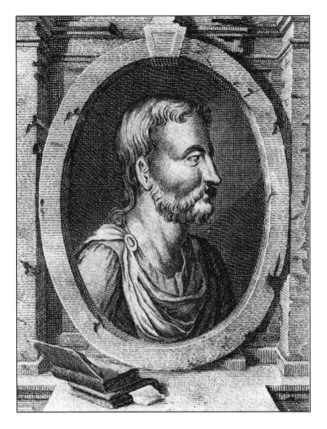

Aulus Cornelius Celsus, Roman writer, flourished during the reigns of Tiberius and Augustus, Rome's "golden age." In the early decades of the first century C.E. he completed an encyclopedia dealing with philosophy, rhetoric, agriculture, military art, law, and medicine. Only the medical section survives. Celsus was not a physician, but he did the research necessary to his task - read everything, cultivated physicians, and regularly attended and closely observed surgical operations and dissections. The result was a masterwork, "De Medicina," the first systematic treatise on medicine that has survived intact. In chapters 5 and 6 of the work Celsus considers skin diseases in some detail. Some of the entities he described some two thousand years ago are recognizable even now; most are not. No dermatologist of today would have trouble identifying his classic description of the two forms of "areae" (shown below, left) as variants of alopecia areata.

Aulus Cornelius Celsus (25 B.C.E.-50 C.E.)

Below: An English translation of the "De Medicina" of Celsus, the earliest systematic treatise on medicine that has survived intact.

BOOK V, CAP. IV. There are two kinds of AREAE. Both agree in this particular, that from the decay of the scarf skin the hair is first thinned and then falls off altogether; and if the part be struck, blood flows, thin and of a disagreeable odor: in either species the progress is rapid in some persons, and slow in others. That is the more unfavorable kind which has rendered the skin dense; fatty; and perfectly smooth. The species denominated alopekia spreads in all sorts of forms. It occurs both in the hair and in the beard. But that which, from its resemblance to a serpent, bears the name ophiasis, begins at the back of the head, does not exceed the breadth of two digits, and extends itself by two points of prolongation towards the ears, and in some cases as far as to the forehead, where they unite. The former affection is common to every period of life; the latter usually occurs in infants: so again the former scarcely ever terminates without medicine, the latter frequently undergoes a spontaneous cure. Some scrape these kinds of areae with a scalpel; some anoint them with caustics mixed up in oil; and, chief of all, with burnt paper: others apply turpentine resin with thapsia: But there is nothing better than daily shaving the part with a razor; because when the cuticle has thus been gradually cut away, the roots of the hairs are laid bare, nor ought one to desist until a thick growth of hair shall have made its appearance; when frequent shaving is had recourse to, it is sufficient to smear the part with common writing ink.

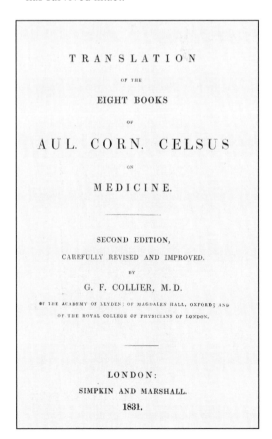

TRANSLATION

OF THE

EIGHT BOOKS

OF

AUL. CORN. CELSUS

ON

MEDICINE.

SECOND EDITION,

CAREFULLY REVISED AND IMPROVED.

BY

G. F. COLLIER, M.D.

OF THE ACADEMY OF LEYDEN; OF MAGDALEN HALL, OXFORD; AND
OF THE ROYAL COLLEGE OF PHYSICIANS OF LONDON.

LONDON:
SIMPKIN AND MARSHALL.
1831.

Hieronymus Mercurialis, one of the most renowned physicians of the late renaissance, practiced first in Rome and later accepted the chair of Medicine in Padua. He also taught at Bologna and Pisa. An erudite and thoroughly educated man, he enjoyed writing and had a special knack for reviewing the medical literature, separating the wheat from the chaff, and reducing large bodies of information to readable paragraphs useful to students and practitioners alike. His impressive list of publications includes monographs on the care of nursing infants, diseases of women, poisons and diseases caused by poisons, diseases of the eyes and ears, the composition of medicines, critiques on the works of Hippocrates, diseases of children, and more. His most influential production was his "Art of Gymnastics" (1569), the first work of its kind, and for many years the model for all subsequent works on the subject.

Unlike many of the eminent physicians of the time, Mercurialis was a warm and friendly man who managed to stay on good terms with everybody, no mean feat in the turbulent world of renaissance Italy.

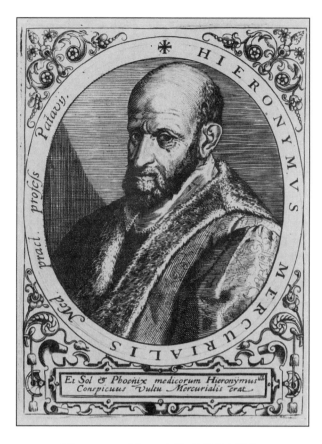

Hieronymus Mercurialis (1530-1606)

The "De Morbis Cutaneis," of Mercurialis (shown to the left) appeared first in 1572. It consists of 16 lectures on skin diseases transcribed by the author's pupil Paulus Aicardius. It is the first work of any size devoted entirely to the subject and is in fact an extended revue of the literature, both ancient and contemporary, in which the opinions of more than 70 authorities are accepted or rejected by the author. The text is wholly Galenical both in its preoccupation with humoral ideas and in its division of the skin diseases into two grand categories, those that affect the head and those that affect the body in general. Therapy is covered in depth.

There would have been no point in delivering these lectures, with their profusion of disease names and treatment recommendations, if Mercurialis were unable to demonstrate in the clinic or at the bedside the proper diagnostic category in which to stow the eruptions observed. But the modern physician in reading this book will see the dermatology of that era only "through a glass darkly." In most cases the inadequacy of the disease descriptions reduces to the level of speculation our ability to identify the conditions considered.

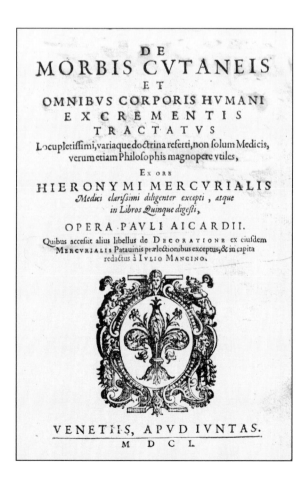

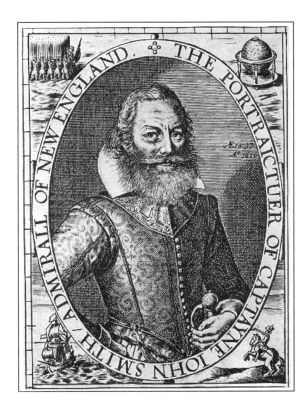

Captain John Smith (1580-1631).
Engraving by Simon Van de Passe.

"The poisonous weed, being in shape but little different from our English yvie; but being touched causeth redness, itchinge, and lastly blysters, the which howsoever, after a while they passe away of themselves without further harme; yet because for the time they are somewhat painefull, and in aspect dangerous, it hath gotten itself an ill name, although questionless of noe very ill nature."

Above: The first account of poison ivy (Rhus toxicodendron) – by Captain John Smith, late of England, then of Jamestown in Virginia (1609).

Below: Powhatan's warriors celebrating the capture of Captain John Smith (1607).

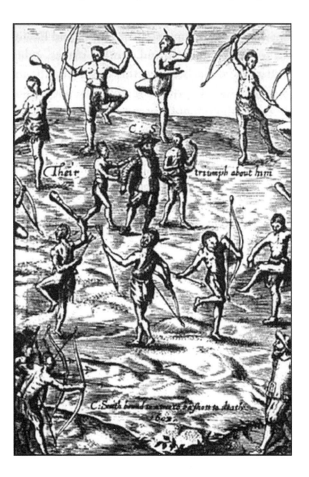

The first mention of poison ivy, the bread and butter friend of North American dermatologists, appears in the 1609 journal of Captain John Smith. Smith headed up the ill fated mercantile colony established in 1607 on the Jamestown peninsula in Virginia. The colony suffered one disaster after another and was finally all but abandoned late in the century.

Captain Smith was not overly concerned about North America's number one sensitizing plant - but remember, a short while before he wrote his account the captain, while exploring the Chickahominy River, had been captured by Powhatan, the area's most powerful Indian Chief. Sentenced to be beheaded, he was saved by the intercession of Princess Pocahontas a moment before the axe was to fall. Next to that, poison ivy is surely "of noe very ill nature."

The first in-depth studies of the plant were conducted by Harvard's James Clarke White and published in his classic monograph, Dermatitis Venenata (1887).

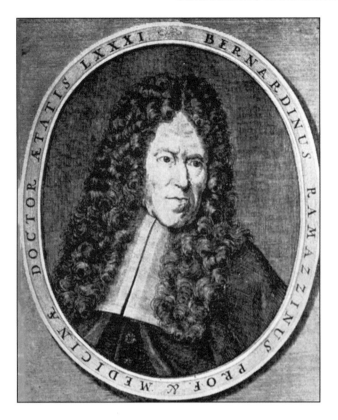

Bernardino Ramazzini (1633-1714)

Bernardino Ramazzini, Italian physician and author of the masterwork, "De morbis artificum diatriba" (Diseases of workers), was born in Modena and received his medical education at Parma. After some years in general practice in Carpi and Modena, he was appointed Professor of the Theory of Medicine at the newly established University of Modena. In 1700, he accepted a professorship at Padua, where he remained for the rest of his life.

Ramazzini wrote a great deal but is remembered today chiefly for his treatise on occupational diseases. It is a fat little book, published in several editions between 1700 and 1713. In it, the author describes the diseases common to some 61 lines of work. A literature review is included in each section, but the enduring value and interest in the work derive from the on site visits and observations of the author himself, who insisted on inspecting everything with his own eyes. His sympathies, which he frequently expressed, lay entirely with the workers, whose working conditions were in fact abysmal. Amiable and at ease with individuals of every social class, he apparently had no difficulty in collecting the data he needed to make his points. The colorful language, conversational tone, personal reminiscences, and intriguing asides survive translation and make the work a pleasure to read.

On his 81st birthday Ramazzini suffered a massive stroke and, to use an expression of his own, "passed over into the ranks of the corpse-goddess, Libitina."

The title page of the 1703 edition of Ramazzini's masterwork is shown to the right.

In truth, Ramazzini was not much of a dermatologist. The few skin conditions included in his text are mentioned by name but never described – scabies, psora, cradle cap, lice and bedbug infestations, and the cutaneous manifestations of syphilis. Leg ulcers appear periodically, along with enough collateral information to identify them as stasis in origin, or ecthymatous. With the exception of an ambiguous reference to hand problems in bakers, examples of allergic and primary irritation contact dermatitis do not appear, although they must have been common in the occupations studied. It is Ramazzini's recognition and documentation of percutaneous absorption disasters that catches the eye of the modern dermatologist and validates the Italian master's presence on these pages. An example of this in the use of mercury ointment to treat syphilis is given below.

"For those who rub in this ointment I can suggest no sounder precaution than that employed by a surgeon of our day who had learned to his cost that his fee did not compensate for his own loss, since he found that the process of anointing did more harm to him than to those he treated; for he was terribly afflicted by diarrhea, colic, and profuse salivation. So he now prepares the mercurial ointment and stays by the patients who are to be treated, but he orders them to rub in the ointment themselves with their own hands and declares that this is better for him and for them. For he runs no risk, while they become heated by the vigorous movements of their arms; this makes the process more penetrating, and they have no reason to be afraid of a remedy which they hope to relieve their torments."

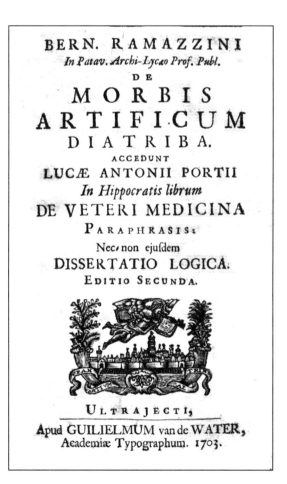

Eighteenth Century "Protodermatologists"

Daniel Turner, London physician and surgeon, wrote the first textbook of dermatology in English - "De Morbus Cutaneis" (1714). He began his professional life as a barber-surgeon, but managed to extract an M.D. degree from Yale College in 1723 (the first ever granted by the American school) in exchange for a collection of books for the school library. Critics said his M.D. really stood for Multum Donavit. Nevertheless, Turner was a remarkable man who in addition to his treatise on the skin published textbooks on surgery and venereal disease that were much admired at the time.

"De Morbus Cutaneis" is a fascinating work and successful in its day, passing through many editions and translated into French and German. In it the reader is yanked along as Dr. Turner hurries from case to case discharging opinions and advice rapid fire with outrageous self-assurance. He destroys his enemies, praises friends, and records the whole bravura performance in a salty, aggressive literary idiom that defies description. An example of his style is given to the right below. It appeared originally in the chapter in "De Morbus Cutaneis" dealing with diseases of the foreskin.

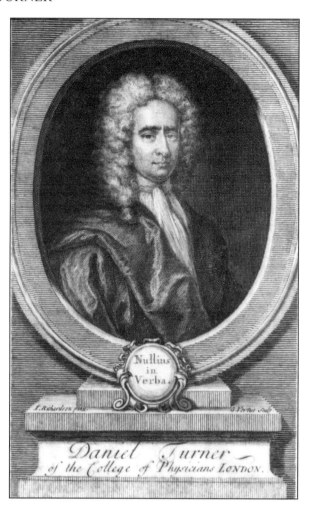

Daniel Turner (1667-1740)

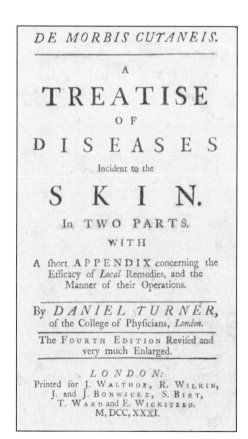

Daniel Turner's treatise on skin diseases, Fourth edition, 1731

"It had been this fellow's misfortune, being drunk, to engage with a foul slut who had not only clapt him, but he unmindful to return the prepuce, the next morning in vain attempted it; and thereupon meeting with this pretender's bills, or seeing them upon some pissing-post, applies for relief; when after a fortnight's pain, well drain'd of his ready money, with his dripping rotten penis came to me; on whom, when I had thus taken off the symptoms, and not able by the common mercurials both inwardly and outwardly to obtain my ends, I hastened a salivation and thereby heal'd his sores: the glans incarn'd, and looks tolerably handsome: the extremity of the prepuce makes a sort of quadrangle, each corner, by reason of the cicatrix having a small knob which hinders it from playing freely over the glans: but from which he may at any time, if so minded, be freed by circumcision. As a martyr in the cause of Venus and unbridled lust, he thinks he has shed blood enough already; and if it now suffice to carry off his water, he talks (at least at present) that he has no other occasion. "

Excerpt from Turner's De Morbus Cutaneis, 1714

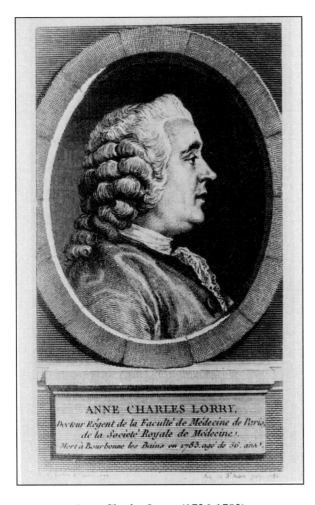

ANNE CHARLES LORRY,
Docteur Régent de la Faculté de Médecine de Paris,
de la Société Royale de Médecine,
Mort à Bourbonne les Bains en 1783, age de 56. ans.

Anne Charles Lorry (1726-1783)

Son of a highly respected professor of law in Paris, Lorry was born on October 10, 1726, near Paris and was graduated from medical school in 1748. The influence of his family and his very real skills as a physician soon resulted in the development of a highly successful practice that included such patients as the Richelieus and Voltaire himself. Darling of the salons and of the ladies, Lorry failed to look after his own health, and at the age of 56 was felled by a stroke that left him partially paralyzed. His practice deserted him, and he had to be rescued by a royal pension, on which he subsisted until his death in 1783.

Lorry made a number of contributions of lasting value to medical science. He was the first to recognize and to localize by means of careful animal experiments the presence of the vital centers in the medulla. He published several well-researched monographs on subjects that interested him, the most famous of which is "De Melancholia et Morbis Melancholicis" (1765), a work recognized both in his own time and now as a milestone in the history of psychiatric medicine.

Lorry's credentials as a dermatologist rest on another of his specialized monographs, an impressive treatise entitled "Tractatus de Morbis Cutaneis," published in Latin in 1777. Much admired by his countrymen, the Tractatus (shown to the right) is in fact a curious production. It deals with all aspects of the skin in a general way - structure, function, relationship to other organs, the influences of diet, climate, exercise, rest, sleep, insomnia, and the like - but with respect to the skin diseases themselves the text fails to live up to the promise of its title. Lorry's descriptions of those entities he considers are imprecise, and his constant immersion in Galenical musings, such as the imagined dangers associated with suppression of certain eruptions, make it a difficult read for the modern physician. Nevertheless, the influence of the Tractatus on French and English dermatology as practiced later was considerable. It was responsible to a significant degree for the excessive use of risky internal medications and futile speculation on the connection between the skin and this or that internal organ that characterized the dermatology of both countries throughout most of the nineteenth century.

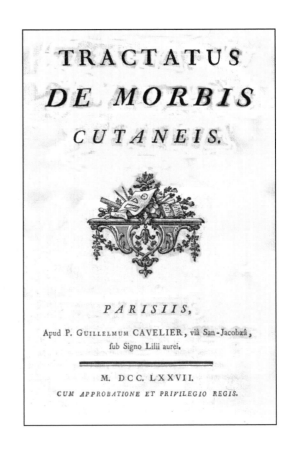

TRACTATUS
DE MORBIS
CUTANEIS.

PARISIIS,

Apud P. GUILLELMUM CAVELIER, viâ San-Jacobæâ,
fub Signo Lilii aurei.

M. DCC. LXXVII.

CUM APPROBATIONE ET PRIVILEGIO REGIS.

11

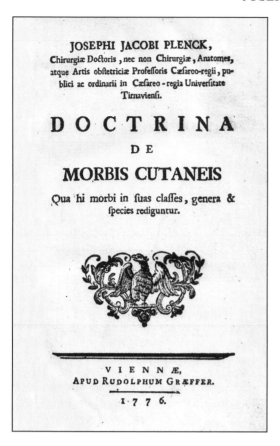

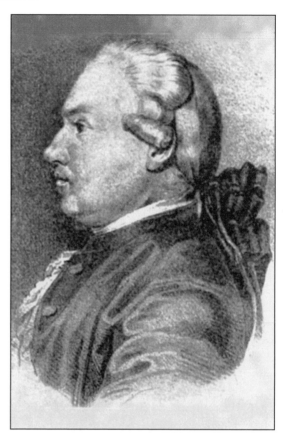

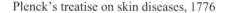

Plenck's treatise on skin diseases, 1776

Joseph Plenck (1732-1807)

Below: Plenck's classification of skin diseases.

Joseph Plenck, a Viennese military surgeon, held a variety of professorial posts in Switzerland, Hungary, and Austria., and wherever he went, he wrote. He seemed determined to compose treatises on every medical subject he taught and, for that matter, on any he might possibly be called upon to teach in the future. Ophthalmology, obstetrics, dentistry, pharmaceutical chemistry, legal medicine, diseases of children, all were grist for his mill, and that list is no more than a sample. The skin's turn to be written up came in 1776. The result was a 128-page monograph in Latin entitled "Doctrina de Morbis Cutaneis," and a fine little book it is. By far the most original of Plenck's efforts, it represented a complete break with the past, a rejection of the classification of skin diseases on the basis of the area of the body involved, and an attempt for the first time to gather into groups those eruptions made up of lesions similar in appearance. The descriptions of the diseases themselves are uninspired and add nothing new, but his classification scheme, shown to the right, was of great importance. It served as the model on which the Englishman Robert Willan two decades later based his great work "On Cutaneous Diseases," the foundation of modern dermatology.

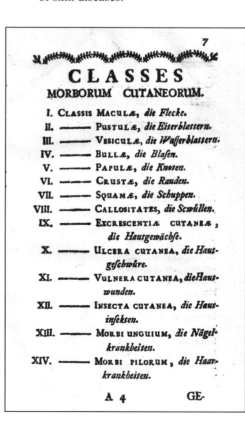

12

Early Nineteenth Century Dermatology:

Founding of the English and French Schools

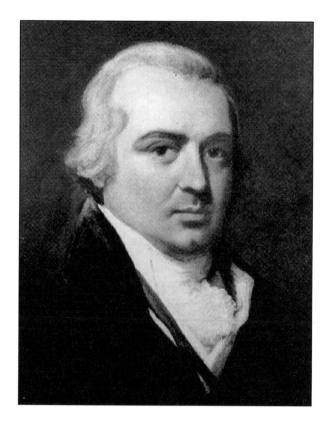

Robert Willan (1757-1812)

Robert Willan, English physician who is regarded properly as the founder of modern dermatology, spent his years at London's Carey St. Dispensary observing and recording the morphology of lesions that appeared on the skin in response to disease – papules, vesicles, wheals, and the like. We now call these varieties primary and secondary lesions; they are the alphabet of clinical dermatology. With this information in hand, he assembled and defined a large set of skin diseases - some old, many new - and classified them on the basis of the morphology of the lesions observed when the disease was at its height. He presented his findings in a masterwork entitled "On cutaneous diseases, Part 1." It appeared in sections from 1798 to 1808. Plate 1 from the work, showing the primary lesions, is the frontispiece of this atlas.

The clarity of the disease presentations in "On cutaneous diseases," and the usefulness of diagnostic tools provided by the lesion definitions brought a measure of order to the field of skin diseases where previously chaos had reigned. The value of the work was further enhanced by the inclusion of 33 hand colored copper plate engravings depicting the diseases described. "On cutaneous diseases" is the first dermatological work that can be read by the modern physician with any degree of comfort.

Willan died of heart disease before he could complete Part 2 of his textbook. It was completed in 1813 by his pupil, Thomas Bateman, in his "Synopsis of cutaneous diseases." The complete classification devised by Willan appears below:

Below: Title page of Willan's "On cutaneous diseases" (1808)

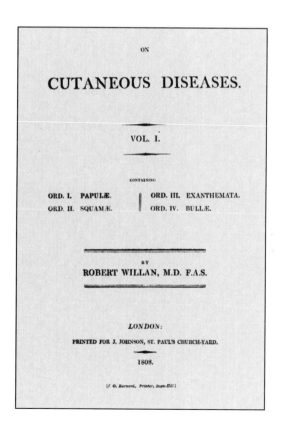

ON

CUTANEOUS DISEASES.

VOL. I.

CONTAINING

ORD. I. PAPULÆ.	ORD. III. EXANTHEMATA.
ORD. II. SQUAMÆ.	ORD. IV. BULLÆ.

BY

ROBERT WILLAN, M.D. F.A.S.

LONDON:

PRINTED FOR J. JOHNSON, ST. PAUL'S CHURCH-YARD.

1808.

[J. O. Barnard, Printer, Snow-Hill.]

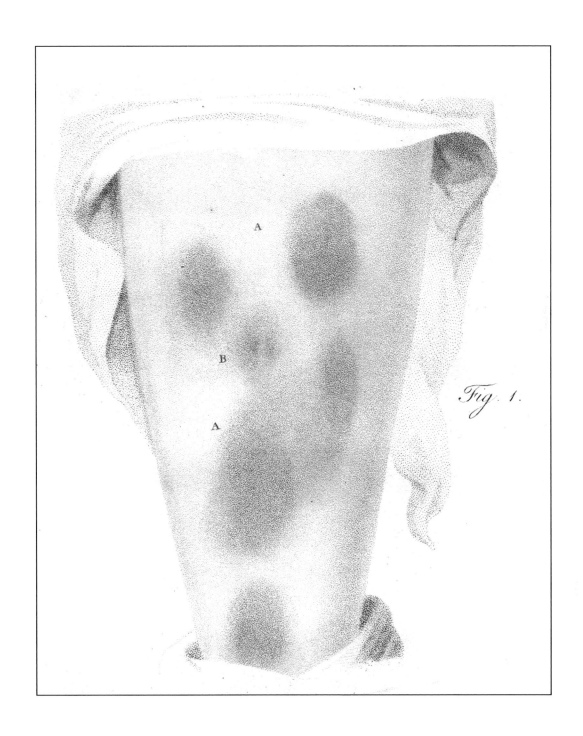

Erythema nodosum, from Robert Willan's "On Cutaneous Diseases" (1808).
The letters A and B are not explained in the text or caption.

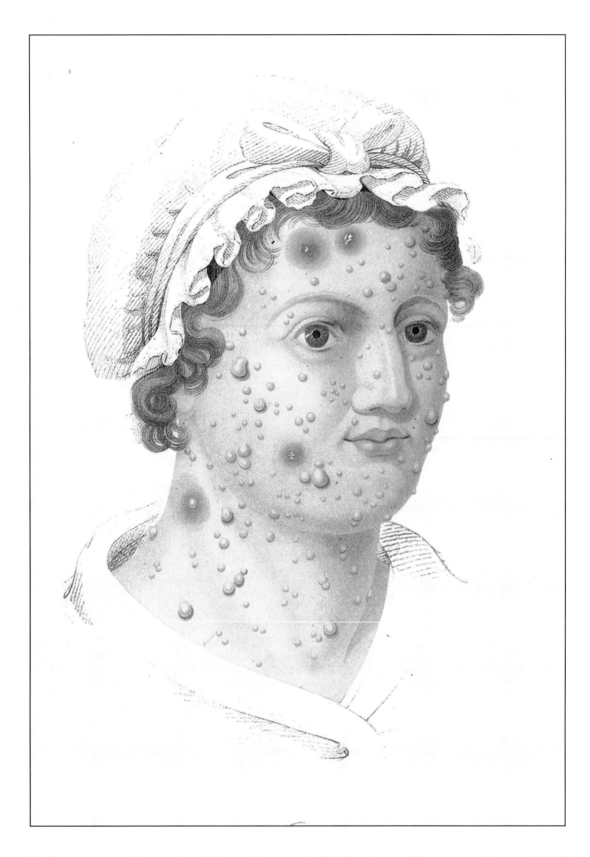

Molluscum contagiosum, from Thomas Bateman's "Delineations of Cutaneous Diseases," 1817.

Thomas Bateman (1778-1821), pupil, friend and associate of Robert Willan, completed Willan's work after the death of his teacher. He published the results in 1813 in his "Practical synopsis of cutaneous diseases," one of the most important books in the history of the specialty. As far as most of the medical world was concerned, modern dermatology began as much with this little volume as with Willan's grander, costly, and narrowly distributed opus, which few physicians ever had the opportunity to see. Bateman added observations of his own to the work, the classic descriptions of lichen urticatus and molluscum contagiosum, for example. The latter appeared in the third edition of the Synopsis, shown to the right. Bateman also completed Willan's collection of plates, added a few of his own, and published the lot in 1817 as "Delineations of cutaneous diseases," the most popular atlas of the day.

During his terminal illness Bateman, who had been an agnostic hedonist with a propensity for wine, women and song in his younger years, underwent a religious conversion that was celebrated by the faithful on both sides of the Atlantic. It is not surprising, therefore, to discover in the bookplates that date from his youth the image of an attractive young lady (below, right). No portrait of Bateman seems to exist.

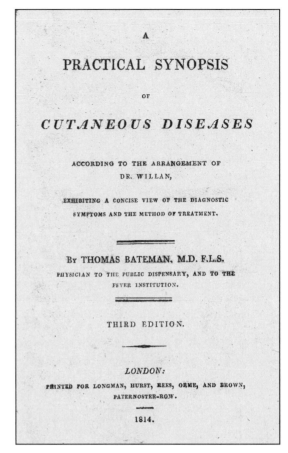

A

PRACTICAL SYNOPSIS

OF

CUTANEOUS DISEASES

ACCORDING TO THE ARRANGEMENT OF
DR. WILLAN,

EXHIBITING A CONCISE VIEW OF THE DIAGNOSTIC
SYMPTOMS AND THE METHOD OF TREATMENT.

BY THOMAS BATEMAN, M.D. F.L.S.

PHYSICIAN TO THE PUBLIC DISPENSARY, AND TO THE
FEVER INSTITUTION.

THIRD EDITION.

LONDON:
PRINTED FOR LONGMAN, HURST, REES, ORME, AND BROWN,
PATERNOSTER-ROW.

1814.

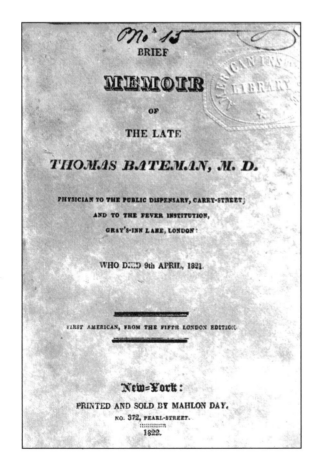

Pamphlet celebrating the religious conversion of Thomas Bateman at the end of his life.

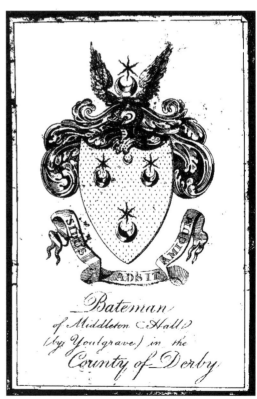

Thomas Bateman's bookplate. Note the hidden symbolism.

Jean Louis Alibert is recognized as the founder of French dermatology and one of the most important figures in the development of the specialty. At l'Hôpital Saint Louis in Paris he established the world's first great dermatologic teaching center (1802), and much of its success was due to the showmanship and oratorical skills of the founder himself. Three days a week Alibert arrived in his magnificent equipage and took his place on the clinic stage. Dressed in satin knee britches and Napoleonic hat he strode back and forth vigorously, exchanging quips with the patients. His speech, exceptionally fluent, bubbled with simile and metaphor. A syphilitic prostitute became "a priestess of Venus wounded by a perfidious dart of love." Patients were placed on display with the names of their disorders in letters two inches high inked on placards across their chest. The clinics became so popular they had to be moved outside to the hospital courtyard. But Alibert was a great deal more than a showman. He was a skillful observer who gave the first descriptions of a number of skin diseases – keloids, and mycosis fungoides, for example, and he recorded his observations in a series of grand and superbly illustrated publications that are much admired even today.

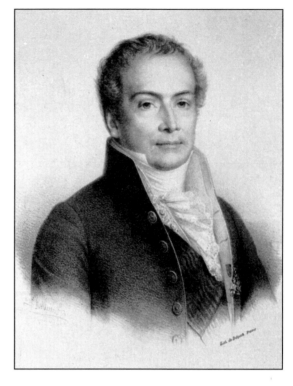

Jean Louis Alibert (1766-1837)

Below: l'Hôpital Saint Louis, Paris, Alibert's base of operations throughout his career.

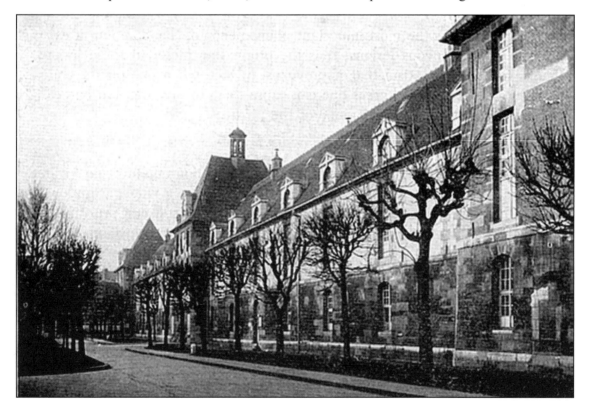

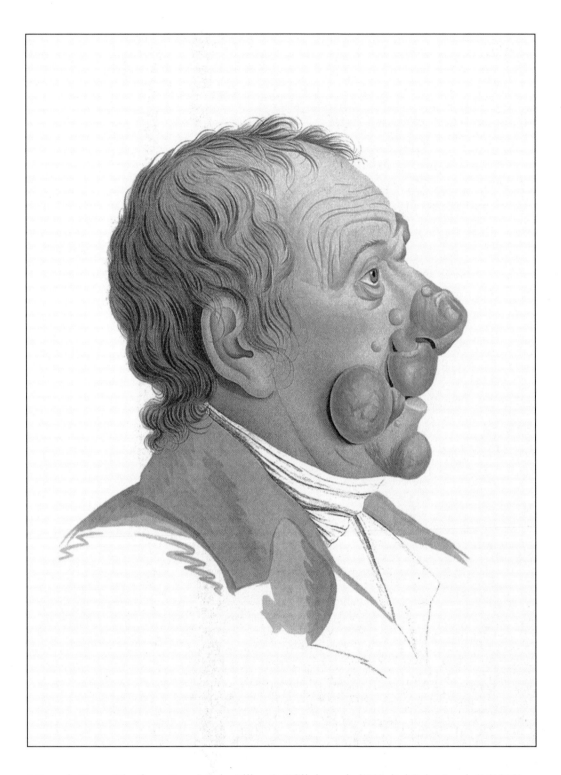

Mycosis Fongoïde, from Jean Louis Alibert's "Clinique de l'Hôpital Saint Louis." (1833).

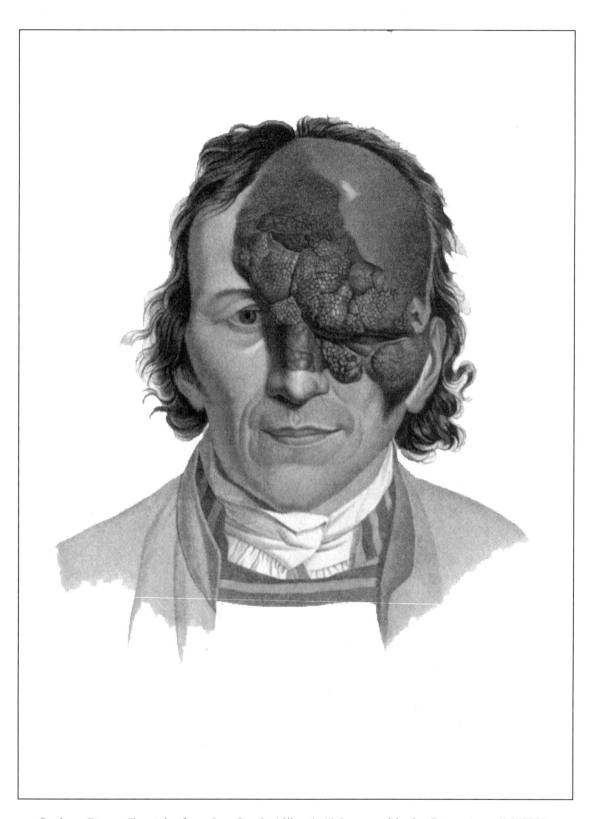

Spalaco-Derma Frontale, from Jean Louis Alibert's "Monographie des Dermatoses." (1832)

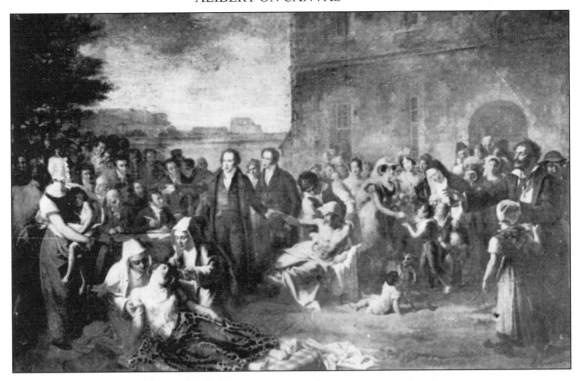

Jean Louis Alibert holding forth in his open air clinic on the grounds of l'Hôpital Saint Louis, Paris. Painting by Berthon. The original hangs in the City Hall of Villefranche-de-Rouergue, Alibert's hometown.

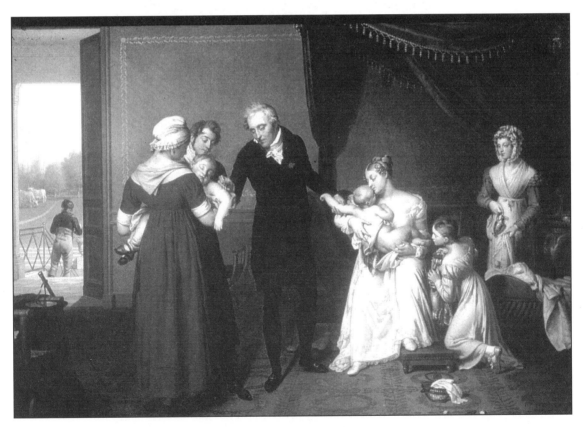

Alibert preparing to vaccinate the child held in the arms of Mme. Desbordes-Valmore (seated). Painting by Constant Desbordes, shown at the Salon of 1822. It hangs now in the Musée de l'Assistance in Paris. Alibert was an ardent proponent of vaccination against smallpox; the procedure was extremely controversial at the time.

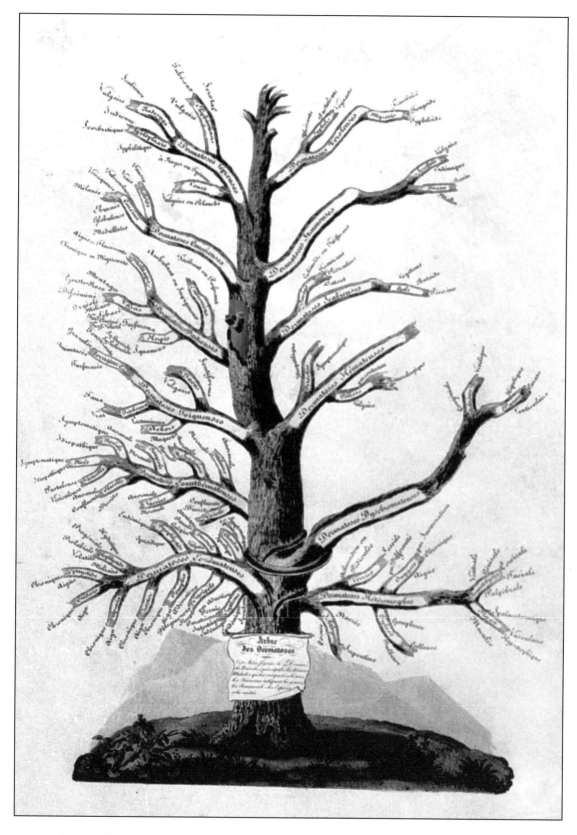

Jean Louis Alibert's famous "Arbre des Dermatoses," a pictorial representation of his "nosologie naturelle," his new classification of skin diseases which he was convinced would triumph over the "unnatural" scheme of Willan that was based on the morphology of the essential lesions. His classification drowned in its own complexity. From the "Clinique de l'Hôpital Saint Louis," Paris, 1833.

22

Laurent Biett, Swiss dermatologist, pupil, friend, and colleague of Jean Louis Alibert, spent his entire professional life at l'Hôpital St. Louis. He was a masterful clinician, hardheaded and precise, and a lecturer of no nonsense skill. His famous 1829 quarrel and debate with his teacher foreshadowed the direction dermatology was to take for the next thirty years.

Alibert had been away tending to the ailments of King Louis XVIII. When he returned to Paris he made an unpleasant discovery. Biett, whom he had left in charge, had been to England, had returned a convert to the Willan system for the identification of skin diseases, and had installed this foreign doctrine at St. Louis. Alibert himself had classified and named skin diseases on the basis of a whole series of shared signs and symptoms, while Willan had named them on the basis of the appearance of the lesions themselves. Alibert was appalled. He wrapped himself in mystery, surrounded himself with scholars and announced that a thorough refutation of the whole Willan business would be forthcoming. Tension mounted when Biett announced that a rebuttal would follow shortly. It was the warm, romantic, Catholic, French extrovert against the cool, scientific, protestant Swiss introvert.

The day was cold when Alibert chose to make his stand, but the clinic was crowded, and Alibert gave the speech of his life, unveiling at the climax, and to tumultuous applause, two huge paintings of his new "natural" system - his tree of dermatoses - trunk, branches, twigs representing interrelationships of the various diseases as he saw them. But his triumph was short-lived. A few days later, before the very same audience, Biett calmly uprooted the newly planted tree, and clearly demonstrated the superiority of the Willan system.

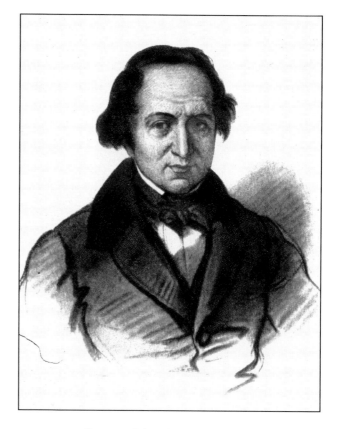

Laurent Biett (1781-1840)

In the majority of cases this form assumes the characters of psoriasis guttata. The spots may be confined to one region of the body, but they generally occupy the neck, back, chest, and abdomen at the same time, or the limbs, face, and scalp. They vary in size from the diameter of a farthing to that of a half-crown piece: they are generally isolated and irregularly circular, a little elevated above the surface, and covered by thin, hard, grayish, tenacious scales, which fall off and expose a smooth, shining surface, of a coppery tint, unlike the red, fissured elevations of psoriasis. Even when more allied to P. guttata, they present a peculiar appearance, which M. Biett considers as pathognomonic; this is a small, white border, surrounding the base of each disc, and evidently produced by laceration of the epidermis.

Biett was not a prolific writer; no textbook bears his name, but his pupils Alphée Cazenanve and Henri (Heinrich) Schedel took care of that. They published his lectures in paraphrase in their "Abrégé pratique des maladies de la peau" (1828). This work, one of the most important in the 19th century, led to the acceptance of the Willan-Bateman morphologic approach to the classification and diagnosis of skin diseases in France and subsequently in the whole of Europe. It contains, among other contributions of note, Biett's classic description of lupus erythematosus.

Shown to the left, buried in a paragraph on the papulo-squamous syphilid, is another "Abrégé" pearl. It is the brief description of the "collarette of Biett," the narrow whitish circle often seen at the periphery of the papular lesions of secondary syphilis, particularly on the palms and soles. It is not pathognomonic, as Biett thought, but none-the-less retains its value as a clinical red flag, a reminder to the examiner that the treponeme may be at work.

In the early decades of the nineteenth century, controversies over the existence of a mite as the cause of scabies swirled around the Alibert clinic in Paris. Monetary prizes, challenges, and fraudulent demonstrations were involved.

Simon François Renucci (birth and death dates unknown), a Corsican medical student at l'Hôtel Dieu, had seen the peasant women of his native land extract the mites from children with "the itch." He was astonished and amused to discover the extent to which this tiny creature had buffaloed the learned professors of Paris. Alibert, a firm believer in the existence of the mite, had been humiliated earlier by unsuccessful attempts to confirm his position. He arranged to have Renucci demonstrate his skills in a clinic at l'Hôpital St. Louis.

The date was August 25, 1834. The notables gathered - believers and non-believers alike. Tensions were running high as Renucci began the proceedings at 10 a.m. A patient was brought in. The young Corsican bent over the man, busied himself with a lesion, straightened, turned, and held aloft the genuine acarus, fixed on the point of a pin. Alibert was vindicated, and the existence of the mite was never questioned again.

Proof that the acarus is the proximate cause of scabies came from an extended series of auto-inoculation experiments conducted by Ferdinand Hebra in Vienna a few years after the Renucci demonstration.

Below, left: KOH preparation, ventral surface of the scabies mite (2001).
Below, right: The Acarus scabiei as depicted in Renucci's Inaugural Thesis (1835). The Corsican was correct.

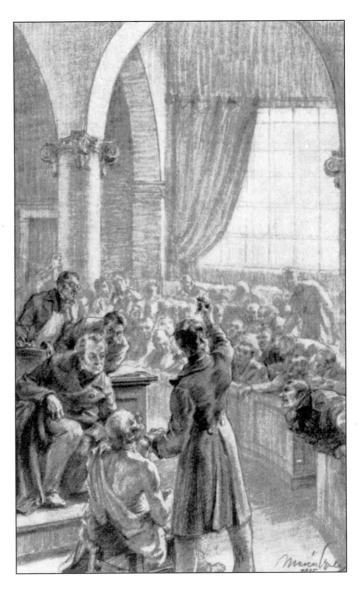

The Renucci demonstration, August 25, 1834.
Charcoal drawing by Jules Meresz.

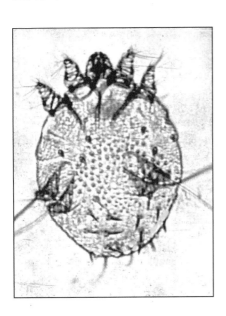

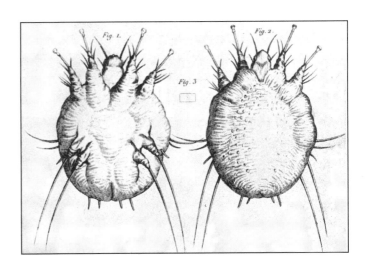

Luca Stulli, multi-talented Croatian physician, was born in Ragusa and received his medical training in Bologna under Uttini, Mondini, and Galvani. Soon after graduation he found it advisable to exit Bologna for political reasons. He took up residence in Florence, where he came under the influence of the renowned naturalist Felix Fontana. He maintained an active interest in the natural sciences throughout his life. From Florence he moved to Rome and Naples, practiced in both cities, and eventually returned to Croatia, where he succumbed to a stroke in 1828.

As a physician, Stulli was best known in his own time as an ardent proponent of cowpox vaccination against smallpox; he was involved in mass vaccination activities, particularly in Dalmatia. He is forever linked now with mal de meleda, the rare inherited condition of palms and soles committed to memory by generations of dermatology students attracted equally by the intriguing nature of the disease and that mellifluous name that rolls so pleasantly off the tongue.

Geology was also of great interest to Stulli, and he was an accomplished classical scholar, a poet, and a successful playwright, as well.

Stulli L. Di una varietà cutanea. Lettera del dottore Stulli. Autologia, Florence 1826;71-72:1-3

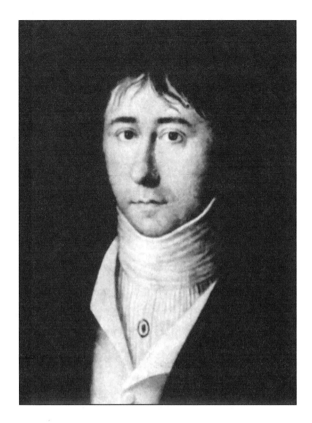

Luca Stulli (1772-1828)

In the classic report cited above, Stulli described 11 individuals in 3 families in a village on the Island of Meleda (Mljet) off the coast of Dalmatia (Croatia). All were afflicted with an eruption of the palms and soles. The condition was present at birth and worsened with the passage of time. The skin was grossly thickened, rough and insensitive to touch. Deep fissures formed, which were bloody and odorous. Knees were sometimes affected. Known now as progressive palmoplantar keratoderma, the condition is characterized by its recessive or variable dominant mode of inheritance.

The location of Meleda is shown on the map below. In former times, dermatologists on vacation sometimes visited the island to view the disorder for themselves, but demographic and environmental conditions on Mljet are much altered now, and mal de meleda has disappeared. It shows up elsewhere only on rare occasions.

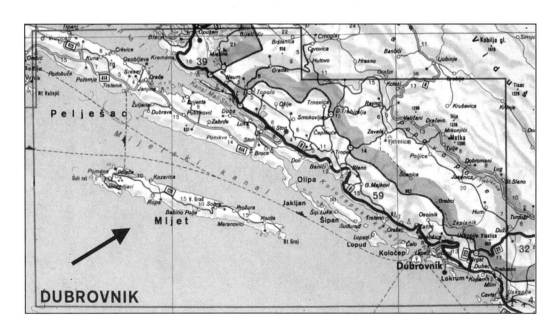

Johann Lucas Schoenlein, German physician, is justly remembered as the man who introduced modern clinical teaching into his homeland. During his years at the Charité in Berlin, he was the first to lecture in the vernacular (1840), and he employed in his clinics the newly developed techniques of auscultation, percussion, chemical analysis of blood and urine, and microscopic examination.

An unlikely exercise in free association on the part of Schoenlein in 1839 led to one of the most important medical discoveries of the 19th century, and one of great significance for dermatology. In perusing the literature he noted that the cause of an epidemic of the silkworm disease which was severely damaging the silk industry in Italy had been shown to be a fungus – the first time a plant had been identified as a cause of an animal disease. He also learned from his reading that a Viennese botanist had observed that the lesions on the leaves of plants attacked by fungi looked very much like the lesions of human skin diseases. Synapses fired, and Schoenlein suspected that he was on to something exciting. He curetted several scutula from a pair of favus patients languishing on his ward, placed them under the microscope, and confirmed his suspicions at once: *no doubt about it, favus is caused by a fungus.*

Schoenlein immediately sent off a letter to Johannes Mueller, editor of *Mueller's Archiv*, describing these events, along with a small drawing of the organism and a desiccated scutulum for the editor himself to inspect. Mueller published the letter in his journal, and henceforth medical mycology was with us for good. The letter was Schoenlein's final word on the subject. He turned the project over to his pupil Robert Remak, who later isolated the causative organism, *Trichophyton schoenleinii*, and named it after his teacher.

The reference and the entire body of the classic letter are shown to the right. The figure that accompanied the report is shown below.

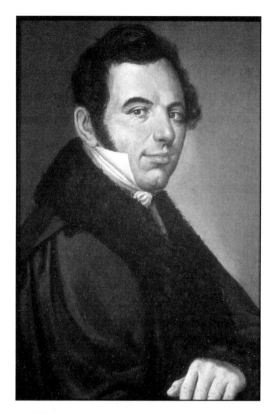

Johann Lukas Schoenlein (1793-1864)

Schoenlein JL. Zur Pathogenie der Impetigines. Arch Anat Phys (Mueller's Archiv), 1839, p 82

Zur Pathogenie der Impetigines.

Von

Prof. SCHOENLEIN in Zürich.

(Auszug aus einer brieflichen Mittheilung an den Herausgeber.)

(Hierzu Taf. III. Fig. 5.)

Sie kennen ohne Zweifel Bassi's schöne Entdeckung über die wahre Natur der Muscardine. Die Thatsache scheint mir von höchstem Interesse für die Pathogenie, obgleich meines Wissens auch nicht ein Arzt sie bisher seiner Aufmerksamkeit gewürdigt hatte. Ich liess mir deshalb zahlreiche Exemplare von Seidenwürmern, die an der Muscardine litten, von Mailand kommen, und meine damit angestellten Versuche haben nicht bloss Bassi's und Audouin's Angaben bestätigt, sondern noch einige andere nicht ganz unwichtige Resultate ergeben. Dadurch wurde ich denn wieder an meine Ansicht von der pflanzlichen Natur mancher Impetigines erinnert, eine Ansicht, die durch Unger's schöne Arbeit über Pflanzen-Exantheme schon früher eine mächtige Unterstützung fand. Da ich gerade glücklicher Weise einige Exemplare von Porrigo lupinosa W. im Hospitale hatte, so machte ich mich an die nähere Untersuchung, und gleich die ersten Versuche liessen keinen Zweifel über die Pilz-Natur der sogenannten Pusteln. Anliegend eine mikroskopische Abbildung eines Pustelstückes. Zugleich sende ich einige mit der grössten Leichtigkeit aus der oberen Schichte der Lederhaut am Lebenden ausgeschälte Porrigo-Pusteln bei. Ich bin eifrig mit weiteren Untersuchungen über diesen Gegenstand beschäftigt, deren Resultat ich bald zu veröffentlichen gedenke.

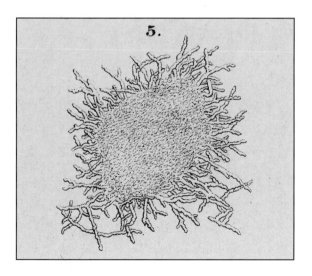

5.

THE FRENCH
WILLANISTS

Pierre François Olive Rayer, a general physician and one of the 19th century's major medical figures, developed a special interest in skin diseases. He learned his dermatology from Biett. He was associated with la Charité hospital in Paris for many years, and it was there that he collected the clinical material that appeared in 1828 in his first major work, the "Traité théorique et pratique des maladies de la Peau." The Traité is a masterpiece, filled with shrewd and accurate clinical observations. Unna considered it next to the texts of Willan and Bateman "the most solid work on dermatology that comes to us from the early part of the [nineteenth] century."

For Rayer, dermatology was only the first stage of a remarkably varied and productive career. In 1837 he discovered that glanders was contagious and could be transmitted from horse to man and back again. His greatest achievement was his "Treatise on diseases of the kidney" (1839), the finest text of the day on renal disease.

Rayer eventually became one of Europe's most celebrated physicians, with a rich and famous clientele, but he was an independent soul who neither sought out these patients nor took any nonsense from them. He often forgot his appointments completely when engaged in experimental work. "Is it true, Doctor, that the Roman physicians were all freed slaves?" asked one patient, a banker who was irked at his independence. "Yes," replied Rayer, "but those were the days when Mercury was the god of bankers and thieves."

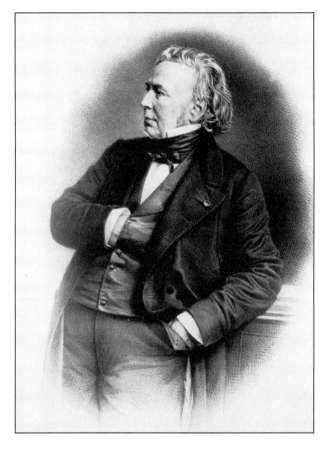

Pierre François Olive Rayer (1793-1867)

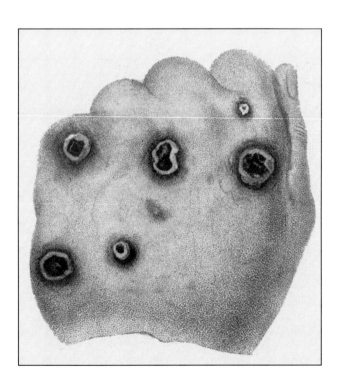

To the left: Ecthyma, figure from Rayer's atlas illustrating his classic description of the disease. Rayer was also the first to describe black hairy tongue and cheilitis exfoliativa. His unerring sense of clinical verismo is evident again in his valuable contributions to the study of the eczematous eruptions. In addition to the acute and chronic designations of previous authors, he furnishes for the first time a description of the peculiarities of eczema as it occurs in certain anatomic locations, the regional eczematous forms that constitute self-contained, highly distinctive entities - pruritus ani, pruritus vulvae, otitis externa, eruptions of the nipple, eyelids, and the like - that demand special attention in matters of diagnosis or management.

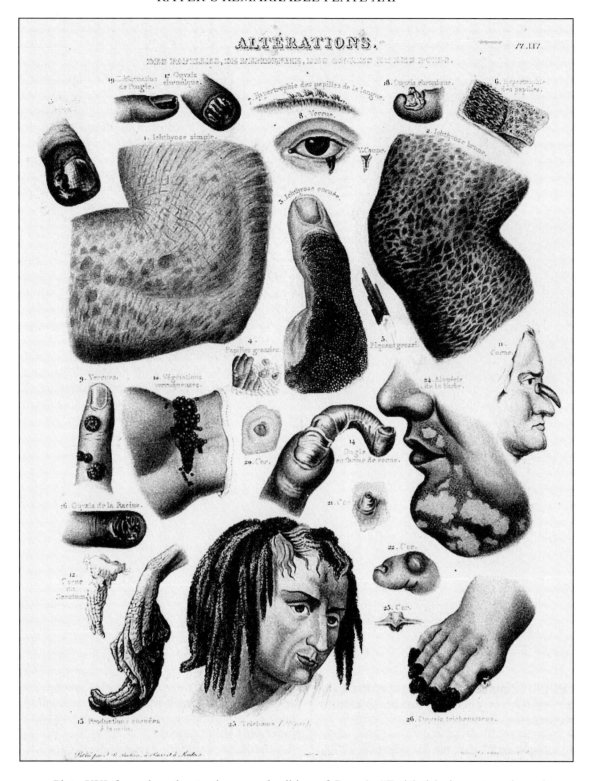

Plate XXI from the atlas to the second edition of Rayer's "Traité théorique et pratique des maladies de la peau," (1835). This plate set a record for "firsts" in medical illustration. Verruca vulgaris, verruca filiformis, alopecia areata of the beard, black hairy tongue, acute paronychia, onychomycosis, onychogryphosis, and corns all make their initial appearance there in recognizable form. The original is in color.

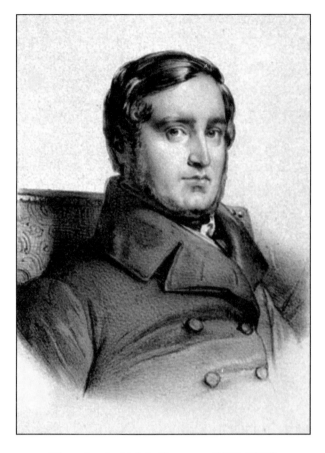

Pierre-Louis-Alphée Cazenave (1795-1877)

Pierre-Louis-Alphée Cazenave, a key figure in the dermatology of France in the middle decades of the 19th century, was a pupil of Biett. Like his teacher, he worked at l'Hôpital St. Louis. He transcribed the lectures of Biett and with a colleague, Henri (Heinrich) Schedel, published them as the "Abrégé pratique des maladies de la peau," He later produced an influential treatise of his own on diseases of the scalp ("Traité des maladies du cuir chevelu"). A peerless morphologist, he brought new levels of precision to the description of the ringworm diseases, expanded on Biett's description of érythème centrifuge and renamed it lupus erythematosus, published the classic description of pemphigus foliaceus, and made notable contributions to the treatment of syphilis and to the study of alopecia areata, linking the latter to vitiligo for the first time. From 1843 to 1852 Cazenave published and edited the first journal in French devoted to dermatology and syphilology, the *Annales des maladies de la peau et de la syphilis*, most of which he wrote himself. It is an impressive curriculum vitae.

Below: the opening of Cazenave's classic description of pemphigus foliaceus as it appeared in 1844 in Cazenave's own journal, the *Annales des maladies de la peau et de la syphilis*. His classic account of discoid lupus erythematosus appeared in the same journal in 1851.

OBSERVATIONS.

PEMPHIGUS CHRONIQUE, GÉNÉRAL; FORME RARE DE PEMPHIGUS FOLIACÉ; MORT; AUTOPSIE; ALTÉRATION DU FOIE.

L..., âgée de 47 ans. me fut adressée à l'hôpital Saint-Louis, le 27 août 1842, pour une éruption qui datait de plusieurs années, qui occupait toute la surface du corps, et dont la persistance avait gravement compromis la santé de cette malade.

La femme L... s'était toujours bien portée, lorsque, à l'âge de 20 ans, elle fut atteinte d'un rhumatisme articulaire qui dura fort longtemps. Depuis, elle eut à deux reprises différentes la *jaunisse*, et, plus tard encore, un érysipèle gangréneux de la jambe.

La maladie actuelle existait déjà depuis quatre ans. Elle aurait débuté, suivant la malade, par un érysipèle de la face, qui s'étendit au sein, puis envahit successivement toute la surface du corps. Les plaques erysipélateuses auraient été alors, dès le début, le siége des élevures du pemphigus. Quoi qu'il en soit, pendant longtemps la face, le ventre, la partie

To the right: The Abrégé of Cazenave and Schedel. One of the most important books in the development of dermatology, it spread the Willanist morphologic approach to the classification and identification of skin diseases throughout continental Europe.

Below left: Cazenave's beautifully written and well illustrated treatise on diseases of the scalp. The first regional dermatologic work of its kind, this treatise served as the model for Sabouraud's grand multi-volume work on the same subject in the early decades of the 20th century.

Below right: Gray patch (Microsporum) tinea capitis, from the Cazenave scalp treatise. Cazenave was the first to point out that ringworm of the glabrous skin and tinea capitis are essentially the same disease. He did so on clinical grounds alone, dismissing the newly reported evidence for the presence of fungi in the lesions as "illusions hatched in the field of a microscope."

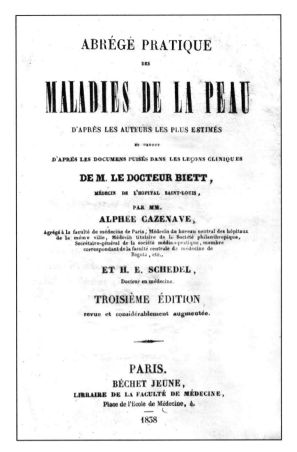

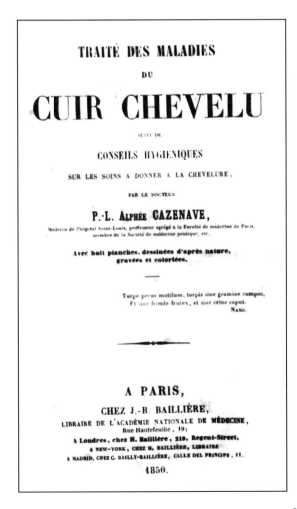

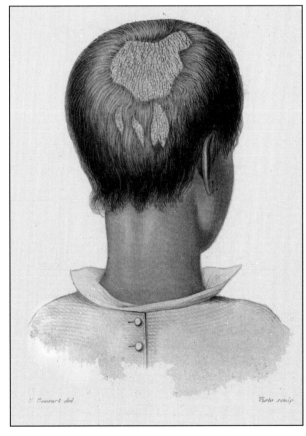

Prescription written and signed by Alphée Cazenave, Paris, 19 August, 1859. Patient's name and diagnosis unknown.

Translation:
1. Monsieur will take, at the moment of going to bed, one of the following pills
    Codeine – six grains
    Extract of valerian twenty-four grains
Monsieur is to have twenty-four pills.
2. He is to take every eight days, one glass, eight grams, from a bottle of Scotch.
3. Every evening after dining he is to take two little cups of an infusion of camomille.

Paris 19 August 1859   Al Cazenave

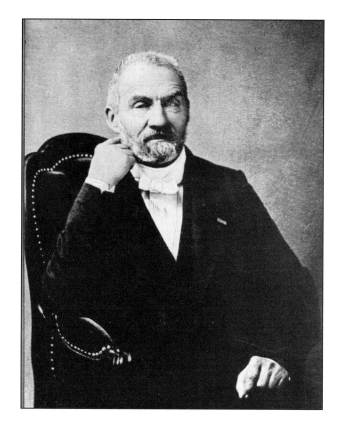

Camille Gibert (1797-1866)

Paris born and educated, Camille Gibert learned his dermatology from Biett, and from 1840 on was associated with l'Hôpital St. Louis. Like Biett, he espoused Robert Willan's morphologic approach to the classification of skin diseases. A prickly colleague, prone to hold a grudge, Gibert was nevertheless extremely popular with students, particularly foreigners, who appreciated his skills as a lecturer and his ability to keep things simple. Both American "protodermatologists," Noah Worcester and Henry Daggett Bulkley spent time in his clinic.

Gibert is remembered now chiefly for his original description of pityriasis rosea (shown below, left), but in his own time he was better known for his demonstration by inoculation experiments that syphilis in its secondary stage is indeed contagious, a fact then doubted by many well known physicians. Gibert died in the Parisian cholera epidemic of 1866.

Below: English translation of the second edition of Gibert's popular textbook.
Left: Gibert's original description of "PR" – short, sweet, and on the money: It appeared in the 1860 edition of the "Practical treatise."

PITYRIASIS: The two most distinctive forms which we have observed in this eruption category are: 1. The one we have described above, the appearance of which recalls that of lichen sometimes, at other times psoriasis. 2. Another variety which one might designate by the name pityriasis rosea, and which presents the following characteristics: small furfuraceous spots which are very lightly colored, irregular, scarcely exceeding a fingernail in size, numerous and close set, although always separated by some interval of normal skin, pruritic, and which appear on the superior parts of the body, with a predilection for the neck, the upper part of the chest, and the upper part of the arms, but which may spread successively from above downwards as far as the thighs in such a way that the total duration of the eruption, which disappears little by little from tine parts first affected as it moves downward, is protracted quite commonly to six weeks or two months. This eruption, which is more common in the female than the male, is observed quite frequently in the warm season of the year. It is seen almost only in young people and in individuals whose skin is fair, fine, and delicate.

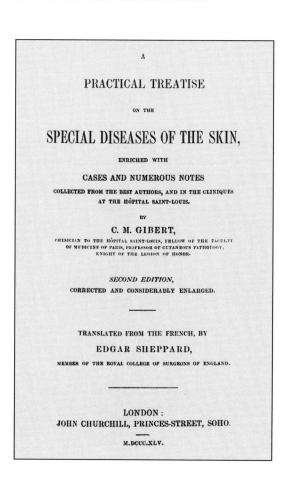

A

PRACTICAL TREATISE

ON THE

SPECIAL DISEASES OF THE SKIN,

ENRICHED WITH

CASES AND NUMEROUS NOTES

COLLECTED FROM THE BEST AUTHORS, AND IN THE CLINIQUES
AT THE HÔPITAL SAINT-LOUIS.

BY

C. M. GIBERT,

PHYSICIAN TO THE HÔPITAL SAINT-LOUIS, FELLOW OF THE FACULTY
OF MEDICINE OF PARIS, PROFESSOR OF CUTANEOUS PATHOLOGY,
KNIGHT OF THE LEGION OF HONOR.

SECOND EDITION,
CORRECTED AND CONSIDERABLY ENLARGED.

TRANSLATED FROM THE FRENCH, BY

EDGAR SHEPPARD,

MEMBER OF THE ROYAL COLLEGE OF SURGEONS OF ENGLAND.

LONDON:
JOHN CHURCHILL, PRINCES-STREET, SOHO.

M.DCCC.XLV.

Successor to Biett at l'Hôpital St. Louis, Marie-Guillaume-Alphonse Devergie was an enthusiastic morphologist who multiplied the species of skin diseases by making overly refined distinctions between elementary forms on the basis of minor variations in color and configuration. Nevertheless, he was a keen observer, the author of the classic description of pityriasis rubra pilaris, and a key figure in the development of the most difficult of all clinical constructs in dermatology to visualize properly, the "eczema" constellation.

First described and named by Willan, eczema started out as a fuzzy designation for vesicular eruptions caused by sunlight and irritants. Devergie pointed out that vesicles need not be present or appeared early and were gone by the time the patient consulted a physician. His four-point route to the diagnosis, noted below, caught on and remained the diagnostic standard for some time. It retains a goodly measure of validity even today, and the term "tenacity" employed in Devergie's classic description of the nummular form of eczema, also shown below, is currently accurate, as well. Dermatologists in Devergie's time tended to think of eczema as a disease *sui generis*, a monolith, but by the end of the 19th century myriad clinical and experimental observations had established eczema as a reaction pattern with many different causes.

Like many physicians of the period, Devergie was expert in more than one specialty. In addition to dermatology he was an authority on medico-legal matters, and many of his publications deal with the daily chores of the morgues of Paris, the detection of poisons, the effects of hanging, gunshot wounds, and the like.

M.G.A. Devergie is not to be confused with his contemporary, Marie-Nicolas Devergie (b. 1784), who authored a superb syphilis atlas.

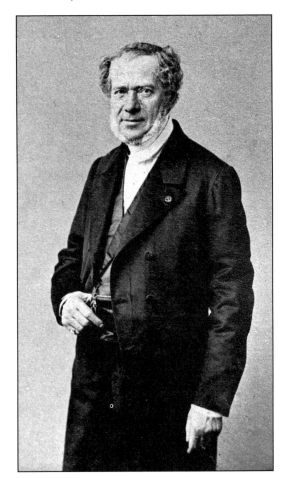

Alphonse Devergie (1798-1879)

Below: Devergie's four-point route to the diagnosis of eczema, with its instructive stiffening simile.
Devergie A. Traité pratique des maladies de la peau, 2nd ed., Paris, Masson, 1857. p 231
Right. Devergie's classic description of nummular eczema.
Devergie A. Traité pratique des maladies de la peau, Paris, Masson, 1854. p 237.

[Eczema is] a superficial disease of the skin characterized by the following four phenomena:1.) redness of the diseased surface; 2.) constant itching that varies in intensity; 3.) secretion of a clear, yellowish, serous discharge that stains linen gray and stiffens it as semen does; 4.) a red and punctate state of the skin made up of the inflamed orifices of canals, myriads of which provide the serous secretion; also, each of these small points when exposed to air shortly gives rise to a series of tiny, extremely scanty serous droplets.

The occurrence together of these four characteristics is so significant that once established it is impossible to mistake eczema for any other disease of the skin.

Nummular eczema has nowhere been described. We observed it for the first time in a post office employee eight years ago, and since that time, having been impressed by its form, we have had occasion to see several examples of it a year. It is less remarkable for its nummular disposition than for its tenacity, and the difficulty experienced in treating it has led us to make it a particular species.

Nummular eczema has the special distinction of developing chiefly on the surface of the extremities, and notably the upper extremities, also on the surface of the trunk. It shows itself there as small plaques which attain immediately the size they are to have; they are rounded, the size of a five franc piece or a little more; they show no thickening, which distinguishes them from herpes; their periphery thins out and merges with the rest of the skin, as in ordinary eczema; they are accompanied, moreover, by redness, a punctate condition of the skin, itching, and serous secretions. They require, in general, several months for cure, and usually yield only to a combination of more or less energetic agents.

EARLY AMERICAN
DERMATOLOGY

A native of New Haven, Connecticut, Henry Daggett Bulkley was born on April 4, 1804. He was educated at Yale, received his M.D. from that institution in 1830, and spent the following year in France, where his studies included a short but important stint at l'Hôpital St. Louis, attending the lectures of Biett and Gibert. He opened an office in New York City and for a few years was interested in dermatology, but as time passed he moved more and more into general medicine. He became one of Gotham's most sought-after diagnosticians. He edited the New York Medical Times, served as president of the N.Y. Academy of Medicine, and involved himself in a host of other non-dermatologic organizational and educational activities which occupied him fully until his death (from pneumonia) on January 4, 1872, at the age of 68.

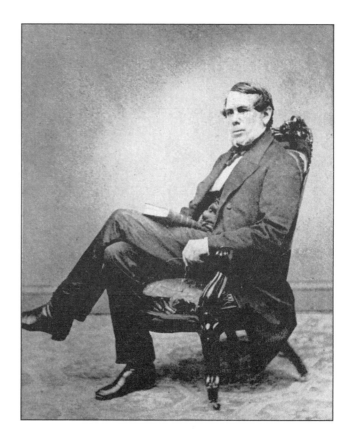

Henry Daggett Bulkley (1804-1872).

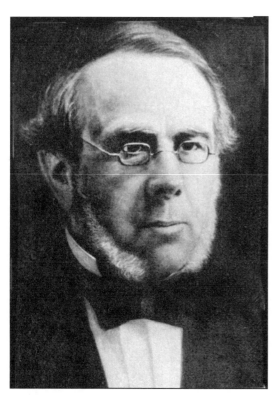

Henry Daggett Bulkley, ca 1870..

Although his time with Biett and Gibert was brief, Bulkley found on his return to New York that he seemed to know more about skin diseases than anyone else – an example of the power of the one eyed man in the land of the blind. He was consulted often by his colleagues.

"As brother physicians and students began to multiply about me," he later reminisced, "the question was asked, perhaps with no very definite object, why I did not lecture on this subject. The idea had not occurred to me, but remembering that the best way to learn is to teach, I began to prepare myself for this, to me entirely new work, and in the year 1837 I gave lectures on Diseases of the Skin, the first, I believe, ever delivered in this country, at an institution established for the treatment of these diseases, known under the name of the "Broome Street Infirmary for Diseases of the Skin"; this had been opened during the previous year and was the first organization for this special purpose, so far as I can learn, in this country - an institution which I had the pleasure of originating and of helping to sustain."

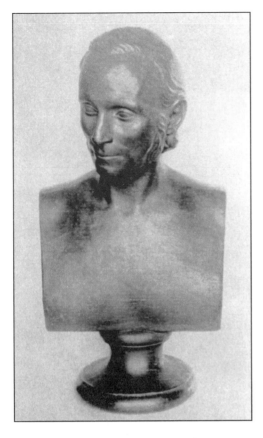

Noah Worcester (1812-1847)
Curiously, no picture of Worcester seems to
exist, and yet this impressive bust is still on
display at the Cincinnati medical school.

A

SYNOPSIS

OF THE

SYMPTOMS, DIAGNOSIS AND TREATMENT

OF THE MORE COMMON AND IMPORTANT

DISEASES OF THE SKIN.

WITH

SIXTY COLORED FIGURES.

BY N. WORCESTER, M. D.,

PROFESSOR OF PHYSICAL DIAGNOSIS AND GENERAL PATHOLOGY, IN THE
MEDICAL SCHOOL OF CLEVELAND, LATE PROFESSOR
IN THE MEDICAL COLLEGE OF OHIO.

PHILADELPHIA:
THOMAS COWPERTHWAIT & CO.
BOSTON, CHARLES C. LITTLE AND JAMES BROWN.
CINCINNATI, DESILVER & BURR.
1845.

"Diseases of the Skin," by Noah Worcester (1845).
America's first textbook of dermatology.

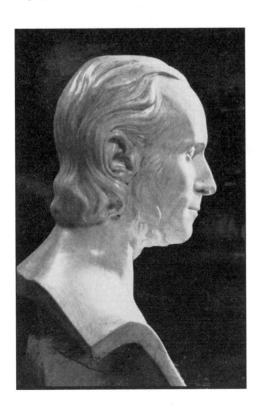

Noah Worcester, author of America's first
authentic dermatologic treatise, was a man ahead of
his time. Dartmouth trained, Worcester spent eight
post graduate months in Europe in 1841, a good
portion of it in Paris in the skin clinics of Cazenave
and Gibert. As a Prof. of Physical Diagnosis and
Pathology at the newly formed Medical School of
Ohio in Cincinnati, he acquired a reputation as a
teacher and practitioner of the first rank, but soon
realized he was suffering from rapidly progressive
pulmonary tuberculosis. In the throes of his disease
he sought relief and refuge in writing, the result of
which was his "Diseases of the Skin" (1845). The
book is a well executed exposition of the French
Willanist approach, and its colored plates are
certainly impressive. Worcester succumbed to his
disease in 1847 at the age of 35. Worcester's treatise
was not a best seller. America at the time was not
ready for the sort of specialization it represented.

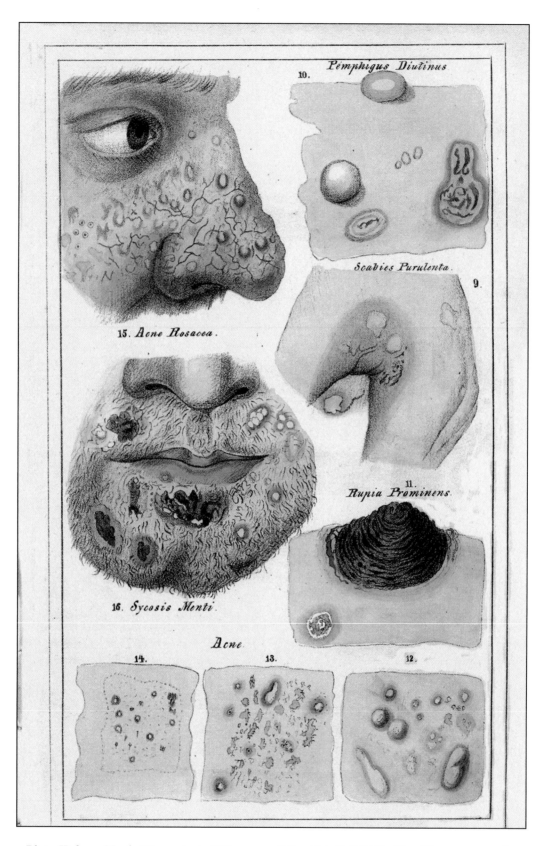

Plate II from Noah Worcester's "Diseases of the Skin" (1845). The Worcester work, America's first dermatologic textbook, was published in Philadelphia, but the remarkably good color plates were produced by the firm of Klauprech and Menzel in Worcester's home base, Cincinnati, a city barely 30 years old at the time.

MID-NINETEENTH
CENTURY LEADERS

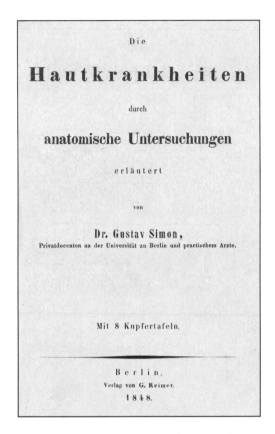

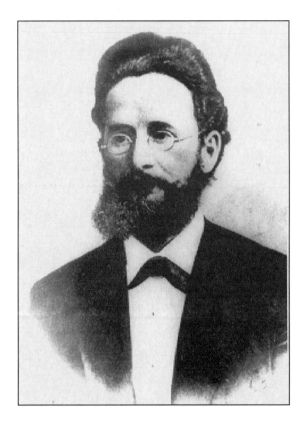

Karl Gustav Theodor Simon (1810-1857)

Simon's textbook of 1848, a key work in the development of dermatology.

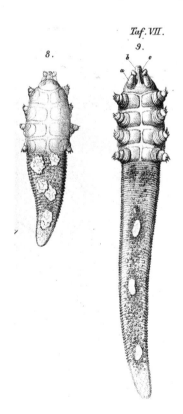

Berlin trained Karl Gustav Theodor Simon entered general practice as a physician to the poor in 1833. Almost as a hobby he began to make little micoscopic studies of skin lesions he observed on his patients. In 1842, while examining follicular tissue taken from a lesion of acne vulgaris, he thought he saw something that looked like a living creature. "Postulation became certainty," he wrote, " when I pressed the object under observation very gently between two glass plates and saw very clearly that it moved." The creature was later named Demodex folliculorum, and the significance of its presence has intrigued investigators ever since. Simon later became chief of the dermatologic clinic at the Charité Hospital in Berlin, and it was in this setting that he completed his most important work, "Die Hautkrankheiten durch Anatomische Untersuchungen Erläutert" (Diseases of the Skin Explained by Means of Anatomical Investigations). The Hautkrankheiten was the first textbook to be devoted entirely to dermatohistopathology and is recognized now as a key work in the development of the specialty.

Simon died of general paresis in 1857, at the age of forty six.

The demodex, as it appeared in Simon's textbook of 1848.

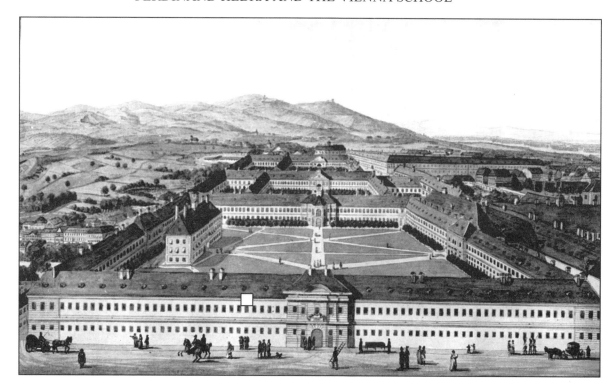

The Allgemeines Krankenhaus, Vienna – professional home to Ferdinand Hebra and his students and spiritual descendants. A good portion of the structure is still standing, although it is much modified and no longer houses skin clinics or inpatients.

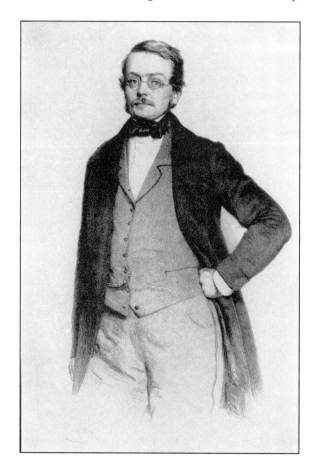

Ferdinand Hebra, Professor of Dermatology at the University of Vienna, was the "Mr. Dermatology" of the world in the middle decades of the 19th century. He began his lecture-clinic series in 1844, and within a few years developed his department into the most efficient and effective center for the teaching of dermatology of its day. Students came from far and wide to be enlightened, and many of them became famous in their own right.

Hebra reclassified skin diseases on the basis of the newer concepts of general pathology. He described several new diseases – tinea cruris, rhinoscleroma, lichen scrofulosorum, and erythema multiforme, for example, - and he augmented and refined with great skill the descriptions of older diseases such as psoriasis and the eczematous eruptions. In a series of topically applied irritant experiments designed to produce "artificial eczema" he laid ground work for experimental dermatology.

To the left: Ferdinand Hebra (1816-1880).
Circa 1850.

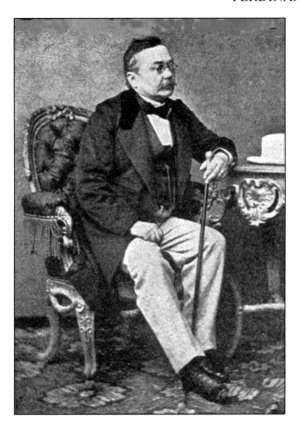

Ferdinand Hebra, mature

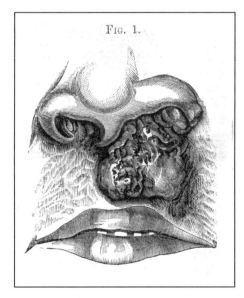

ON

DISEASES OF THE SKIN,

INCLUDING THE

EXANTHEMATA.

BY

FERDINAND HEBRA, M.D.

PROFESSOR FÜR DERMATOLOGIE AN DER UNIVERSITÄT, PRIMARARZT DER ABTHEILUNG FÜR
HAUTKRANKHEITEN IM K. K. ALLG. KRANKENHAUSE IN WIEN, ETC. ETC.

VOL. I.

TRANSLATED AND EDITED BY

C. HILTON FAGGE, M.D.,

MEMBER OF THE ROYAL COLLEGE OF PHYSICIANS;
ASSISTANT-PHYSICIAN TO, AND LECTURER ON EXPERIMENTAL PHILOSOPHY AT,
GUY'S HOSPITAL; PHYSICIAN TO THE ROYAL INFIRMARY FOR THE
DISEASES OF CHILDREN AND WOMEN.

THE NEW SYDENHAM SOCIETY,
LONDON.

MDCCCLXVI.

Volume I of the influential five volume English translation of the second edition of the Hebra textbook.

"Hebra was a most remarkable man and in his daily clinics showed a keenness of observation which was simply wonderful. He rarely asked his patient any questions, but a hasty glance would usually enable him to tell more about the case than any one of his students would elicit by a lengthy catechism. Taking the patient's hand in his and looking straight at the class he would say "this man is a tailor" and we soon found that he discovered this fact by feeling the needle pricks on the roughened forefinger. A hatter he would recognize by some peculiar callous on the ball of the thumb…" observations by the American, George Henry Fox, who studied with Hebra in 1871.

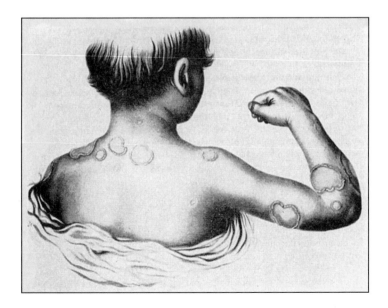

Erythema multiforme, from the Hebra atlas. Hebra saw that the endless series of erythemas described by older authors were merely variants of this single disease (1860).

Rhinoscleroma, from Hebra's textbook (1860)

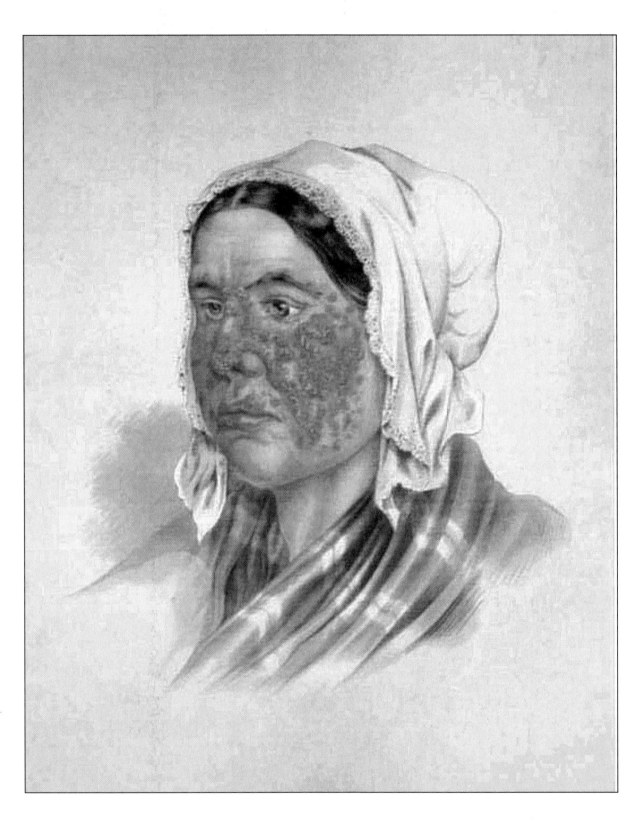

Lupus erythematosus. Plate 6 from Volume I of the Ferdinand Hebra "Atlas der Hautkrankheiten" (1856-1876). Chromolithograph by Anton Elfinger.

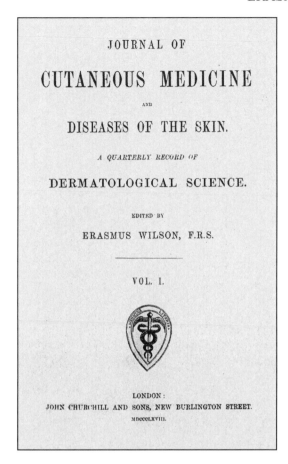

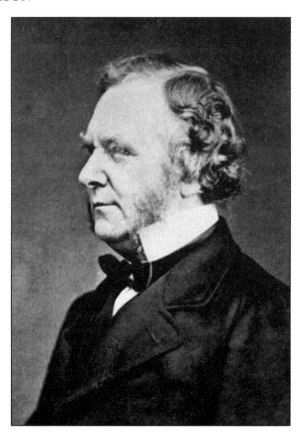

Erasmus Wilson (1809-1884)

Volume 1 of the Journal of Cutaneous Medicine, 1868 – the first dermatologic journal in English.

Erasmus Wilson, England's answer to Ferdinand Hebra, and the most famous English dermatologist in the middle decades of the 19th century, began his professional life as an anatomist, but in the 1840s switched his allegiance to diseases of the skin. He annoyed his colleagues by his propensity and ability to draw attention to himself, but his contributions to the specialty were many and significant. He was a marvelous clinician with an eye for the new. He published the classic descriptions of lichen planus, exfoliative dermatitis, infantile eczema, neurotic excoriations, delusions of parasitism, and nevus araneus. He founded and edited the *Journal of Cutaneous Medicine* (1868), the first journal in English devoted to the specialty. His "On Diseases of the Skin" (1847) remained the most popular textbook on the subject in English for many years, and his atlas ("Portraits of Diseases of the Skin") contains some of the most striking color plates ever published. Wilson's enormously popular "Practical Treatise on Healthy Skin" (1845), written for the general public, did a great deal to inform the man in the street of the benefits to be derived from consulting a dermatologist when skin becomes a problem.

Right:Erasmus Wilson's "Healthy Skin."
First American edition , 1846.

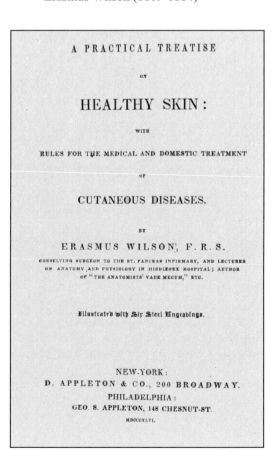

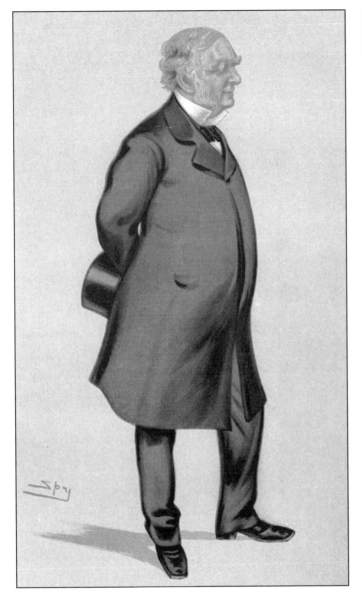

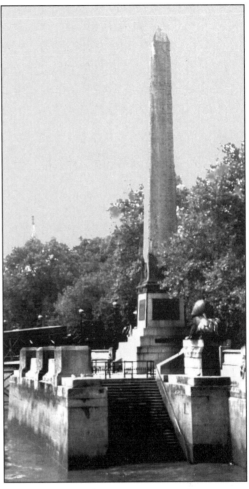

Erasmus Wilson, shown above left in an 1880 Vanity Fair magazine caricature, became a wealthy man, largely through shrewd investments in gas and railroad companies. He was active in many charitable enterprises.

Above, right: The obelisk, Cleopatra's Needle, mentioned in the caption to the caricature, below.

VANITY FAIR. London, December 18, 1880. Man of the Day – No. CCXXXIV.
 Mr. Erasmus Wilson, M.R.C.S.. He is one-and-seventy years of age and a great doctor.

The son of a naval surgeon he made himself first known as an anatomist, and finally settled down into the greatest authority on the difficult and complex subject of diseases of the skin. He is the senior Vice-President of the College of Surgeons. He travels during his holidays and has written many things besides medical works. During one of his travels he saw the Egyptian obelisk called "Cleopatra's Needle" which had been given to England but never reached its destination. He made therefore and carried out the patriotic resolve to bring home and set up the obelisk at his own expense. This he did, and the stone after many adventures reached London and now stands on the Thames embankment – a relic of an immodest cult, and a testimony to the public spirit of an excellent surgeon. He is a man of merit and modesty: and he declined to become a knight bachelor. (signed) Jehu Junior.

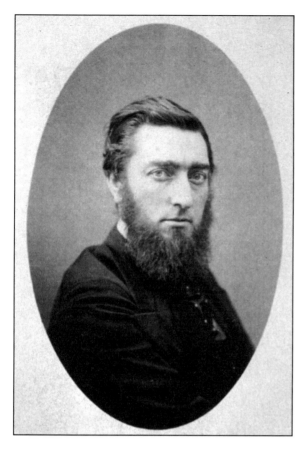

William Tilbury Fox (1836-1879)

(William) Tilbury Fox, the chief dermatologic counterweight to Erasmus Wilson in Victorian England, began his professional life as an obstetrician, but switched to dermatology in 1863. He was associated with the Charing Cross and University College Hospitals. His textbook, "Skin diseases," which appeared in 1864, was an instant success, and he soon built up an enormous private practice. Fox was in fact the very model of the complete dermatologist. Along with his clinical skills he immersed himself in the new discoveries in histopathology, bacteriology, and mycology emanating from the continent and was among the first to import them into England. Fox also had a good eye for the clinically new. Impetigo contagiosa,. dyshidrosis, and kerion ringworm were all first described by the London master. His busy schedule took its toll. He died of a massive coronary in 1879 while vacationing in Paris. He was just 43 years old.

Below: Impetigo contagiosa, from Fox's "Atlas of skin diseases," 1877. The original is in color.

Below: Fox's summary of the disease impetigo contagiosa, as it appeared in the 1877 atlas. He first described the disease in 1864.

Diagnostic features are - its apparently epidemic character in many cases; the antecedent febrile condition; its attacking children; the origin from isolated vesicles which tend to enlarge into blebs and to become pustular, the bleb having a depressed centre and, it may be, a well-defined, slightly raised, rounded edge; the isolation of the spots; the uniform character of the eruption and its general and scattered condition; its frequent seat and commencement about the face or head; the circular, flat, granular, yellow crusts looking as if stuck on; its contagious nature and inoculability; its frequently following in the wake of vaccination; the absence of pain, and especially troublesome itching at night.

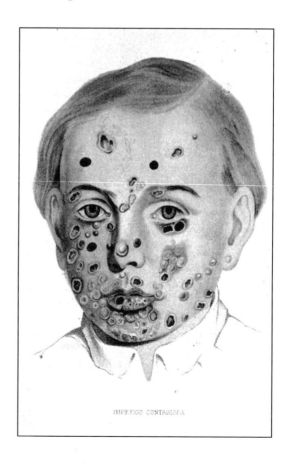

IMPETIGO CONTAGIOSA

Ernest Bazin, the dominant figure in French dermatology in the 1850s and 60s, was outspoken, easily irritated, and brilliant. Trained as an internist, he came to l'Hôpital St. Louis in 1847 after a dozen years in general practice and immediately lashed out at the local followers of Willan whose preoccupation with morphology he considered to be hopelessly superficial. To Bazin it seemed obvious that the great majority of skin lesions were merely external manifestations of various whole body disorders, which he called diatheses or constitutional diseases. Two of these creations, the syphilitic and scrofulitic diatheses, were valid to a certain extent, but herpetism, arthritism, and others were largely imaginary.

Along with his like-minded friend, Alfred Hardy, Bazin was the recipient of devastating criticism for his diathetic constructions, most of it emanating from the pen of Alphonse Devergie. It is evident in the published versions of these heated exchanges between Willanists and non-Willanists (which make enjoyable reading) that both Bazin and Hardy gave as good as they got. The quarrels were, in fact, salutary dialectics that resulted by the end of the 19th century in a more sensible and flexible attitude toward the relationship of skin lesions to problems in the inner corpus.

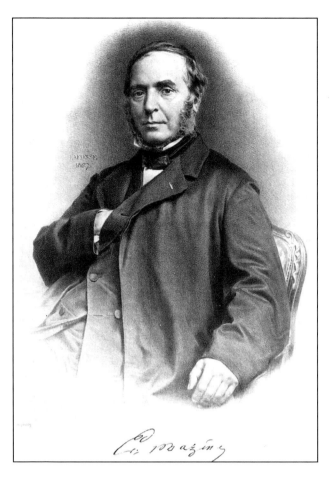

Ernest Bazin (1807-1878)

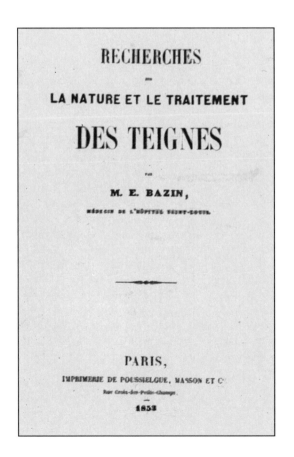

Despite his immersion in diathetic murkiness, Bazin was a first class clinician. He gave us the classic descriptions of erythema induratum, malignant syphilis, and hydroa vacciniforme. Early in his career he became interested in mycology. He confirmed for himself the contentions of Schoenlein, Gruby, and Remak that favus and ringworm are caused by fungi, and in 1853 published a fine little book on the subject. The title page of the work is shown to the left. His own contributions were largely therapeutic and practical, but his establishment of St. Louis as a center for mycologic study had far reaching consequences. It is a straight line from Bazin through Lailler and Besnier to Sabouraud. The splendid French contributions to the study of the ringworm fungi were and are a source of pride for the dermatologists of that country, and rightly so.

Bazin retired from St. Louis in 1872 and spent his remaining years taking care of his private patients and writing articles in defense of his diathetic system for publication in the medical encyclopedias of the time. He died from pulmonary congestion in 1878. He had been in poor health for a year, but was tough enough to make a house call the day before his death.

Alfred Hardy, Parisian dermatologist and a chief at l'Hôpital St. Louis, joined his friend Bazin in resisting the Willan and Bateman morphologic approach to the classification of skin diseases. A former internist and pupil of Alibert, he revived his teacher's "natural system" without its outlandish terminology and refurbished it in accordance with the latest ideas in internal medicine. Unfortunately, the data necessary to arrange the majority of skin diseases in accordance with whole body concepts did not yet exist, and Hardy's system bogged down in abstruse etiologic concepts such as his "dartrous diathesis" that were in fact intellectual blind alleys. Despite his excursion into diathetic folly, Hardy was the steadiest French dermatologist of his day and the closest to the mainstream. He was also the key figure in the final resolution of the Willan and Alibert conflict, which he defused by retaining the best ideas of both camps.

Hardy was a lively, vivacious man, even a little brusque in manner. George Henry Fox remembered him as "extremely nervous." A marvelous speaker with a sonorous voice, he achieved in his lectures that magic mix of mordant wit and information that medical students have always found irresistible.

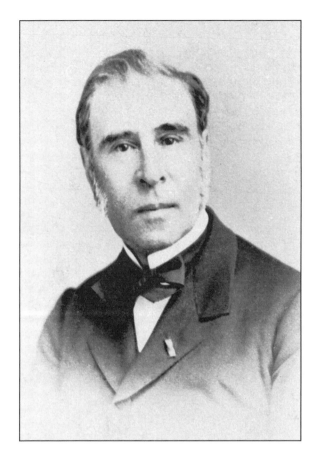

Alfred Hardy (1811-1893)

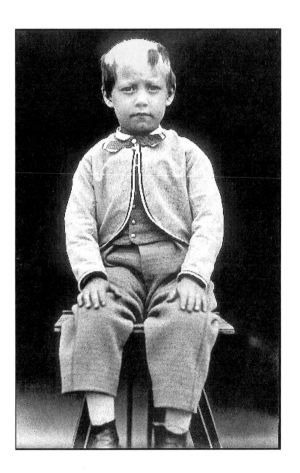

Hardy's instinctive feel for what was important and his gift for the composition of simple, transparent prose combine to make his published works the best source of information on the French attitudes and activities of his time. One of his publications, the "Clinique photographique de l'Hôpital St. Louis," is classic. It is an impressive collection of 50 clinical and histopathologic photographic prints taken and processed by Hardy's student A. de Montmeja and mounted on pages containing explanatory text by Hardy himself. The work appeared in 14 sections in 1867 and 1868. The quality of the images, some of which are hand tinted, is excellent. The appealing little boy with alopecia areata (shown to the left) is a typical example. Individual prints had been tipped in to publications earlier, but the Hardy-Monteja opus is the first true photographic atlas.

Historians interested in skin diseases also owe Alfred Hardy a special debt of gratitude for the reminiscences of his student days at St. Louis, which he committed to print in 1885. Without the details and human touches supplied in that fine little memoir, much of the romance and drama of the era of Alibert and Biett would have been lost forever.

Late Nineteenth Century British Dermatology

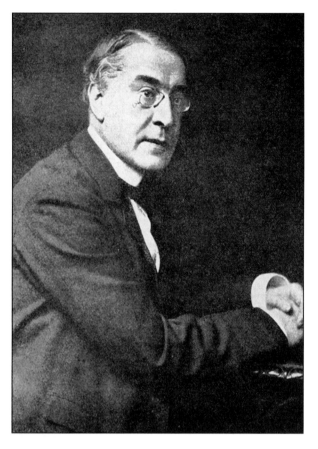

Henry Grundy Brooke, dermatologist, talented musician, art aficionado, and mordant wit, dominated the dermatology of the Midlands and northern England to such an extent that he was known throughout his career by the territorial designation "Brooke of Manchester." Along with Malcolm Morris, he founded the British Journal of Dermatology in 1888 and co-edited the publication during its early years. In a classic 1892 report, cited below, he described the first cases of the multiple and often familial form of trichoepithelioma that continues to be known by the name he assigned to it, epithelioma adenoides cysticum.

Brooke was a member of "the big five," the group of dermatolgists who more or less reigned over British dermatology late in the nineteenth century and early in the twentieth. The others were Radcliffe Crocker, Colcott Fox, Malcolm Morris, and J.J. Pringle.

Brooke HG.Epithelioma adenoides cysticum. Brit J Dermatol 1892;4:269-76

Henry Grundy Brooke (1854-1919)

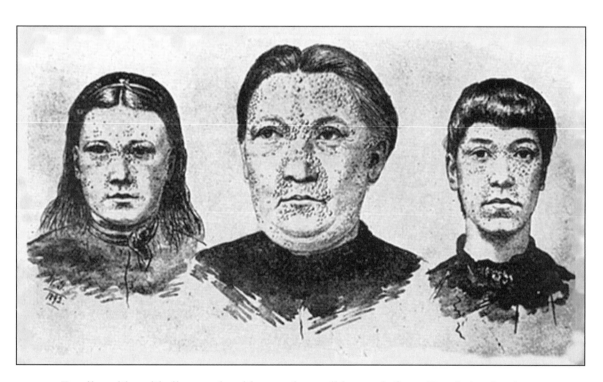

Family with epithelioma adenoides cysticum, lithograph from Brooke's classic paper, 1892

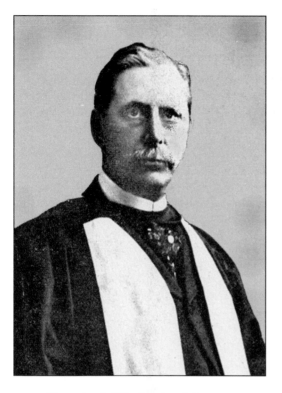

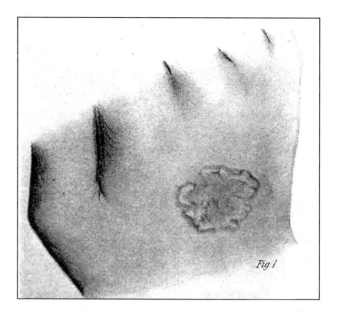

Granuloma annulare, from Radcliffe-Crocker's classic paper.

Radcliffe-Crocker H. Granuloma annulare. Brit J Dermatol 1902;14:1-6

Henry Radcliffe-Crocker (1845-1909)

Henry Radcliffe-Crocker, England's most influential dermatologist in the final quarter of the 19th century, succeeded Tilbury Fox as chief of the skin department at London's University College Hospital (1876). The eclectic views of Fox were embraced enthusiastically by Crocker. He was the first to establish micrococci as the cause of impetigo, and unlike many of his contemporaries, took the time to master the new science of histopathology. He was also a superior clinical dermatologist - responsible, for example, for the original descriptions of granuloma annulare (cited above) and erythema elevatum diutinum (cited below) - and as much as any man in his generation concerned himself with everything new in therapy. All of these streams are united happily in Crocker's "Diseases of the Skin" (1888-1903), the finest magisterial dermatologic work in English in the final decades of the 19th century. The work established its author at once as Britain's premier specialist in the field.

Crocker died of a heart attack while vacationing in Switzerland in August 1909.

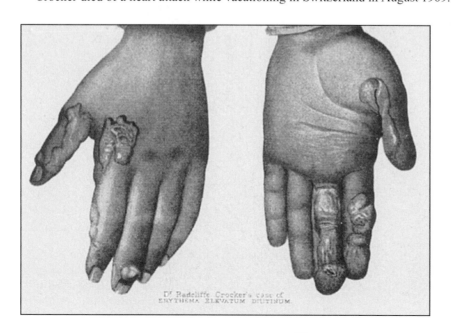

Radcliffe-Crocker H. Erythema elevatum diutinum. Brit J Dermatol 1894;6:1-7

Left: Erythema elevatum diutinum, from Radcliffe-Crocker's classic paper.

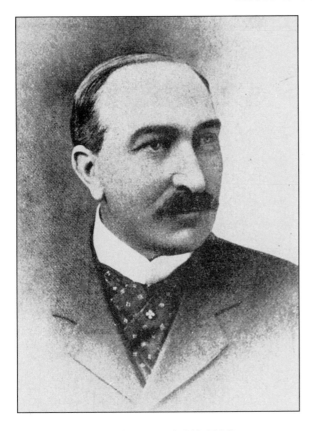

Thomas Colcott Fox (1849-1916)

Thomas Colcott Fox, the younger brother of Tilbury, was associated with London's Westminster Hospital An omnivorous reader on both cutaneous and general medical subjects, Fox developed into Britain's finest dermatologic diagnostician. "No one can make a better diagnosis," the French master Ernest Besnier declared. More than the other members of the "big five," Fox also had a genuine flair for investigative work. His contributions to mycology - the clarification of the microsporum family - were notable, and simultaneously with Thibierge of Paris he established the tubercle bacillus as the cause of erythema induratum.

It was as a remarkable teacher that Fox was best remembered by the generation that followed. "Genial and kindly to all," Arthur Whitfield wrote, "he took a very special interest in the young men and did his utmost to help them win their spurs." Whitfield went so far as to characterize his teacher as "the rock upon which the modern English School of Dermatology is founded."

Fox TC. Erythema gyratum perstans. Internat atlas rare skin diseases, Hamburg, 1891, Part XVI

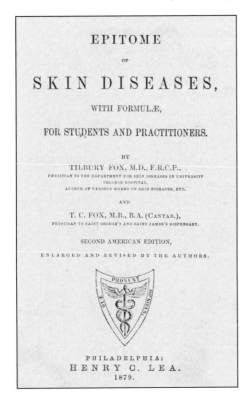

Second American edition of the very successful student handbook written by Colcott Fox in collaboration with his brother Tilbury. (1878).

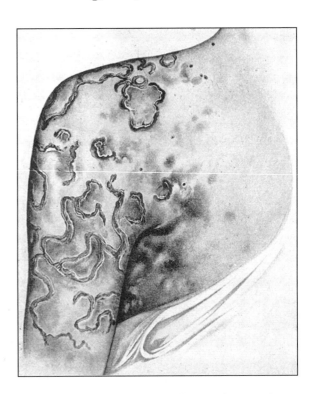

Erythema gyratum perstans, from Colcott Fox's classic 1891 paper, cited above. It is an early example of the gyrate erythemas that have caused so many taxonomic difficulties over the years.

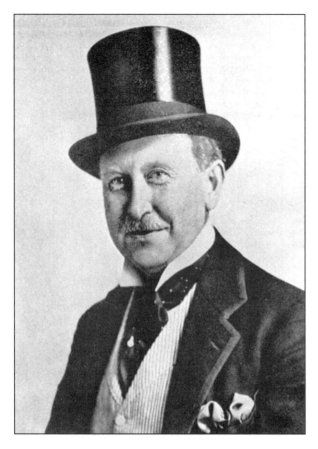

John James Pringle (1855-1922)

Another member of Britain's 'big five," John James Pringle was a short, cherubic bachelor type, patient and tolerant. Throughout his life he cultivated an exquisitely refined style in speech and literary output. He was a connoisseur of music, wine, and art, cosmopolitan and bilingual - his French having been perfected by six months of assiduous attendance at celebrated Parisian nightspots. Pringle was also at all times an exemplar of sartorial perfection. But he was of course a great deal more than aesthete combined with dandy. Born in Scotland and an Edinburgh graduate, he spent two years in Vienna, Paris, and Berlin studying dermatology and joined the staff of London's Middlesex Hospital in 1883.

Pringle was perhaps Britain's most effective teacher at the postgraduate level; five of his students eventually became chiefs of university hospital dermatology sections. A fine clinician, the describer of adenoma sebaceum, he served as editor of the British Journal of Dermatology from 1891 to 1895, and because of his remarkable literary ability, he was called upon constantly to correct, edit, and rewrite society transactions, congress proceedings, and the like.

Pringle JJ. A case of congenital adenoma sebaceum. Brit J Dermatol 1890;2:1-4

Pringle's classic description of adenoma sebaceum appeared in the *British Journal of Dermatology* in 1890. Rayer had described and depicted the entity earlier, but the French master's efforts went unnoticed. It was Pringle's paper, published in a widely read journal and accompanied by a better picture (shown to the right) that called the attention of the dermatologic world to the condition.

It has been pointed out repeatedly that Pringle named the eruption badly, the lesions being neither adenomata nor of sebaceous origin. Nevertheless, the term remains in common use even now, along with other obvious misnomers: Kaposi's sarcoma and *Histoplasma capsulatum*, for example, none of which seem to have interfered with medical progress. The remaining manifestations of the syndrome, now known as tuberous sclerosis, were described here and there in dribs and drabs over the years, and it is likely that the catalogue is not yet complete.

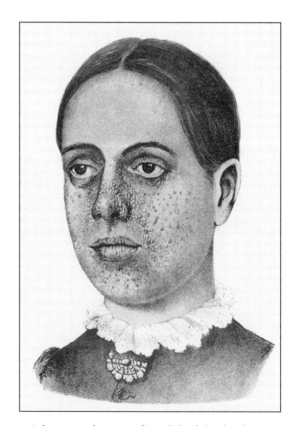

Adenoma sebaceum, from Pringle's classic paper, 1890.

53

Malcolm Morris, the most serious minded of Britain's "Big Five," came up the hard way, troubled in his early days by financial difficulties and nameless personal problems, which he overcame by grim determination. He received his dermatologic training in Berlin and Vienna. Appointed in 1882 to head the newly created skin department at St. Mary's Hospital in London, he remained with that institution until his retirement in 1902.

Morris was a born organizer and reformer, whose dermatologic interests lay chiefly in skin problems associated with public health and social questions – tuberculosis, leprosy, syphilis, and the like. In 1913 he agitated for the creation of a Royal commission on venereal disease, a problem neglected in Britain at the time, and he served on the commission when it was created.

A sharp eyed clinician, a successful practitioner and colorful teacher, Morris was the first to describe xanthoma diabeticorum. He was noted for his ability to handle VIPs and difficult patients, including King Edward VII, who knighted Morris for professional services rendered.

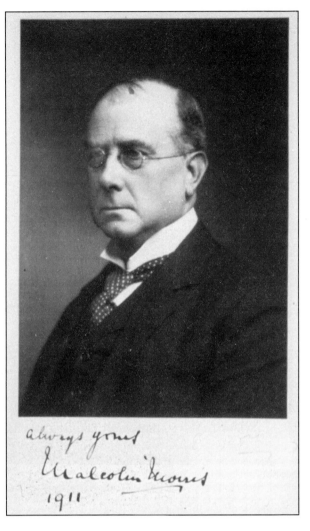

Malcolm Morris (1849-1924)

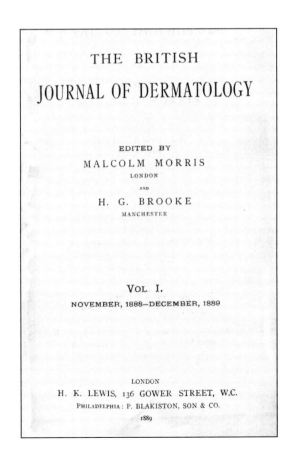

As important as any of the contributions of Malcolm Morris was his part in founding *The British Journal of Dermatology*. The year was 1888, and he was joined in the enterprise by his friend H.G. Brooke ("of Manchester"). The title page of the first issue is shown to the left.

Morris and Brooke co-edited the organ for the first few years of its existence, and from the beginning they showed themselves to be in full possession those sine qua nons for success in the publishing world - an understanding of the needs and wants of the readers and a skin thick enough to deflect the barbs of the benighted who commonly occupy seats on editorial boards. The "BJD" is still in print and retains the distinctive blend of readability and appreciation for both the clinical and the basic instilled in it by Morris and Brooke in its earliest years.

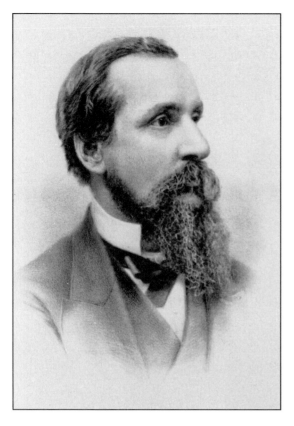

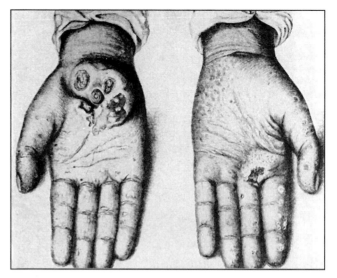

Arsenical keratoses, plate from Hutchinson's atlas. In the classic report cited below, Hutchinson was the first to call attention to this dangerous, pre-malignant consequence of the systemic administration of arsenic, a medication much overused in the treatment of psoriasis, eczematous eruptions, and other conditions in the 19th century.

Jonathan Hutchinson (1828-1913)

Hutchinson J. Arsenic cancer. Brit J Dermatol 1887;2:1280-1

Jonathan Hutchinson was an odd, peripatetic, English genius with an encyclopedic knowledge of the medicine of his day and an astonishing ability to extract from his memory bank, when called upon to do so, the details of the thousands of cases he had seen. He considered himself a surgeon, operated skillfully, and published much on surgical subjects, but he was also perfectly at home as an ophthalmologist, syphilologist, and journal editor, and over the years became as much a dermatologist as anything else. He frequently attended the skin clinics both in England and on the Continent, and his many publications - papers, journals, atlases - are filled with accounts and plates of skin diseases, especially bizarre, rare, and "casus pro diagnosi" examples. His name is associated with the notched teeth common in congenital syphilis and the triad of signs he considered pathognomonic of that disease – the teeth, 8th nerve deafness, and interstitial keratitis. Among other things, he was the first to give a decent account of melanotic whitlow, and published the classic descriptions of arsenical keratoses, hydroa aestivale, and angioma serpiginosum.

Hutchinson J. A peculiar form of serpiginous and infective naevoid disease. Arch Surg 1890;1:Plate IX.

Right: Angioma serpiginosum, plate from Hutchinson's classic description, cited above.

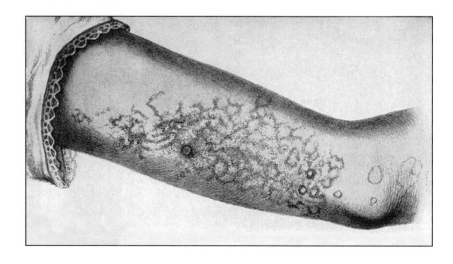

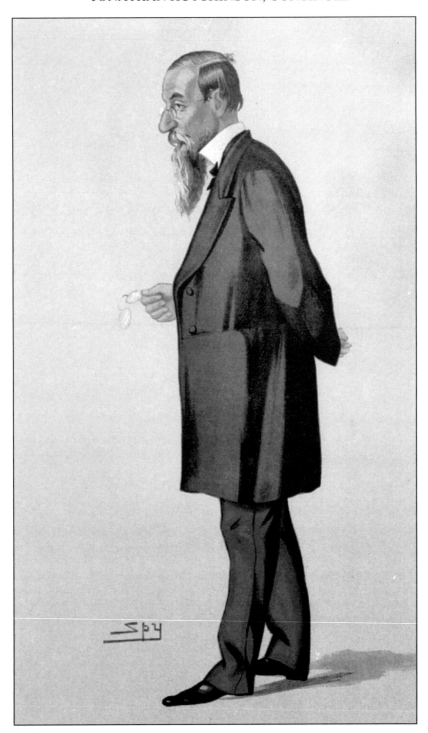

Chromolithograph of Jonathan Hutchinson by Leslie Ward, English caricaturist who under the pseudonym Spy published in the popular magazine Vanity Fair a series of portraits of famous people in the last quarter of the 19th century.

"He is a quiet, very sensitive man," the caption stated, "who treats his patients with quite fatherly care and with exceeding skill. He is a specialist of more than one kind, being a great authority upon defective or diseased eyes. His study is the whole of medicine, as Bacon's was the whole of Nature; and of him a great medicine man once said: 'I do not believe in specialists, but I believe in Hutchinson because he is a specialist in everything.' And being so, he has well earned the gratitude of thousands.

He has a pretty place at Haslemere; and he always carries with him four pairs of spectacles."

Late Nineteenth Century Austrian Dermatology

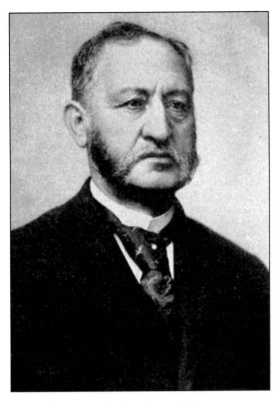

Isidor Neumann (1832-1906)

Below, left: Neumann's classic 1873
monograph on the lymph vessels of the skin.
Below, right: Psoriasis, woodcut from
Neumann's 1869 textbook.

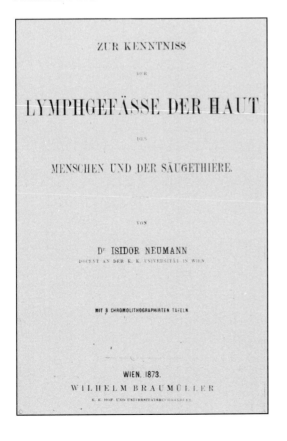

Isidor Neumann, Moravian born pupil of Hebra and a professor at the University of Vienna, was a pioneer in cutaneous histopathology. He studied microscopy with the Viennese pathologist Carl Wedl in the early 1860s and soon after put to use his newly acquired skills in a series of histologic studies on senile degeneration of the skin, argyria, and the syphilids. It was also the inclusion of histologic material, carefully described, unprecedented in detail, and accompanied by numerous microanatomic illustrations that marked Neumann's highly successful "Lehrbuch der Hautkrankheiten" (1869) as something new and special. The woodcut from this work shown below appears to be the first representation of the histopathologic changes in psoriasis. Still a bit primitive, it nevertheless represents a quantum leap forward from the images of Gustav Simon, thanks to the newly available carmine stain. Neumann's 1873 monograph on the lymph vessels of the skin, the title page of which appears below, is also the first of its kind.

A strong clinician as well, Neumann was responsible for the classic description of pemphigus vegetans and set the seborrheic keratosis apart as a distinct clinical entity. In his day, Neumann was even better known as a master syphilologist. He succeeded Carl Ludwig Sigmund in the Second Chair at Vienna, headed up the Syphilisabteilung, and set forth his enormous experience in dealing with the treponeme in 1896 in "Syphilis," a massive, state of the arts tome on the disease.

While studying in Vienna in 1871, the American dermatologist George Henry Fox was a little put off by the didactic style of Neumann's lectures, but later had this to say: "In Prof. Wedl's laboratory where I studied microscopy I found him working daily, and as I was able to secure a seat next to him at the table, I became somewhat better acquainted and found him to be a most affable, helpful, and friendly man."

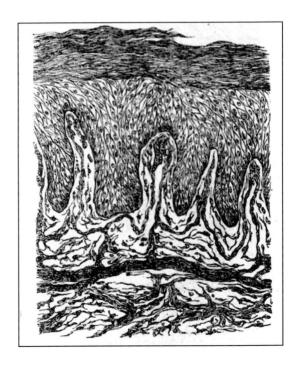

Moriz Kaposi, Hebra's son-in-law and the most famous of the older master's pupils, served as the chair of the dermatology department in Vienna from 1881 until his death in 1902. Born Moriz Kohn in Kaposvár, Hungary, he later changed his name and his religion (from Judaism to Catholicism), no doubt to circumvent the anti-semitism of the day that commonly interfered with career advancement.

Under Kaposi, the Vienna clinic continued to draw students from all over the world.

"He is an impressive lecturer," wrote one attendee, "fluent, never hesitating for a word, enlivening what he says by frequent touches of humor. He does not forget the mustard in his sandwiches, and true to his nationality – for he is Hungarian by birth – makes them extra pungent now and then."

Like most of Hebra's students, Kaposi mastered the new science of microscopy early in his career, and histopathology is prominently displayed in his 1880 masterwork, "Pathologie und Therapie der Hautkrankheiten in Vorlesungen." Popular and influential, the Vorlesungen is nothing if not forthright; the reader is never left in doubt with respect to the author's opinions on the controversial issues of the time.

The present day familiarity of Kaposi's name rests largely on its association with diseases he described - his pigmented sarcoma (shown below), his varicelliform eruption, dermatitis papillaris capillitii, systemic lupus erythematosus, and xeroderma pigmentosum, all of which are with us still.

Right: reference citation and title page of Kaposi's classic 1872 paper on his pigmented sarcoma.

Below: Kaposi's sarcoma from Kaposi's atlas

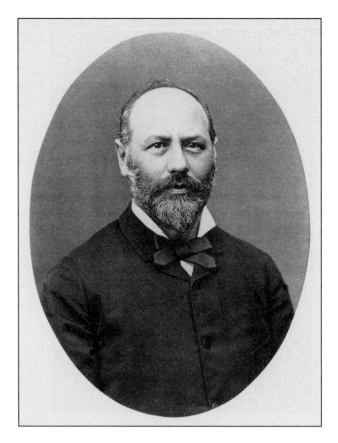

Moriz Kaposi (1837-1902)

Kaposi M. Idiopathisches multiples Pigmentsarkom der Haut. Arch f Dermatol

Idiopathisches multiples Pigmentsarkom der Haut.

Von

Dr. Kaposi,

Docent an der Universität in Wien.

Mit Recht hebt Köbner in einem über Sarkome der Haut handelnden Aufsatze *) hervor, dass diese Neubildung auf der Haut an und für sich selten vorkommt, und bisher mehr Object anatomischer als klinischer Aufmerksamkeit gewesen ist. Daselbst werden zwei Krankheitsfälle mitgetheilt, in deren erstem Hautsarkome in grosser Anzahl als metastatische Bildungen, wahrscheinlich von den Lymphdrüsen der Leistengegend her, entstanden waren, während im zweiten Falle die allgemeine Sarkomatosis von einem seit Kindheit bestandenen Naevus des linken Zeigefingers ausgegangen war, der primär in ein pigmentirtes Spindelzellensarkom sich umgewandelt hatte. Beide Fälle endigten innerhalb drei Jahren tödtlich. Die Section war in einem derselben gestattet worden.

Ich glaube eine Form des Pigmentsarkoms der Haut als eine *typisch-klinische* von denjenigen absondern zu können, welche unter allen Umständen als *consecutive* (metastatische) Eruptionen und demnach von den verschiedensten Primärherden ausgehen können, und deren Beispiele in den Fällen von Köbner gegeben sind.

Ich will die hier zu beschreibende Form deshalb als *idiopathisches multiples Pigmentsarkom* der Haut bezeichnen.

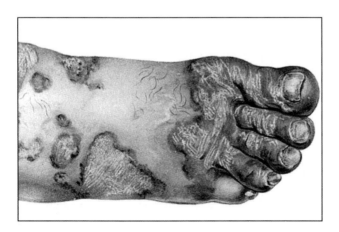

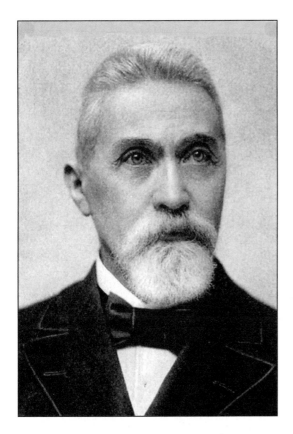

Filipp Joseph Pick (1834-1910)

Considered by some to be the most brilliant of Hebra's students. Filipp Pick eventually became the Professor of Dermatology at Prague. A much published and inventive therapist he introduced or popularized many new topical medications, including iodoform and the salicylic acid plaster. Pick functioned equally well as a clinical investigator. He identified tinea cruris as a mycotic infection (1869), demonstrated the contagiousness of molluscum contagiosum by inoculation experiments (1892), and independently described lepothrix. In 1900 he published the classic description of a mysterious malady, erythromelia (Pick's disease) - a livid redness of the extensors of the arms and legs accompanied by venous dilatation – which seems not to have been seen by anyone anywhere since.

In 1889, Pick, along with Albert Neisser, founded the Deutsche Dermatologische Gesellschaft (the "DDG"), Germany's first and most important dermatologic organization at the national level. Pick presided over its first meeting, held in Prague in June of that year.

Among the most significant of Pick's accomplishments was his collaboration with Heinrich Auspitz in launching the *Archiv für Dermatologie und Syphilis* (1869). The two men co-edited the journal until the death of Auspitz in 1886, after which Pick continued alone. Published in several different cities at various times the Archiv also appeared at times as the *Vierteljahresschrift für Dermatologie und Syphilis*. Under the steady hand of Pick the Archiv became the most prestigious dermatologic publication in central Europe, the repository for the best papers by the best authors. "The heart of the entire enterprise was F.J. Pick," historical researchers Sebastian and Scholz concluded, "He loved the Archiv as a father loves his child. "

ARCHIV

FÜR

DERMATOLOGIE UND SYPHILIS.

HERAUSGEGEBEN

von

Dr. Heinrich Auspitz, und Dr. Filipp Josef Pick,
Docent an der Universität   Docent an der Universität
WIEN   PRAG

unter Mitwirkung von

Dr. M'CALL ANDERSON Londou, Prof. BAZIN Paris, Dr. BERGH Kopenhagen, Dr. BIDENKAP Christiania, Prof. BIESIADECKI Krakau, Prof. BOECK Christiania, Dr. BURCHARDT Cassel, Prof. DITTRICH München, Prof. FRIEDREICH Heidelberg, Prof. HALLIER Jena, Prof. HEBRA Wien, Prof. KLOB Wien, Dr. KÖBNER Breslau, Docent M. KOHN Wien, Prof. LANDOIS Greifswald, Prof. LEWIN Berlin, Prof. LINDWURM München, Docent LIPP Graz, Dr. MICHAELIS Wien, Prof. MOSLER Greifswald, Dr. OEWRE Christiania, Docent NEUMANN Wien, Prof. PETTERS Prag, Prof. REDER Wien, Prof. RINDFLEISCH Bonn, Prof. v. SIGMUND Wien, Dr. SIMON Hamburg, Hofrath v. VEIEL Cannstatt, Dr. VEIEL jun. Cannstatt, Prof. v. VINTSCHGAU Prag, Prof. WALLER Prag, Docent WERTHEIM Wien, Prof. ERASMUS WILSON London, Prof. ZEISSL Wien und vielen anderen Fachmännern.

Erster Jahrgang.

MIT VIER LITHOGRAPHIRTEN TAFELN UND VIER HOLZSCHNITTEN.

PRAG, 1869.

J. G. CALVE'SCHE K. K. UNIV.-BUCHHANDLUNG.

OTTOMAR BEYER.

Brilliant, erratic, impatient, and combative, Heinrich Auspitz was an Austrian dermatologist, a pupil of Hebra who worked in his younger years at the Allgemeines Krankenhaus in Vienna. His name is remembered now largely in connection with his "bleeding points" sign that facilitates the diagnosis of psoriasis, but he contributed much more than that to his chosen specialty. His outstanding work in dermatologic histopathology is noted below, and yet he was vehemently opposed to the classification of skin diseases on the basis of pathology put forward originally by Hebra. He attempted instead throughout his career to the integrate the entire body of clinical cutaneous knowledge and all of the pertinent observations recorded in the literature of pathology, physiology, and experimental medicine into a grand pathogenetic design, a sort of unified field theory for dermatologic disease. He failed, of course, for want of sufficient data, but it was a brilliant failure that anticipated the dermatologic approach of our own time.

Auspitz was the odds-on favorite to fill the professorial vacancy in Vienna that arose with the retirement of Carl Ludwig Sigmund, but at the last minute the job went instead to Isidor Neumann. Auspitz was appointed later to a similar although somewhat less prestigious position, but he was bitterly disappointed and died soon after, in 1886, at the age of 50.

Auspitz H, Unna P. Die Anatomie der syphilitischen Initial-Sclerose. Viertelj Dermatol Syph 1876;9:161-200

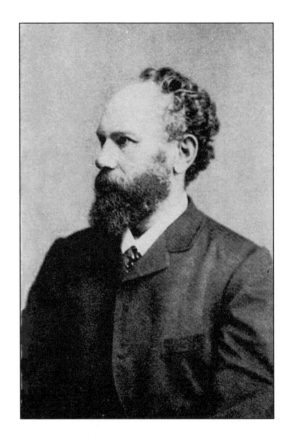

Heinrich Auspitz (1835-1886)

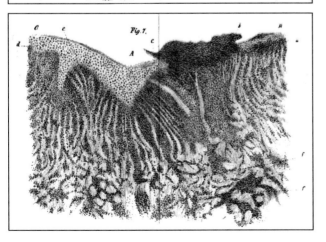

Auspitz learned the fundamentals of pathology from Carl Wedl in Vienna and soon excelled his master in the study of the pathologic changes associated with skin diseases. He coined the terms acanthoma, acantholysis, and parakeratosis and published a classic account of the anatomy of the dermal-epidermal junction and important studies on the infiltrates of syphilis, lupus vulgaris and scrofula. His brain was wired in that special way that allows a really fine histopathologist to convert a static two dimensional tissue section into an animated three dimensional panorama that enables him understand and communicate to others the essential message that lesional changes are works in progress.

Shown to the left are the beginning and Figure 7 from his classic 1877 study of the pathology of the syphilitic chancre. Note that the co-author was Paul Gerson Unna, Auspitz's most famous and successful pupil.

LATE NINETEENTH CENTURY GERMAN DERMATOLOGY

Heinrich Koebner, renowned German dermatologist, was a restless experimenter with an unusual turn of mind. He received his dermatologic training in Vienna and Paris, following which he opened a practice in Breslau, his hometown. After years of agitation he succeeded in convincing the government to create a university skin clinic in that city. He was appointed chief of the new facility but was forced by illness (tuberculosis) to resign shortly after it opened. In 1877 he founded a true polyclinic in Berlin and remained there until retirement.

His postgraduate time in Paris was largely spent at l'Hôpital St. Louis working with Ernest Bazin, who was then involved in ringworm research, and the French master stimulated in Koebner a life-long interest in mycology. Koebner made important contributions to the field. He was the first to inoculate lower animals with human fungi (rabbits), and in the paper cited below gave us the classic description of mycotic sycosis barbae. Ever the enthusiast, he once appeared at a medical meeting proudly exhibiting on his arms and chest three different fungus infections self-inoculated to prove the infectiousness of the organisms being studied.

Koebner also left us the classic description of epidermolysis bullosa simplex.

The description of the phenomenon that bears his name appears below, to the right.

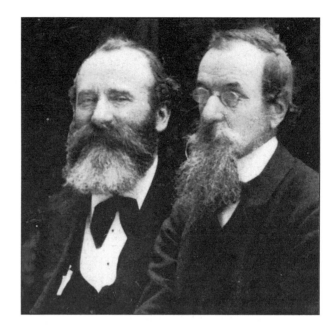

Heinrich Koebner (1838-1904), left, with his friend Jonathan Hutchinson (1828-1913) at the 1892 meeting of the International Congress of Dermatology in Vienna.

Koebner H. Zur Aetiologie der Psoriasis, Viertelj Dermatol Sypn 1876;8:559-61

Below: Translation of Koebner's classic description of his phenomenon as it was reported in the reference cited above. It was included in an address on the cause of psoriasis delivered by Koebner before the Silesian Society for National Culture.

Koebner H, Michelson P. Ueber parasitäre Sykosis. Arch f Dermatol Syph 1869;1:7-17

Below: Mycotic sycosis barbae - Figure from the classic paper cited above. The letters a and b refer to superficial and deep lesions.

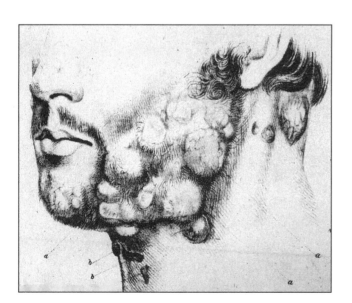

"At the meeting of the medical section on May 3rd, 1872, Dr. Koebner spoke on the etiology of psoriasis. Earlier he had demonstrated a case in which 5 and 6 years after the appearance of an isolated plaque, various traumatic influences on widely separated areas of the body (excoriations from riding, suppuration from a co-existing lymphadenitis, a horse bite, and lastly, a tattoo) had been followed by the outbreak of psoriasis limited almost exactly to the damaged skin area, with generalized spread later. The horse bite had exerted the greatest influence on the eruption, and the strict localization to the points and lines of artificial wounds was very evident in the figures and letters in an area that had been tattooed a few weeks previously."

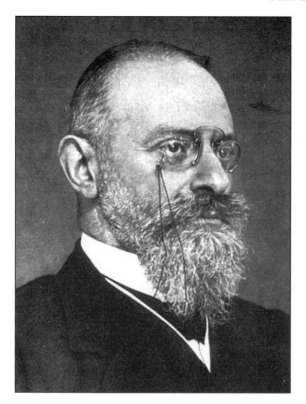

Albert Neisser (1855-1916)

Neisser A. Ueber eine der Gonorrhoe eigentümliche Micrococcusform. Centralblatt Med Wissenschft 1879;17:497-500

Albert Neisser, preeminent German research dermatologist and archrival of Unna, receiced his M.D. from the University of Breslau in 1877 and his dermatologic training under Oscar Simon at the same school. He succeeded Simon as chief of dermatology at the Breslau clinic in 1882.

Neisser's remarkable talent for investigative dermatology became evident early in his career when at the age of twenty-four, two years into his dermatologic training, he identified the gonococcus as the cause of gonorrhea. His description of the organism is referenced and shown below. A year later he confirmed the existence of the leprosy bacillus, discovered six years earlier by Armauer Hansen but, unfortunately, Neisser failed to give the Norwegian the credit he deserved. The rest of his career was largely devoted to the study of syphilis. He was a coauthor with August Wassermann of the classic paper on the "Wassermann reaction," and following the successful inoculation of chimpanzees with *Treponema pallidum* by Metchnikoff and Roux (1903), spent several years in Java inoculating a colony of these animals, working out in great detail the incubation period, lymphatic routes of dissemination, and other parameters of the disease.

Neisser was a cultured man, an attentive father, and an accomplished pianist. He lived very well, traveled everywhere with his charming wife Toni, appreciated and collected objets d'art, hob-nobbed with the rich and famous, and entertained them lavishly in his beautiful Breslau villa.

Individual elements are circular and surprisingly large, with a strong affinity for methyl violet and dalia. They may also be stained in concentrated solutions of eosin, but they do not then contrast so markedly with the many granules in the pus corpuscles called eosinophile cells by Ehrlich as they do when the methyl violet stain is used. They do not stain with methyl green or indulin. With objectives of lower power they appear to be girdled by a ring of light that probably represents a mucus capsule. They are, however, seldom seen as solitary individuals; almost always they appear as two micrococci packed close together, so close in fact that they give the observer the impression of a single organism shaped like a figure 8, a biscuit, or a German dinner roll [Semmel].

Right: Albert Neisser's renowned dermatology clinic in Breslau (1894). Breslau (Wroclaw), then in Germany, is now within the boundaries of Poland.

More than 30 future heads of university dermatologic clinics or major hospitals trained with Neisser in this facility.

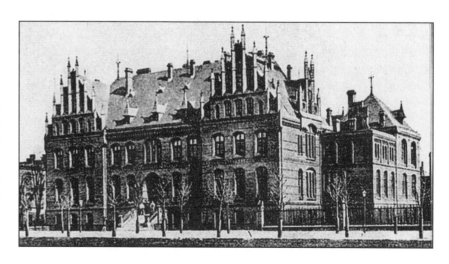

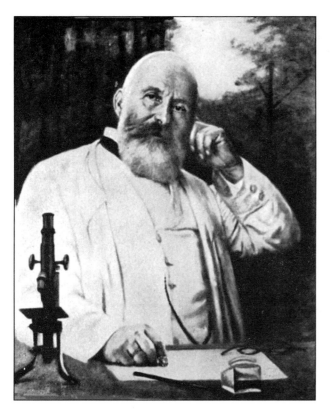

Paul Gerson Unna, the best known dermatologist in the world in the early decades of the 20th century, was a pupil of Hebra and Auspitz. In the 1880s he opened a private clinic in the Hamburg suburb of Eimsbüttel. Over the years he added laboratories, accommodations for inpatients, and a fine new home for his family. He called the complex the "Dermatologikum," and the name soon became familiar in medical circles everywhere. Within this private compound he carried on successfully the sort of clinical, investigative, and pedagogical activities that would normally be found only at a great university center. In 1886 he opened its doors to postgraduate students, particularly those who were interested in sharpening their skills in histopathology.

Because he held no university appointment (until late in life), Unna's freelance activities generated a considerable amount off resentment in German academia. It is perhaps the best measure of the man that he was able to battle the officially anointed on equal terms and even, after years as the target of the harshest criticism, win the universal admiration and respect of that privileged class.

Paul Gerson Unna (1850-1929)

It is difficult to catalogue Unna's contributions to the specialty, because he had irons in virtually every dermatologic fire. His name is remembered for the most part now for a pair of therapeutic innovations – the Unna gelatin boot and Unna's paste – two minor items in a constant stream of treatment modalities that emanated year in and year out from the wards and laboratories of the Dermatologikum. Eucerin, ichthyol, and adhesive tape were also among the most successful of the products he developed.

It was as a master of histopathology and a teacher of the same that Unna was best known in his day. Examples of his contributions are noted below.

The classic description of ballooning degeneration (plate shown to the right) appears in Unna's monumental textbook, "Histopathologie der Hauthrankheiten" of 1894 (English translation, 1896). Other major contributions include description and naming of the plasma cell, development of the tissue stains acid orcein, polychrome methylene blue, and pyronin methyl green, in depth investigations of keratohyalin and the structure of the stratum corneum, and the identification of mast cells in the infiltrates of urticaria pigmentosa.

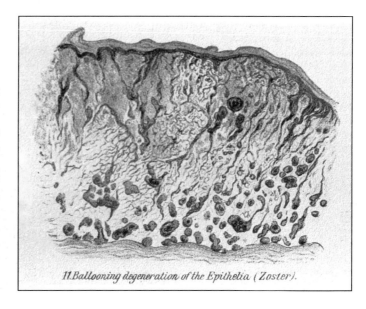

11.Ballooning degeneration of the Epithelia (Zoster).

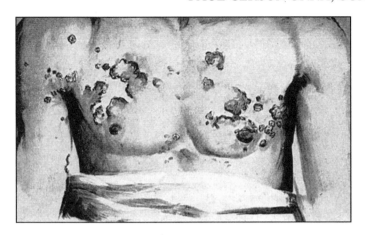

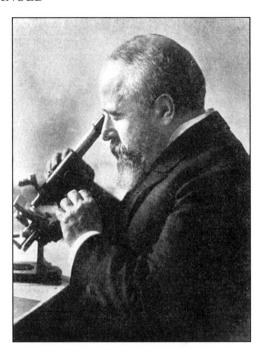

Unna P. Seborrhoeal eczema. J Cutan Genit Urin Dis 1887;5:449-459

Unna maintained a career-long interest in "eczema," although the bacteria he isolated and proposed as the cause were rejected out of hand by his colleagues. The demonstration by others that redness and scaling can in some instances be the only visible manifestations of the condition set the stage for the detachment of a sizeable portion of the eczema monolith, and the perception of morphologic interrelationships that led to the detachment can be counted as another of the 19th century's great clinical syntheses. The synthesizer in this instance was Paul Gerson Unna. He called his startling new arrangement seborrhoeal eczema, and he exploded it in 1887 at a meeting of the International Medical Congress in Washington, D.C. The concept caught on immediately and stands as a splendid example of an idea whose time has come. The plate shown above, the "petaloid seborrheid of Unna," is from his classic paper on the subject (cited above).

Paul Gerson Unna at work. The man was unique - superior clinical skills, laboratory expertise, investigational talent, and a devotion to teaching combined in a single individual, and with it all a genuine concern for the most homely and practical aspects of the specialty.

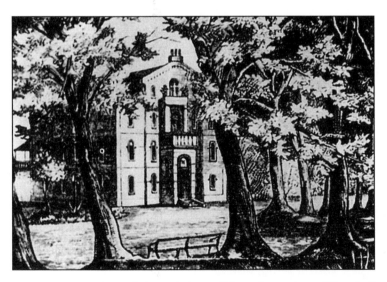

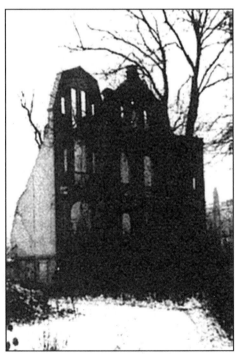

Above, left: Artist's rendition of a portion of Unna's Dermatologikum (1884).
Above, right: Dermatologikum ruins following a World War II aerial bombing raid.

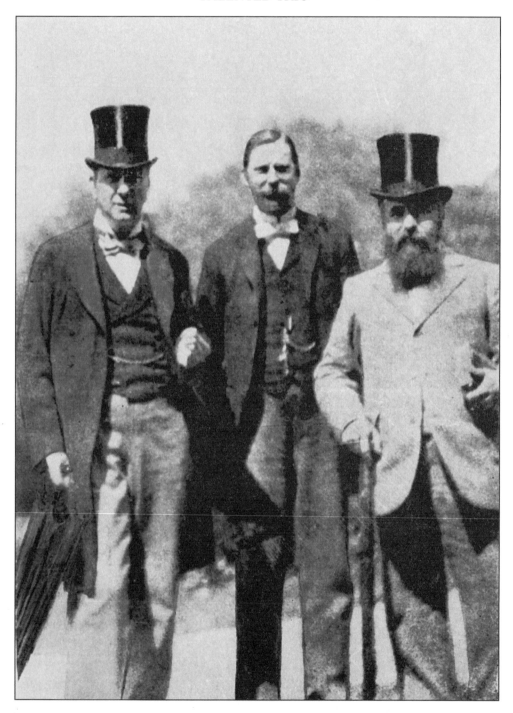

L to R: Malcom Morris (1849-1924), Henry Radcliffe-Crocker (1845-1909),
Paul Gerson Unna (1850-1929). London meeting, ca. 1896.

LATE NINETEENTH CENTURY FRENCH DERMATOLOGY

An underrated figure in the development of French dermatology in the latter half of the 19th century was Charles Lailler. Paris born and educated, and a chief of service at l'Hôpital St. Louis, he was an important bridge between the old dermatology of Bazin and Hardy and the new. An expert morphologist, he took on and successfully handled the diplomatically difficult task of bringing Ernest Besnier up to speed on clinical dermatology when Besnier took over as a chief at St. Louis after years in internal medicine.

Lailler also set up on the grounds of St. Louis a school for tinea capitis children who were routinely excluded from the regular school system. This school served later as a training ground for Raymond Sabouraud whose *fin de siècle* mycologic discoveries revolutionized the field.

It was also Lailler who discovered and employed the master craftsman, Jules Baretta, whose amazingly life-like moulages of skin diseases were important teaching aids at the time.

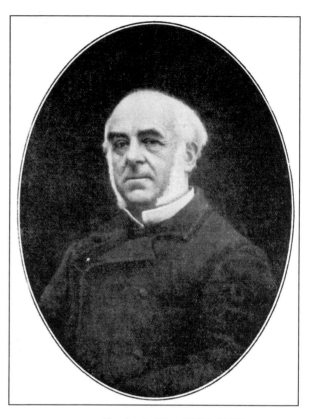

Charles Lailler (1822-1893)

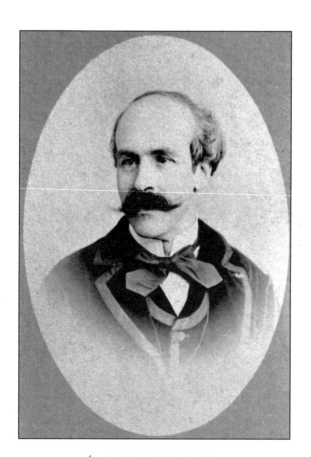

Émile Vidal (1825-1893)

The stylistic star of the St. Louis faculty in the latter half of the 19th century was Émile Vidal. Paris born and trained, he was one of the most appealing physicians of his generation and enormously successful in practice.

"The penetration of his mind was truly marvelous," Brocq observed, "He examined the patient with a vivacity and dexterity not soon forgotten. He left nothing unexplored, discovering the decisive point with almost uncanny rapidity. He pronounced a word and the diagnosis was made. His pupils had on numerous occasions admired this almost infallible diagnostic ability. One felt himself to be in the presence of a born clinician."

Vidal was particularly interested in lupus vulgaris and the lichens; he described the neurodermatitis circumscripta form of the latter that continues to be associated with his name. He was more than a clinician; he concerned himself with all aspects of the dermatology of his time, introduced his colleagues and pupils to the German histopathologic and bacteriologic techniques and discoveries, and was a pioneer in the study of infectious skin diseases by inoculation experiments.

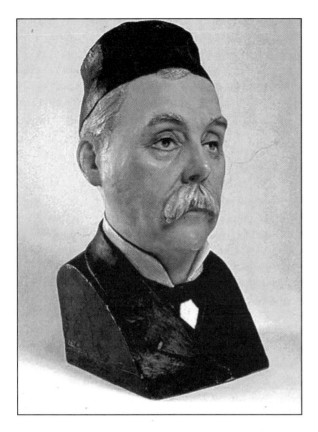

Jules Baretta was a Parisian master moulage craftsman associated with l'Hôpital St. Louis. Charles Lailler first observed Baretta making cardboard paste models of fruit in Jouffroy Street, was impressed by his remarkable talent, and imported him into St. Louis. He provided the young man with a subsidy - out of his own pocket - and taught him the dermatologic aspects of his craft. Baretta's moulages were made available for student teaching purposes, along with graphics and models of skin diseases from many other sources, in the famous musée at St. Louis, the organization and maintenance of which fell not surprisingly to Lailler in his capacity as departmental workhorse and perpetual volunteer. As noted below, other moulage makers of great skill appeared on the scene in the 19th century, some working with wax and others with cardboard paste, but it is generally agreed that Baretta's workmanship is unexcelled. Two examples of his more than two thousand creations are shown below.

It is fitting that the image of Baretta himself is preserved in moulage form in the bust shown to the left, crafted by Stéphane Littre and on display in the St. Louis musée, where much of Baretta's work has been preserved.

Jules Baretta (1834-1923)

The unbelievably realistic moulages of Baretta and equally talented artists, such as Joseph Towne in England and Anton Elfinger in Vienna, were highly prized anatomic and dermatologic teaching aids in the latter half of the 19th and early decades of the 20th centuries. Expensive, fragile, and difficult to show to large groups, they morphed gradually from teaching aids into museum curiosities following the development of color photography, particularly Kodachrome and the projectable 35 mm slide. The latter in turn is yielding now to computer stored and projectable digital images. Such is the nature of progress.

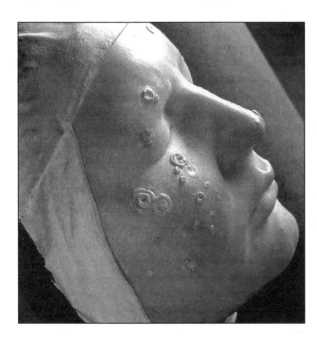

Tinea favosa, moulage by Jules Baretta.

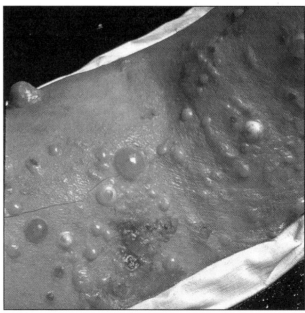

Bullous pemphigoid, moulage by Jules Baretta

Ernest Besnier, the most important French dermatologist in the final quarter of the 19th century, was born in the northern town of Honfleur, trained in Paris, and following the retirement of Bazin took over as a chief at l'Hôpital St. Louis (1873).

Besnier's published works are few in number, but choice. His exposition of the atopic dermatitis constellation (1892) is classic, and his essay on "eczema" in the massive "Pratique Dermatologique" of 1900 is a blend of scholarship and common sense that can be recommended even now as a model for prospective authors of monographs in depth. Besnier himself can also be recommended as a model for departmental chairmen – a superb and well informed teacher, endowed also with the ability to evaluate the talents of his young charges and point them in the right direction. Such was the case in his management of Raymond Sabouraud, who after a rocky tour with Émile Vidal transferred to Besnier's service and had this to say, " I felt that I had finally found the teacher of my dreams." It was Besnier who suggested that Sabouraud take up the study of fungi and supported him when his early results were regarded by others with grave suspicion.

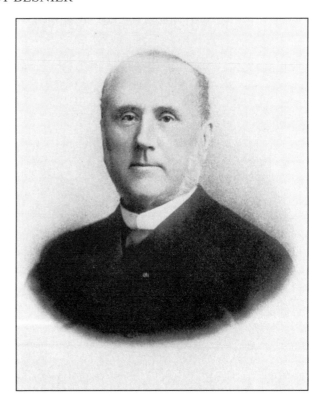

Ernest Besnier (1831-1909)

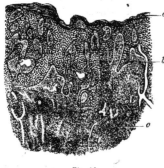

From the beginning Besnier was smitten with the urge to reform. He was convinced that under Bazin and Hardy, French dermatology was bogged down, had failed to assimilate the many advances being made, particularly in Austria and Germany. As a first remedial step, he commissioned his bilingual friend Adrien Doyon to translate Kaposi's "Vorlesungen" into French (1881), and took advantage of his own perfect command of the current French and English literature to add extensive and extremely perceptive commentaries to Kaposi's original text. The result was the "Pathologie et Traitement des Maladies de la Peau," a felicitous hybrid that reinforced the best in Kaposi and enriched the Austrian work with the insights provided by the new generation of French dermatologists. The Kaposi-Besnier-Doyon opus remained the most influential textbook in French for more than 20 years, and it was a key factor in blurring the nationalistic differences that had characterized the practice of the specialty for the first 80 years of the 19th century. A typical page of the classic is shown to the left, Kaposi at the top of the page, Besnier at the bottom.

Besnier also sent Doyon to study in depth the organization of the dermatology department in Vienna, and used the Doyon report to reorganize and modernize his own. Others at St. Louis followed his lead, and the result was that as the twentieth century began, the French were as well equipped as any to deal with the future.

Adrien Doyon, French dermatologist and venereologist, studied medicine in Lyon and was affiliated with l'Hospice de l'Antiquaille in that city. In 1858 he was appointed *médecin-inspecteur* of the spa at Uriage, a position he maintained until his death in 1907.

Early in his career Doyon collaborated with the renowned venereologist Paul Diday in the publication of several valuable studies on genital herpes and on the teaching and treatment of skin and sexually transmitted diseases. He is best remembered now for his key role in the modernization of French dermatology, which had fallen behind its Austrian counterpart in the middle decades of the 19th century. A significant portion of the modernization can be attributed to France's premier dermatologic journal, the "Annales," founded by Doyon, as noted below.

Also of great importance was Doyon's collaboration with Ernest Besnier in instituting much needed reforms. In 1882, Besnier, newly installed as a chief at St. Louis, commissioned Doyon to travel to Vienna to discover the secrets of the Hebra-Kaposi success story. Doyon, who was fluent in German, sent back an insightful and extraordinarily detailed report that provided Besnier with the ammunition he needed to extract from the bureaucracy the power and the means to bring Parisian dermatology up to speed.

It was also Doyon who, at Besnier's request, translated Kaposi's "Vorlesungen" into French. The publication of this work, thoroughly annotated by Besnier, did much to blur the nationalistc differences and misunderstandings that had previously divided French and Germanic dermatology to the detriment of both.

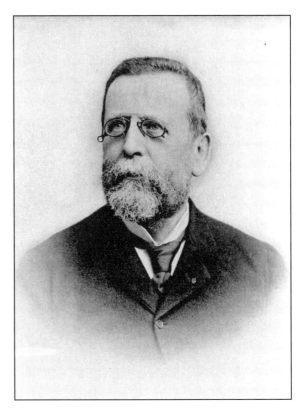

Adrien Doyon (1827-1907)

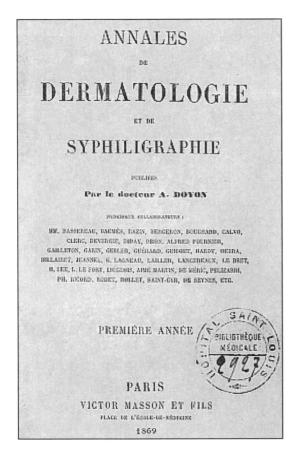

Volume 1 of the *Annales de Dermatologie et de Syphiligraphie*, brain child of Doyon, arrived on the scene in the years 1868/69. It was not the first journal in France devoted to skin and sexually transmitted diseases (STDs). From 1843 to 1852, Alphée Cazenave published and edited the *Annales des Maladies de la Peau et de la Syphilis*. In it Cazenave made some effort to review other literature, foreign and domestic, but his Annales was for the most part a one-man show, a repository for his own thoughts and observations. Doyon had something quite different in mind. From the beginning he enlisted the help of a large staff of contributing editors, all of whom were recognized authorities. The masthead of Volume No. 1, shown to the left, lists the names of 35 of these illuminati. The first issue appeared in November 1868. Most of the articles dealt with the STDs, diseases that were a substantial part of dermatologic practice well into the 20th century, particularly syphilis, which in the absence of laboratory tests could only be diagnosed early from its skin and mucous membrane signs. .In addition to the magisterial papers, abstracts of domestic and foreign literature, translations of foreign reports, accounts of medical conferences, and the comings and goings of the officially anointed were recorded in considerable detail.

Now in its 133rd year of publication the journal is strikingly similar in form to the original issues, confirming both the foresight and the percipience of its remarkable founder. A list of the classic reports and important discoveries that have made their debut on the pages of the Annales would be impressive indeed.

Dermatology never produced an observer with a sharper eye than Jean-Louis Brocq. Born in the south of France, he received his dermatologic training at l'Hôpital St. Louis. Chief at the Broca Hospital in Paris for many years and later at St. Louis, he was best known for his detailed studies on exfoliative dermatitis, pseudopelade, dermatitis herpetiformis, congenital ichthyosiform erythroderma, lichen simplex chronicus, and parapsoriasis, and for his numerous contributions to the monumental "Pratique dermatologique," France's magnificent summation of the entire field at the beginning of the 20th century. His skills are evident in the deftly executed miniature cited and noted below. It is the classic description of the fixed drug eruption, wrapped up in a single paragraph with such precision that physicians since have had no trouble recognizing its occurrence in association with drugs other than antipyrine. Antipyrine, new at the time, was a popular antipyretic-analgesic.

Brocq, a tall, thin man with flashing black eyes, was inclined to be feisty. His pupil, Lucien Pautrier, described his teacher in this manner: " He impressed those seeing him for the first time as being cold and distant; he retained from his southern origin a pungent Gascon accent and a vivacity of spirit and almost petulance in discussions that made him a remarkable speaker and a formidable opponent in debate."

In poor health most of his life, Brocq retired in 1921, continued to write, and died in 1928.

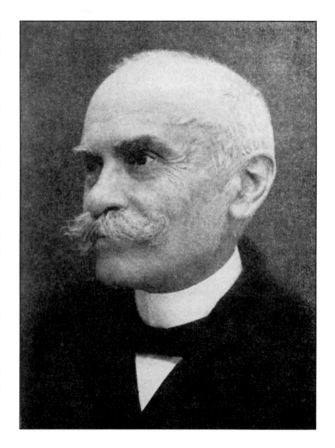

Jean-Louis Brocq (1856-1928)

Antipyrine can produce eruptions characterized by plaques that are round or rather oval in shape, and sometimes very large; the major axis may be as long as 8 cm. The lesions are separated one from another and occur here and there on the body with no tendency at all to symmetry; they are ordinarily few in number. In the beginning they are brownish red in color and are accompanied only by sensations of smarting or tension, rarely by itching. Later they become completely asymptomatic; the redness disappears little by little, leaving a brownish color that varies in its degree of darkness, even approaching black after repeated attacks. Sometimes they become phlyctenular and resemble the bullous eruptions previously described. When the erythema disappears a lamellar desquamation almost always occurs at the sites involved. The borders are very sharply demarcated; the lesions are sometimes accompanied by a pronounced tumefaction of the integument, which then has a thickened appearance, although it can always be moved over the deeper parts. With the passage of time the pigment tends to disappear, and in the small plaques this may take place rather quickly so that it is gone by the end of two or three weeks, providing the patient takes no more Antipyrine. But when the plaques are large, the pigment has a tendency to persist for a longer period of time, and if the subject is unlucky enough to take the medication again, he suffers a new erythernatous and congestive attack at the sites of the previous plaques. They once again become red and increasingly pigmented. These are, in short, the noteworthy characteristics of the lesions: they are circumscribed, pigmented, and fixed.

Brocq L. Éruption érythémato-pigmentée fixe due à l'Antipyrine. Ann Dermatol Syphiligr 1894;8:308-313

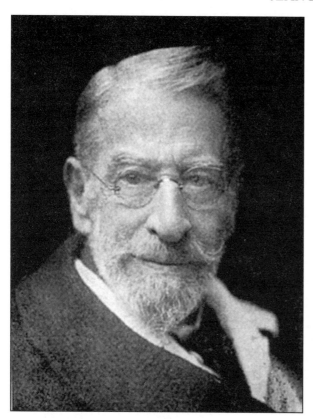

Jean Darier (1856-1938)

It is given to only a few of us to excel in both in the laboratory and the clinic. Jean Darier, French dermatologist whose career spanned the later decades of the nineteenth century and the early decades of the twentieth, moved between the two worlds deftly and with consummate ease. Born in Budapest of French parents, he began his professional life as a microscopist, a histopathologist, and his international fame was based mainly on his skills along these lines. He was also endowed with the "Willan eye," able to recognize the clinically new as new and in many cases confirm his judgment by demonstrating the uniqueness of his discoveries at the microscopic level. The best known of the entities described by him is keratoses follicularis (1889), routinely referred to even now as Darier's disease. He gave us the classic descriptions of pseudoxanthoma elasticum (1896), and erythema annulare centrifugum (1916), as well. Also of lasting value are his studies of hypodermic sarcoidosis and the tuberculides.

Darier worked at a number of different hospitals in Paris early in his career, but headed a service a l'Hôpital St. Louis from 1909 until his death in 1938.

Darier J. De l'Érythème annulaire centrifuge. Ann Dermatol Syph 1916;6:57

Right: erythema annulare centrifugum, from the Darier classic paper cited above.

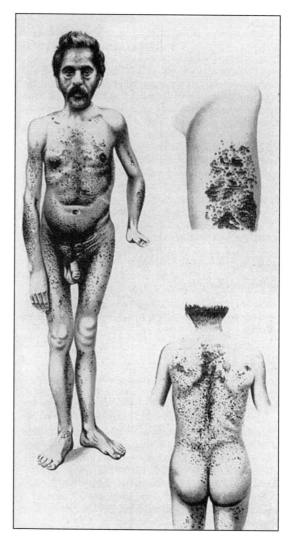

Darier J. De la psorospermose folliculaire végétante. Ann Dermatol Syph 1889;10:597

Above{ keratoses follicularis, from the Darier classic paper cited above.

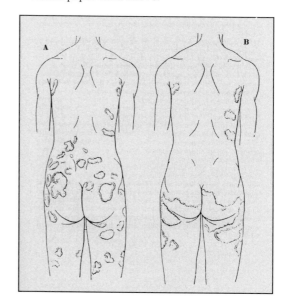

LATE NINETEENTH CENTURY AMERICAN DERMATOLOGY

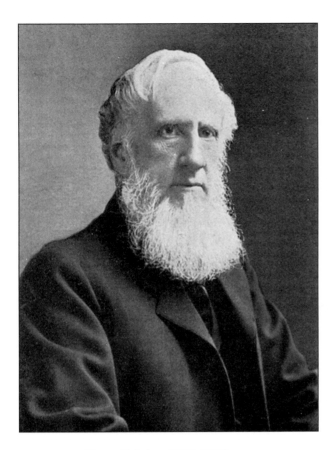

Louis Duhring (1845-1913)

Louis Duhring was America's first dermatologist with clout. Philadelphia born, and a graduate of the University of Pennsylvania medical school, he spent two post graduate years in the intensive study of skin diseases in Vienna, Paris, and London. He returned to Philadelphia, set up practice, and in 1876 at the age of 31 became Professor of Skin Diseases at his alma mater.

Duhring was a tireless worker. The classic description of pruritus hiemalis (1874) was followed by an atlas of skin diseases (1876-80), the "Practical Treatise on diseases of the skin" (1877) - the first American dermatologic textbook to be translated into foreign languages, including French - and the classic dermatitis herpetiformis synthesis described below. The shrewd observations and insights evident in these works impressed the Europeans, and from then on Duhring's opinions on the dermatologic problems of the day were routinely noted and treated with deference in European journals and texts. American dermatology had arrived.

Duhring amassed an enormous fortune through canny investments. He never married, and on his death in 1913 left the sum of one million dollars to his university. It was the largest bequest to a school by a single individual up to that time.

**Duhring L. Dermatitis herpetiformis.
JAMA 1884;3:225-9**

Duhring's description of dermatitis herpetiformis represents one of dermatology's finest clinical syntheses. It united under one title a great many grouped, pruritic, papular, vesicular, bullous, and urticarial eruptions that had rattled around in the literature as independent entities for years, poorly described and saddled with a host of confusing names. Modern immunologic investigative techniques have confirmed the accuracy this insightful synthesis. Duhring also showed us the proper way to extract the maximum mileage from a winner. He published 18 papers on the subject.

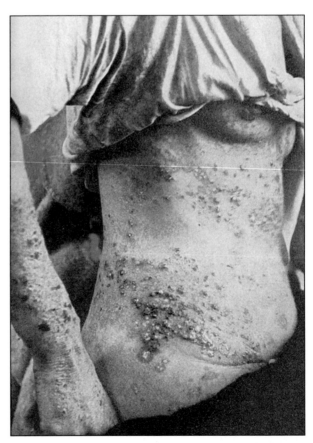

To the right: Dermatitis herpetiformis (Duhring's disease), one of Duhring's original patients.

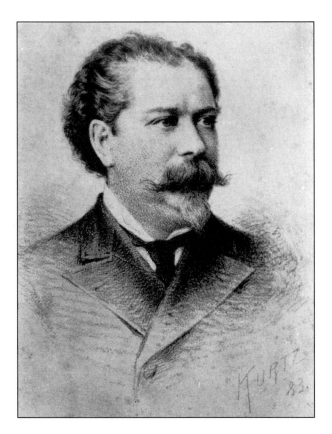

Morris Henry Henry (1835-1895)

Morris Henry Henry, an immigrant from England, arrived in the United States as a teenager. He received M.D. from the University of Vermont in 1860, served as a naval surgeon under Admiral Farragut during the American Civil War, and at the conclusion of the conflict entered practice in New York. Although primarily a surgeon, Henry involved himself heavily in matters pertaining to dermatology and syphilology during the decade between 1865 and 1875. In 1870 he founded the the *Americal Journal of Syphilography and Dermatology*, the first journal in North America devoted to the specialty (described below). In 1872, he published a monograph, "Treatment of venereal diseases," that was widely read and much admired. The monograph was, as Henry noted, a summary of the methods being used at the time in Vienna. An early member of the New York Dermatological Society, the oldest such society in the world (founded 1869), Henry made a lasting impression on the membership, as noted below.

Henry's outstanding achievement was his journal. He founded it and served as the editor in chief during the five stormy years of its existence (1870-1875). The masthead of Volume I is shown to the right. In a set of reminiscences of the New York society, George Henry Fox left us this revealing vignette:

"Another prominent, if not as popular a member of the society, was Dr. Morris H. Henry, editor of the Americal Journal of Syphilography and Dermatolog*y*. He was a red-faced gentleman of affable appearance, but extremely bluff and aggressive in both speech and manner. Whether intentionally or unconsciously, he succeeded in irritating the older and terrorizing the younger members of the society, and although his conduct of the journal was most creditable to himself and to the profession, his petty squabbles with his contributors seemed to take much of the joy out of their lives....For many a year after I joined the society, Dr. Henry's peculiar eccentricities formed a never ending subject as we were gathered around the table after our regular monthly meeting."

Whatever his problems in dealing with his contributers, Henry succeeded in putting together a first class journal. For historians interested in the dermatology and syphilology of the 1870s, both European and North American, the AJSD is a resource goldmine.

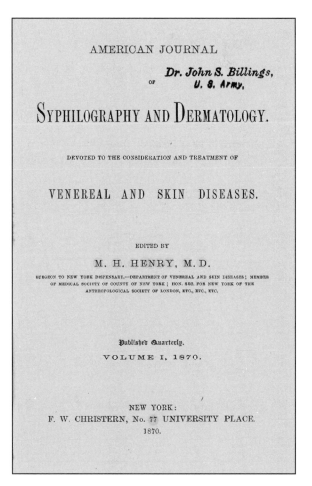

James Clarke White, formidable Bostonian and America's first professor of dermatology, taught at Harvard and ran the skin department at the Massachusetts General Hospital for many years. He learned his dermatology in the Hebra clinic in Vienna. One of a handful of dermatologists to write an autobiography, White filled his with a staggering array of personal details and opinions that show him as a keen observer with the gift of total recall and no disposition whatever to hide his light under a bushel. He wrote constantly, eight books and 200 papers, uniformly high in quality and covering nearly every aspect of dermatology. He was, along with Louis Duhring, a member of the earliest group of scholarly and thoroughly professional dermatologists who elevated the American version of the specialty to a level approaching parity with European departments by the end of the 19th century.

White's clinical skills are evident everywhere in his writing and are particularly well demonstrated in his paper on what is now called "Darier's disease," but which, considering the dates of publication, might with equal justice be called "White's disease."

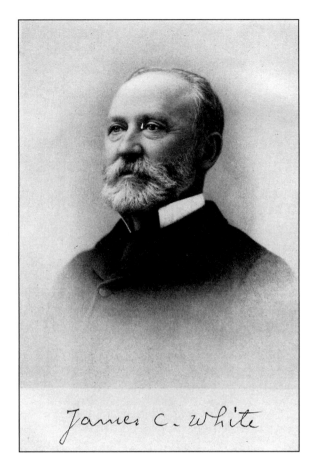

James Clarke White (1833-1916)

DERMATITIS VENENATA:

AN ACCOUNT

OF

THE ACTION OF EXTERNAL IRRITANTS UPON THE SKIN.

BY

JAMES C. WHITE, M.D.,

PROFESSOR OF DERMATOLOGY, HARVARD UNIVERSITY; PHYSICIAN TO OUT-PATIENT DEPARTMENT FOR SKIN DISEASES, MASSACHUSETTS GENERAL HOSPITAL.

BOSTON:
CUPPLES AND HURD,
Medical Publishers.
1887.

"My book on "Dermatitis Venenata," published in 1887, was written to fill a gap in dermatological literature, in the preparation of which I was much aided by my special knowledge of chemistry and field botany."

The quote is from White's autobiography. The work, the title page of which is shown to the left, is the first monograph on the condition we now call contact dermatitis. It is a well-written literature review, accompanied by White's own experimental efforts in the investigation of the nature and effects of the poison ivy resin. As in all works on the subject in that era, the selectivity of many forms of contact dermatitis, the fact that some individuals exposed to contactants developed dermatitis while others exposed in exactly the same way did not, confounded the author. The solution to that mystery was a long way off. White, as he indicated, did have a special knowledge of chemistry, acquired in his undergraduate days at Harvard. He was in fact offered a professorship in chemistry at his alma mater earlier in his career.

A figure of great importance in the development of American dermatology, Lucius Duncan Bulkley was the son of the Henry Daggett Bulkley who delivered the first lectures on skin diseases in the United States. Bulkley Jr. received his dermatologic training in Vienna, Paris, Berlin, and London. He practiced in New York City.

In 1874, Bulkley arranged for the publication of a new periodical, a quarterly which he called the *Archives of Dermatology*; he edited it until its demise in 1882. During this period it was the only journal in English, in either Europe or the United States, devoted to dermatology. In 1883 he founded New York's Skin and Cancer Hospital, the first such institution in North America concerned exclusively with the care of skin diseases. This institution has, of course, been the stage for a number of the finest moments in American dermatology and the home base for many of the specialty's best-known figures. Bulkley also deserves recognition for his continuing advocacy and successful organization of the section on dermatology and syphilology of the American Medical Association, work in which he was ably assisted by the then young William Corlett of Cleveland.

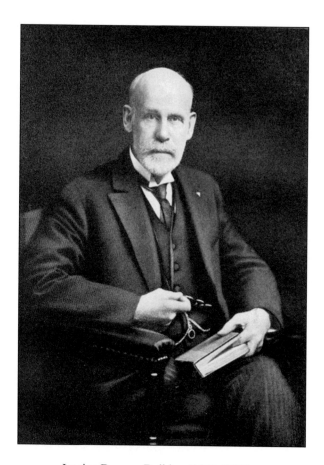

Lucius Duncan Bulkley (1845-1928)

It was the fashion late in the 19th century and early in the 20th for American dermatologists to review the foreign literature thoroughly, add their own experiences, and publish monographs in depth on a variety of subjects. Bulkley excelled in this sort of endeavor. He turned out monographs on eczema, dermatologic nursing, the relationship of diet to skin disease, cancer, the relationship of cutaneous problems to internal disease, and more. Shown to the left is one of his best, a mini-treatise on acne vulgaris, the first of its kind. Bulkley from his earliest years was preoccupied with dietary fancies, so it is not surprising that the interdiction of "sweets" and similar delights played an important part in his management of the disease. He eventually became a dietary fanatic, convinced that cancer, skin cancer included, could be cured or prevented by adherence to dietary regimens to which he was privy. In the end his fanaticism destroyed his credibility, blinded the younger generation to the marvelous contributions he had made to the specialty in its formative years, and reduced him to a pathetic figure sitting silently and by himself at the medical meetings he attended during his final days.

A C N E

ITS

ETIOLOGY, PATHOLOGY AND TREATMENT

A PRACTICAL TREATISE BASED ON THE STUDY OF
ONE THOUSAND FIVE HUNDRED CASES
OF SEBACEOUS DISEASE

BY

L. DUNCAN BULKLEY, A.M., M.D

PHYSICIAN TO THE NEW YORK SKIN AND CANCER HOSPITAL; ATTENDING
PHYSICIAN FOR SKIN AND VENEREAL DISEASES AT THE NEW
YORK HOSPITAL, OUT-PATIENT DEPARTMENT, ETC

NEW YORK & LONDON
G. P. PUTNAM'S SONS
The Knickerbocker Press
1885

TRANSACTIONS

OF THE

AMERICAN DERMATOLOGICAL ASSOCIATION.

REPORTED BY DR. L. DUNCAN BULKLEY, SECRETARY.

First Annual Meeting, held at the Cataract House, Niagara Falls, New York,
September 4th—6th, 1877.

Present Drs. ATKINSON of Baltimore, BRODIE of Detroit, BULKLEY of New York, CAMPBELL of New York, DUHRING of Philadelphia, FOX of New York, HARDAWAY of St. Louis, HEITZMANN of New York, HYDE of Chicago, TAYLOR of New York, VAN HARLINGEN of Philadelphia, WHITE of Boston, WIGGLESWORTH of Boston, and YANDELL of Louisville.

The President, Dr. James C. White of Boston, in the chair.

FIRST DAY, MORNING SESSION.

THE Council presented a report of the work done by the officers in preparing for the present meeting. All the members of the Association had been communicated with in reference to the presentation of papers, and when all the titles had been sent in, their place upon the programme was decided by lot.

The Council had also invited a number of gentlemen in this country who were interested in Dermatology, to be present at the sessions of the Association, and a number of Dermatologists in other countries to take part in the exercises by their presence, or the presentation of papers. Responses were received from Professors Hebra, Sigmund, and Zeissl of Vienna, Köbner of Breslau, Profeta of Palermo, Italy, Englested of Copenhagen, Guibout of Paris, and Anderson of Glascow, also from Drs. Güntz of Dresden, Tilbury Fox, Hilton Fagge and Dyce Duckworth of London. A written communication was received from Dr. Duckworth, and printed pamphlets from Drs. Sigmund, Zeissl, Köbner, Güntz and Profeta; a telegram of congratulation was received from Dr. Güntz just before the opening of the session.

The appointment of the Nominating Committee being next in order, Drs. Van Harlingen, Wigglesworth and Hardaway were chosen by ballot.

Drs. Atkinson and Brodie were appointed to audit the Treasurer's accounts.

The President then delivered his Annual Address, reviewing the progress of Dermatology in America during the past twenty-five years, and the gradual recognition of the branch in the Colleges of the Country.

Transactions of the first day of the first meeting of the American Dermatological Association. This prestigious organization, which is still in existence, is the oldest functioning national dermatological society in the world. Over the years it has exerted a profound influence on the development of the specialty in North America. The founders were I.E. Atkinson (Baltimore), Thomas R. Brown (Baltimore), L. Duncan Bulkley (New York), Samuel C. Busey (Washington), Louis A. Duhring (Philadelphia), Carl Heitzmann (New York), Edward L. Keyes (New York), John A. Ochterlony (Louisville), Henry C. Piffard (New York), Robert W. Taylor (New York), Arthur Van Harlingen (Philadelphia), Faneuil D. Weisse (New York), James C. White (Bosyon), and Edward Wigglesworth Jr. (Boston). The first meeting was held at the Cataract House, Niagara Falls, NY. The archives of the ADA are an invaluable resource for those investigating the history of North American dermatology.

George Henry Fox, beloved doyen and Nestor of American dermatology, whose 91 year life span carried him from the beginning of the specialty in the United States to its maturity, practiced in New York and taught at the Skin and Cancer Unit of the Post-Graduate Medical School in that city. He studied in Europe, mastered German, and spent a great deal of time in Hebra's clinic. Fox wrote with skill, insight, and sometimes humor, on many clinical subjects, the most enduring example of which is his classic description of the troublesome apocrine gland disturbance that continues to be known as Fox- Fordyce disease. Fordyce, a fellow New Yorker, handled the histopathologic section of the report.

Fox was best known in his day for his successful publishing ventures. For years he conducted interesting cases from his office to a nearby photographic studio to be recorded for posterity, and in 1880 and 1881 published his collection in two great atlases, one on skin diseases and one on syphilis. These works were the first of their kind to make use of the new publishing techniques that allowed the pictures to be printed directly on the pages with ordinary non-fading printer's ink.

Fox was also the author of an autobiography, "Reminiscences" (1926), that is both a joy to read and a valuable historical resource.

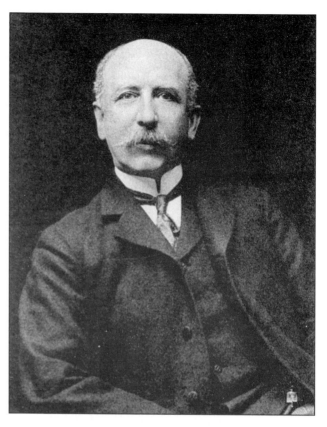

George Henry Fox (1846-1937)

Below, left: Keloid, from Fox's "Photographic Illustrations of Skin Diseases" (1880).
Below, right: An annular syphilid, from Fox's "Photographic Illustrations of Cutaneous Syphilis" (1881).

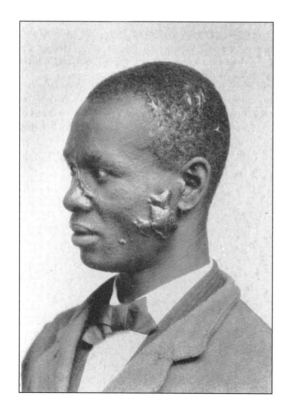

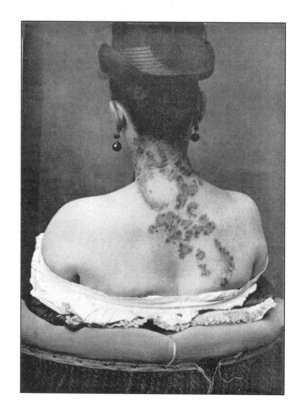

Henry Granger Piffard, the consummate bustling New Yorker, energized the Gotham scene for nearly forty years. A graduate of the College of Physicians and surgeons, he received his dermatologic training in the clinics of London, Paris, and Vienna, and later became Professor of Diseases of the Skin at N.Y. University. In 1875 he organized the first postgraduate course in dermatology in North America, which from 1882 on he conducted with great success at N.Y. Postgraduate Medical School.

Piffard published his "Elementary treatise on diseases of the skin" in 1876, the second such textbook by an American (Worcester's was first), and followed it with a treatise on materia medica and a beautifully turned out new text "Practical treatise on diseases of the skin" (1891). The latter featured many fine flash powder illuminated photographs taken by the author himself, who introduced the technique to his colleagues.

He was known as "Brains" Piffard to his friends, who regarded him as omniscient. A perpetual enthusiast for the something new, he worked his way ardently through botany, fishing, watercraft design, Esperanto, medical politics, mushrooms, shooting, bicycling, electrical devices, radiotherapy, and the design and manufacture of medical instruments.

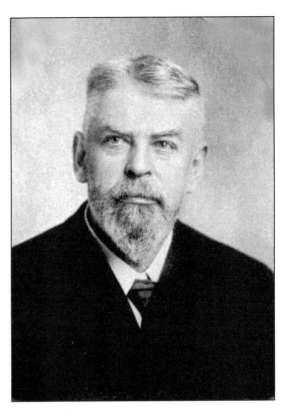

Henry Granger Piffard (1842-1910)

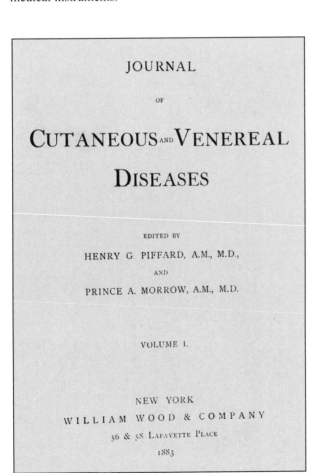

In 1882, the ever-entrepreneurial Piffard joined with his New York friend and colleague Prince Morrow to found a new dermatologic journal. The first issue appeared in 1883 under the title *Journal of Cutaneous and Venereal Diseases*. Piffard himself bailed out after four years, but the journal remained the most important repository for North American dermatologic contributions for 36 years. During this time it underwent several name changes and eventually became the official organ of the American Dermatological Association (ADA). Like many medical journals then and now it suffered from chronic financial difficulties that generated internal conflicts, often heated. Members of the ADA grew weary of the assessments levied for its maintenance, and in 1919 William Allen Pusey, the most politically powerful figure in American dermatology at the time, convinced the American Medical Association to take it over. The name was changed to the *Archives of Dermatology and Syphilology* , which journal is published now as the *Archives of Dermatology*.

Sigmund Pollitzer, much admired New York dermatologist and intellectual gadfly, was trained first in physics and mathematics and received his medical degree from Columbia in 1884. Following a tour of the medical clinics in Europe and a stint as a medical officer with the Serbian army in the 1885 war between Serbia and Bulgaria, he returned to New York and opened a medical office. Bored with general practice and interested in dermatology, Pollitzer journeyed back to Europe where he studied with Unna, Malcolm Morris and Jean Darier. He was one of Unna's favorite students, and it was during his stay with the Hamburg master that he published the classic description of acanthosis nigricans noted below. Back in the United States, he taught for many years at the New York Post-graduate Medical School and Hospital.

Pollitzer was not a prolific writer, although in addition to his work on acanthosis nigricans he made significant contributions to the study of hidrademitis suppurativa, parapsoriasis, the xanthomata, and the treatment and serodiagnosis of syphilis. He was a lively participant in discussions at dermatologic meetings. His early rigorous training in the hard sciences limited his tolerance for cerebral mushiness, and his comments were always pertinent and often a little sharp. A founding member of the Society for Investigative Dermatology (SID), he was one of the stalwarts who put their reputations on the line in defense of the new organization when it was under attack by the forces of reaction during its formative days. He died in 1937, the SID's inaugural year.

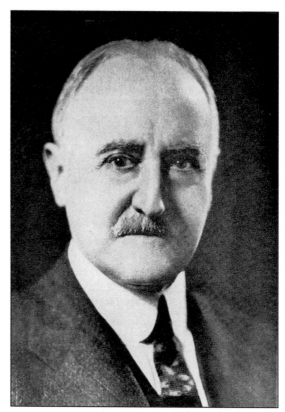

Sigmund Pollitzer (1859-1937)

Pollitzer S, Acanthosis nigricans. International atlas of rare skin diseases, Hamburg, 1891, Part X

Shown below are the plates from Pollitzer's classic description of acanthosis nigricans. The patient was a 65 year old widow who 8 weeks prior to admission to Unna's clinic had developed a soft, slightly elevated eruption, dirty grey and brown in color, on the upper extremities, neck, perioral areas, oral cavity, genital-crural areas, and part of the trunk. Her skin lesions improved on topical treatment, but her general medical condition declined, and she died 9 months later. Autopsy was refused, but all signs pointed to carcinoma occultum.

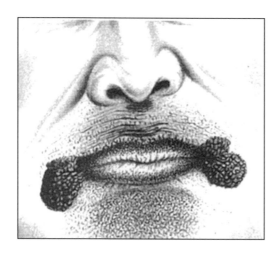

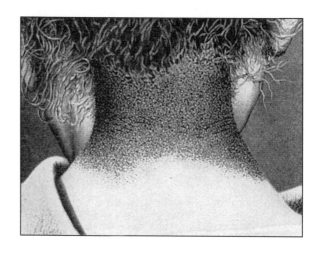

Born and educated in England, Thomas Casper Gilchrist came to the United States as a young man in 1882. He studied dermatology with Duhring in Philadelphia and later worked with Robert Morrison, professor of dermatology at Johns Hopkins in Baltimore. He succeeded Morrison to the chair at Johns Hopkins in 1897.

Gilchrist was a much published author. The most significant of his contributions, noted below, was his classic description of North American blastomycosis, often called Gilchrist's disease. He described his first case at a meeting of the American Dermatological Association in 1894. A biopsy of the patient's hand lesion had been sent to him by Louis Duhring. Gilchrist first thought the organisms he observed in tissue were protozoa, but later noted that some were budding and identified them correctly as yeast forms. A second case, recorded by Gilchrist in 1896, is shown below. In 1898 he and his coauthor W.R. Stokes succeeded in culturing the organism from the lesions in this case. They named their new discovery *Blastomyces dermatitidis*, and differentiated it clearly from the cryptococcus described at the time by Busse and Buschke as the cause of European blastomycosis.

Sigmund Pollitzer remembered Gilchrist as "a man of slender build, possessed of a fine sense of humor, (who) delighted in telling droll stories, which he delivered with a broad Scottish accent."

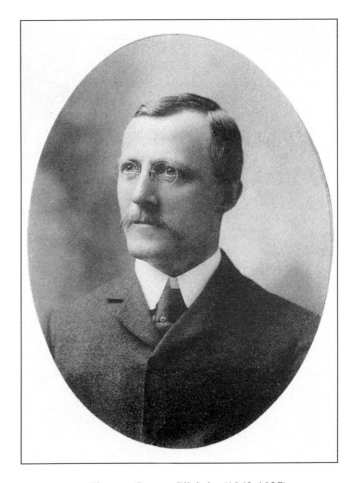

Thomas Casper Gilchrist (1862-1927)

Gilchrist TC. Protozoan dermatitis. J Cutan Dis 1894;12:496
Gilchrist TC, Stokes WR. A case of pseudo-lupus vulgaris caused by a Blastomyces. J Exp Med 1898;3:53-78

Right: Gilchrist's second case of blastomycosis – a 33 year old man with slowly progressive lesions of 11 years duration. Far right: budding forms of *Blastomyces dermatitidis*, figure drawn by Gilchrist for his 1898 report.

Gilchrist was a skilled medical artist; many examples of his work appeared as illustrations in the dermatologic textbooks of his time.

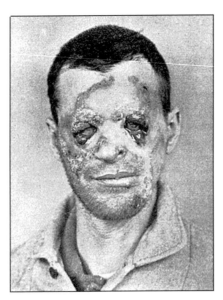

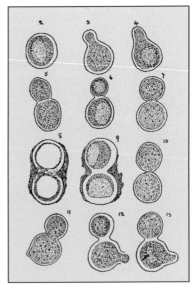

An Ohio native, John Addison Fordyce was graduated from Northwestern Medical College in 1881 and completed three years of postgraduate training in Europe, much of it in the clinic of Moriz Kaposi in Vienna. He opened an office in New York, where for many years he conducted an extremely busy dermatologic practice. Always active in teaching and dermatologic organizational activities, he became chief of the skin department at Bellevue, and later at Columbia..

Fordyce was a prolific writer, making many contributions to his favorite fields of interest – histopathology and syphilology. In 1896 he published the classic description of the angiokeratomata that commonly occur on the scrotum of older men, and in the same year described the sebaceous gland condition shown below.

"He lived," his friend George Miller McKee wrote, "in an atmosphere of culture and refinement, surrounded by etchings and paintings and a voluminous and varied library, all of which were very dear to him."

Fordyce died of acute appendicitis in 1925 at the age of 67.

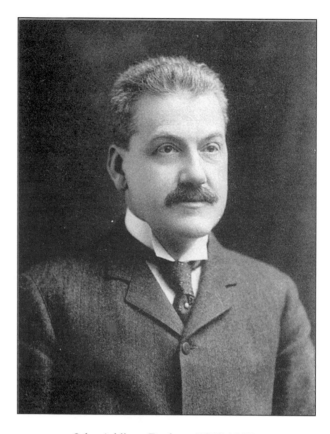

John Addison Fordyce (1858-1925)

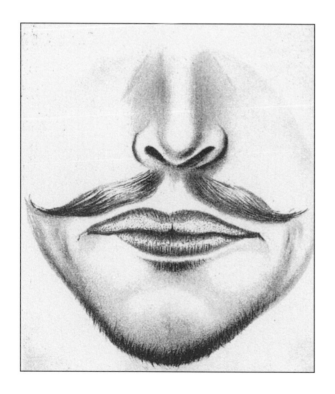

Fordyce JA, A peculiar affection of the mucous membrane of the lips and oral cavity. J Cutan Dis 1896;14:413

In the report cited above, Fordyce described the condition often called "Fordyce's glands" as a disease state, but it is now regarded as no more than a variant in the distribution of sebaceous glands. Nevertheless, when the whitish yellow papules that characterize the condition occur in profusion on the lips and extend onto the buccal mucosa they can confound the uninitiated and bother the patient, as well. We appreciate the effort put forth by JAF to call it to our attention. The plate from his report is shown to the left. The original is a life-size chromolithograph. Similar lesions have since been described on the labia minora, glans penis, and inner surface of the foreskin.

LATE NINETEENTH CENTURY ITALIAN DERMATOLOGY

Domenico Majocchi, Italy's first dermatologist of note, was born in Roccalvecce, a small town near Rome. He received his M.D. from la Sapienza and after a brief period in private practice in his home town retuned to Rome to study dermatology under Scillingo at the Ospedale di S. Galliano. Here he was exposed to a large amount of clinical material, which he studied assiduously. In 1880, he was appointed Professor of Dermatology at Parma and later held the same position at the University of Bologna.

Largely self taught, Majocchi was particularly interested in dermatopathology, the cutting edge of dermatologic technology and the hallmark of the progressive in the 1870s and 80s. The detailed histological material included in his clinical reports demonstrates his mastery of the subject as it existed at the time. His publications on granuloma tricofitico (Majocchi's granuloma), osseous syphilis, and purpura annularis telangiectodes are especially well known. The latter, sometimes called Majocchi's disease, is noted below. Dermatologic history also appealed to him; he published a scholarly account of the ill-starred campaign of Charrles VIII in Italy and essays on Marcello Malpighi and prehistoric medicine, as well.

Majocchi was by nature a kind and generous man, highly esteemed by his many pupils. He was a popular figure at social gatherings. Fond of music, he was particularly devoted to the works of Richard Wagner. Majocchi retired in 1924 and died in Bologna in 1929 at the age of 80.

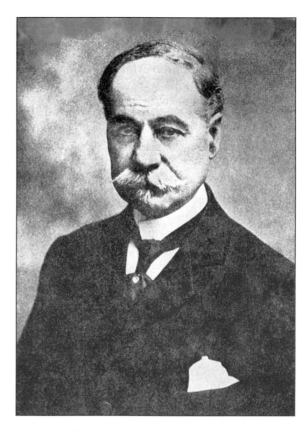

Domenico Majocchi (1849-1929)

Majocchi D. Purpura annularis telangiectodes. Arch f Dermatol Syphilol 1898;43:447-68

Majocchi's summary: "1) Rose-colored and livid red spots made up of capillary ectasias with subsequent hemorrhages, without preceding hyperemia, without perceptible infiltration of the skin, and usually in association with the hair follicles. 2) Slow extension of these. 3) Constant eccentric growth of the spots. 4) Symmetrical distribution of the dermatosis. 5) Primary location always on the extremities, particularly on the lower. 6) Usually absence of itching and disturbances of sensation. 7) Termination in slight atrophy and achromia of the skin, together with alopecia."

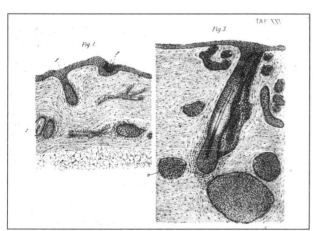

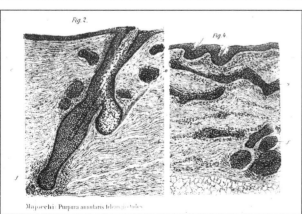

Left: Figures 1-4, from Majocchi's classic report: Fig. 1. Vertical section through an atrophic lesion showing the disappearance of capillary ectasias. Fig. 2. Longitudinal section of a follicle showing early vascular ectasia – f. Hair follicle showing small-cell infiltration in the papillary area. Fig. 3. Longitudinal section of a follicle showing progressive vascular ectasia development. Fig. 4. Vertical section through a skin lesion showing a moderate amount of telangiectasia. – v. capillary ectasia of the papillary vascular network; small-cell infiltration in the dermis. – f. cross section of a follicle.

Augusto Ducrey, distinguished Italian dermatologist, was born in Naples and received his medical training in that city. He did his dermatologic training with Tommaso De Amicis, chief of the Neapolitan clinic. He was associated with De Amicis from 1884 to 1894, and it was during this period that he discovered the causative organism of chancroid, the *Haemophilus ducreyi*. The unusual route followed by Ducrey to make the discovery is noted below.

Ducrey later became chairman of the dermatology department at Pisa and in 1911 accepted a similar post at Genoa. In 1919 he was elevated to the chairmanship in Rome, which position he occupied until retirement. He died in 1940 in Rome, at the age of 79.

Ducrey was not a prolific writer, but seemed equally at home in clinical and research settings. His expertise in microbiology is demonstrated in his contributions to the study of the leprosy bacillus and the causative organism of trichomycosis axillaris. He was the first to recognize the presence of "grain itch" in Italy and added new forms to the clinical catalogues of the dermatophyte infections and cutaneous tuberculosis.

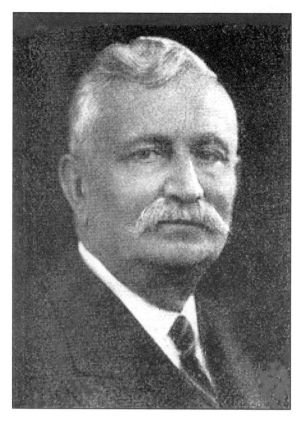

Augusto Ducrey (1861-1940)

Ducrey A. Recherches expérimentales sur la nature intime du principe contagieux du chancre mou, Ann Dermatol Syphilig 1890;1:56-57

1 do not believe that soft chancre can be produced by the inoculation of ordinary, banal pus. My experiences have convinced me that ordinary isolation methods using nutritive gelatin or artificial culture media and pus from the surface of a soft chancre have produced no satisfactory results. But I have succeeded in isolating the pathogenic organism on natural cultural terrain, by which I mean the skin of man himself, and I have also succeeded in purifying the chancre of all the other microorganisms that accompany it. This was accomplished by a special method involving repeated passages through a certain number of generations in a perfectly antimicrobial medium

***

The bacterium is 1.48 p in length and 0.5 p in width, short and thick, with very rounded ends, and it usually shows the lateral notching characteristic of microbes that have the ∞ configuration. Sometimes the notching is slight, or not present at all, in which case the microorganism appears as a short, thick bacillus. It is found in abundance in some preparations and is absent from others.

Ducrey's classic report on the cause of chancroid, excerpts of which are shown to the left, appeared in the French literature of 1890. It had been known for a long time that unlike the "hard chancre" of syphilis, the lesions of chancroid ("soft chancres") are auto-inoculable. Material taken from a chancroid lesion and inoculated into normal skin elsewhere on the same individual is capable of producing a new lesion identical to the source. Bacterial smears from chancroid lesions typically contain many different bacteria, but Ducrey noted that in performing multiple sequential auto-inoculation procedures only one organism persisted, a small bacillus which he described and presented as the cause of chancroid.

The unorthodox approach to the isolation of the organism cast doubt on the validity of Ducrey's discovery; it was not until Unna confirmed the presence of chains of the bacterium in tissue sections taken from typical cases of chancroid (1892) that Ducrey was given the credit he deserved. Culture on artificial media did not take place until much later, and even with today's superior technology, the *Haemophilus ducreyi* is not an easy microbe to isolate.

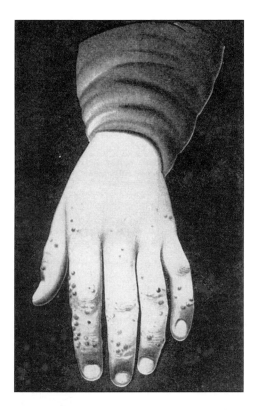

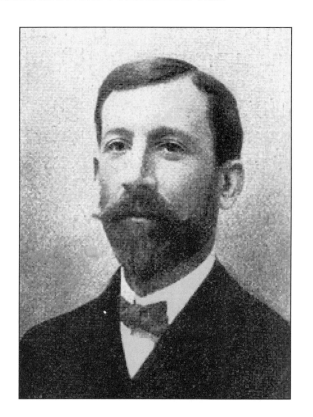

Angiokeratoma, plate from Mibelli's classic account.

Vittorio Mibelli (1860-1910)

Born on the Island of Elba, Vittorio Mibelli received his medical trainung in Siena and Florence and his dermatologic training with Unna in Hamburg. In 1901 he took over the chair in Parma.

A complete dermatologist, Mibelli was a member of the new generation, determined to bring home to Italy the *wissenschaftliche Dermatologie* of the German-speaking world, and he succeeded. His work in histopathology and mycology was thoroughly modern, and like his Hamburg teacher he carefully cultivated his clinical skills as well. He contributed cogently to the literature of urticaria pigmentosa, alopecia areata, and geographic tongue. Two of his clinical contributions are classic – the description of angiokeratoma (figure shown above to the left), and the description of porokeratosis, figure shown below. Both figures appeared with text in the 1891 International atlas of rare skin diseases (Parts 5 and 27), and both diseases continue to be linked with his name in everyday dermatologic parlance.

Mibelli was an able teacher, especially skilled in handling beginners. His careful, well-organized presentations, free from histrionics and verbosity, made him the easiest of lecturers to understand.

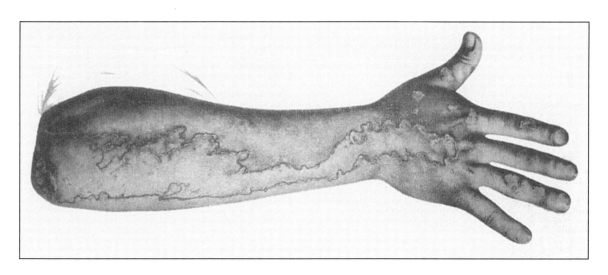

EARLY SCHOOLS IN OTHER COUNTRIES

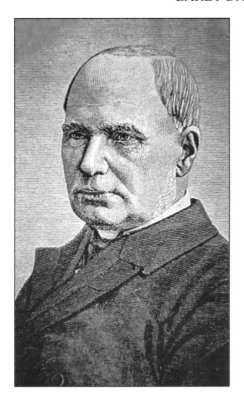

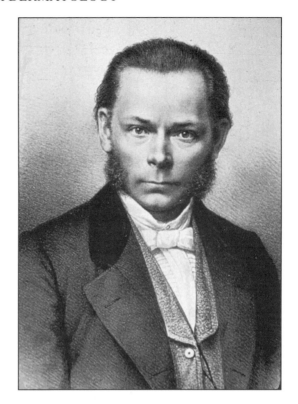

Above: Sophus Engelsted (1823-1914), Denmark's first Professor of Dermatology.

Rudolph Bergh (1824-1909)

Below: Alexander Haslund (1844-1906)

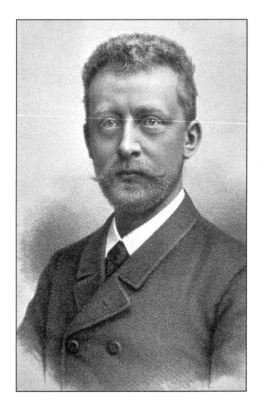

Sophus Engelsted, Danish internist who trained in Berlin, Paris, and Vienna, participated in a government sponsored reorganization of the Copenhagen medical school curriculum in 1873. He set up a course in syphilis and skin diseases, subjects not previously taught as specialties, and became Denmark's first professor of dermatology. His broad knowledge and teaching skills made him a favorite with students.

Alexander Haslund, successor to Englested, received formal dermatologic training in Vienna. He was interested in dermatologic rarities; his teaching was a bit too sophisticated for the medical students, but sharpened the skills of his assistants and prepared them to develop Danish dermatology in the next generation as a truly scientific discipline.

Prominent in the early development of Danish venereology was Rudolph Bergh. Bergh was also renowned zoologist and among the earliest to investigate thoroughly the scabies mite demonstrated so dramatically by Renucci in Alibert's clinic a few years earlier.

94

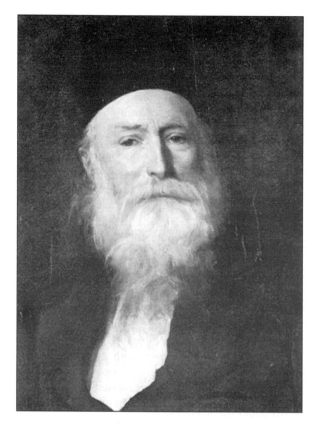

Daniel Cornelius Danielsen (1815-1894)

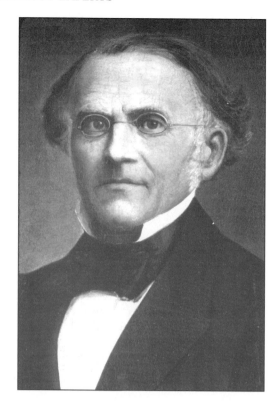

Carl Wilhelm Boeck (1851-1875)

Below: Gerhard Armauer Hansen (1841-1912)

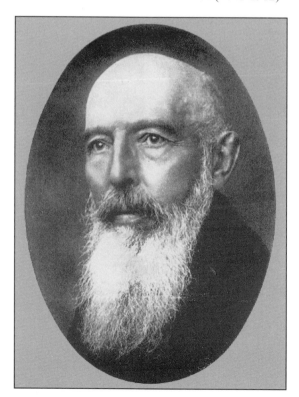

Daniel Cornelius Danielsen, Norwegian dermatologist, created Pleiestiftelsen on the outskirts of Bergen, the great center for the study and care of leprosy patients. He is the acknowledged founder of leprosy research, and an observant clinician who was the first to describe scabies crustosa. The disease was later named "Norwegian scabies" in his honor. The term has never been popular in Norway, and is now obsolete.

Carl Wilhelm Boeck was Norway's first professor of dermatology and syphilology. He was the uncle of Caesar Boeck, who succeeded him. Carl worked and taught at the Rikshospitalet in Oslo. His interests lay mainly in the study of leprosy and syphilis, both of which were public health problems of considerable significance in Norway at the time. In 1848, together with Danielsen, he wrote the "Traité de la Spedalskhed,," the first modern treatise on leprosy.

Gerhard Armauer Hansen, the discoverer of the leprosy bacillus, was also associated with the Bergen leprosy institution. He was the son-in-law of Danielsen, but unlike his father-in-law, who believed that leprosy is a hereditary disease, Hansen was convinced of its contagiousness and worked diligently to discover the cause. As early as 1872 he observed the presence of small rods lying within the "lepra cells" in tissue taken from leprosy lesions. His methods were primitive and his findings not well publicized, so it was some time before they were universally accepted. To Hansen his discovery was proof enough that leprosy was transmissible, and he instituted case isolation regulations that resulted in the reduction of the number of leprosy cases in Norway from 2800 in 1875 to 300 in 1912.

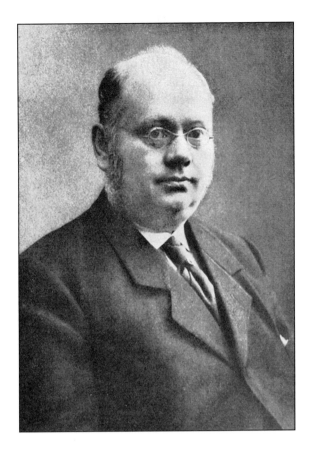

Caesar Peter Boeck (1845-1917)

Caesar Peter Moeller Boeck, renowned Norwegian dermatologist, received his medical training in Christiana (Oslo) and his dermatologic training in Vienna. He became associated with the Rikshospitalet in Oslo, joined the faculty of the University of Norway, and in 1895 took over the chair of dermatology at that school.

An enthusiastic teacher with a special knack for effective therapy, his clinics soon became extremely popular. He was particularly interested in tuberculosis and was among the first to work out the clinical and histologic pictures of the tuberculides. In later years he devoted much of his time to the study of sarcoidosis, his classic account of which is noted below.

During the twenty-year period from 1891 to 1910, Boeck decreed that with rare exceptions no patient with primary or secondary syphilis who came under his care would be treated with mercury or any other anti-syphilitic medication. All were hospitalized to prevent additional contagion and were placed on supportive care until all signs of the disease had disappeared. Boeck had come to believe that mercury was too dangerous and that treatment of any kind interfered with the development of host resistance. His successor Edvin Bruusgaard later tracked down a large number of these patients, and his findings stood for many years as the only data-based evidence for the natural course of syphilis.

Boeck was an unselfish kindly man. He was a connoisseur of fine paintings and possessed a magnificent collection himself.

Boeck C. Multiple benign sarkoid of the skin. J Cutan Genitourin Dis 1899;17:543-50

Left: Figure from Boeck's classic paper on sarcoidosis, cited above. The original is in color. The paper was published simultaneously in the American and Norwegian literature. The patient was a 36 year-old policeman with no signs or symptoms other than the skin lesions and lymphadenopathy. Bluish red papules and nodules with yellowish borders were evident on the face, scalp, back, buttocks, arms, and to a lesser extent the legs. Enlarged cubital, axillary, and femoral nodes were present. Years later the patient died at the age of 80 and at autopsy was found to have no trace of sarcoidosis.

Besnier and Hutchinson had reported cases earlier that were probably examples of sarcoidosis, but Boeck gave the condition a name, furnished clear clinical and histologic descriptions, and a graphic image in color. That potent combination established the entity as a disease *sui generis*.

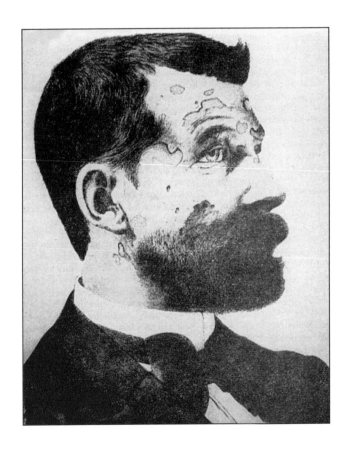

James Elliot Graham, Canada's first dermatologist, was born in Toronto and received his M.D. from the university in that city. He worked for a year in the Brooklyn General Hospital and served (unranked) with the Prussian army during the 1870 war. Several years of study in the European dermatologic clinics followed, after which he returned to Toronto to practice. He was made professor of clinical medicine at the University of Toronto in 1887, and five years later was appointed lecturer on dermatology at that institution.

Graham was elected to the American Dermatological Association in 1879, the first Canadian to be so honored, and served as president of the society in 1888. Among his published works were papers on congenital syphilis, scleroderma, molluscum contagiosum, and hydroa aestivale – case reports combined with mini-literature reviews, all set down in the conversational style of medical writing of that era in which personal interactions among dermatologist, patient, and referring physician are described in enjoyable detail.

Graham, a diabetic, also contracted pulmonary tuberculosis, and died from complications of the two diseases in 1899 at the age of 52.

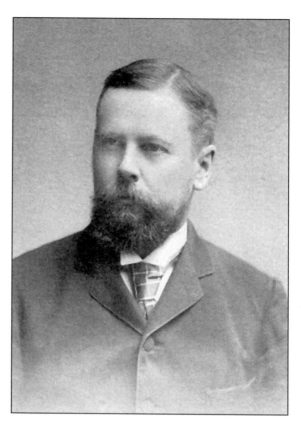

James Elliot Graham (1847-1899)

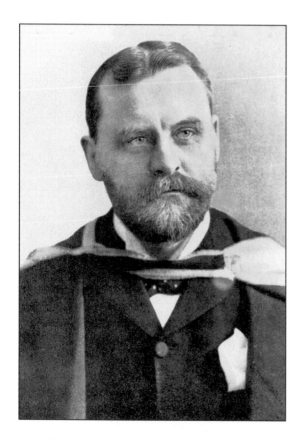

Francis John Shepherd (1851-1929)

Francis John Shepherd, Canadian surgeon, anatomist, and sometime dermatologist, received his M.D. from McGill University in 1873. He did two years of postgraduate work in London, Paris, and Vienna and returned to Montreal, where he became professor of anatomy. His real love was general surgery, at which he excelled and which he practiced for many years with great success. Like many others, Shepherd had fallen under the spell of Hebra during his stay in Vienna, and he somehow managed to combine his surgical activities with a life-long interest in skin diseases. He organized the department of dermatology at the Montreal General Hospital (his surgical home base) and secured for it a separate clinic, which he attended.

Shepherd was an early member of the American Dermatological Association, president in 1900. He attended its meetings regularly, and because he brought with him medical skills apart from the study of skin diseases, was a valued contributor to the lively discussions that were then the hallmark of that organization.

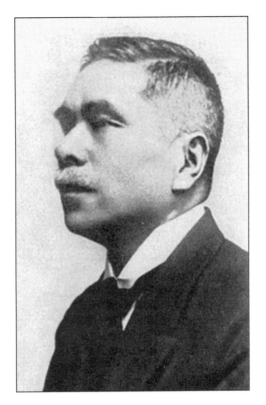

Keizo Dohi (1866-1931)

Izuko Toyama (1877-1951)

Below: Masao Ota (1885-1945)

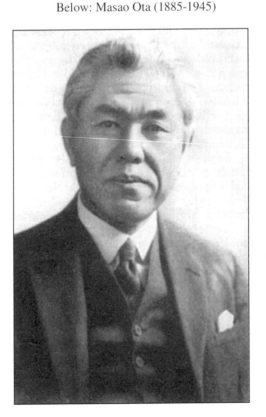

Japan under the shoguns had been completely cut off from the West for two hundred years. Following the famous 1853 visit to Edo bay of the armed fleet commanded by the American Commodore Matthew Perry, an agreement was signed to open Japan to trade with America. Conservatives were outraged that the shogun had capitulated to the barbarians. The result was a devastating civil war, and in 1868 victorious forces restored the emperor Meiji to power.

Ito Hirobumi, Japan's first prime minister and the power behind the throne, convinced his colleagues and the emperor that the best way to handle the barbarians was to master the technology of the West and beat them at their own game. A decision was made to modernize virtually all Japanese institutions, including medicine. The model of the latter to be followed was the medicine of the German-speaking nations, and the talented young Keizo Dohi was chosen in 1893 to study dermatology under Moriz Kaposi in Vienna. Within 20 years the remarkable Dohi had succeeded in establishing a dermatologic program in Tokyo on a par with others in the West. His successors, Izuko Toyama (1932) and Masao Ota (1937) continued the tradition of excellence.

José Eugenio Olavide, founder of Spanish dermatology, received his M.D. from the San Carlos Hospital in Madrid and did two years of postgraduate work in Paris, none of it apparently specifically concerned with skin diseases. Back in Madrid, he found himself in 1860 in charge of the 120 beds in the San Juan de Dios Hospital devoted to cutaneous problems and he began the difficult task of teaching himself dermatology on the job. Greatly influenced by the writings of the Parisian master, Ernest Bazin, who was then at the height of his powers, Olavide set up a teaching program at San Juan de Dios and eventually became Spain's first de facto professor of dermatology. His successor, Juan de Azúa (1858-1922) was the first officially to occupy the newly created chair of dermatology in Madrid.

Olavide's work is a strange mixture of abstruse pathogenetic speculations similar to the diathetic ruminations of Bazin, combined in his 1871 textbook with descriptions of the skin diseases equal in interest and accuracy to any that emanated from the more advanced European centers. Olavide also had a talent for investigational and experimental dermatology. He was among the first to inoculate the dermatophytes into the skin of lower animals, and as early as 1872 was engaged in attempts to isolate the microorganisms airborne in hospital environments.

From 1871 through 1880, Olavide published his most impressive and important work, the magnificent atlas of skin diseases, noted below.

Recognized and honored everywhere as the rock upon which Spanish dermatology was founded, Olavide died in 1901, at the age of seventy.

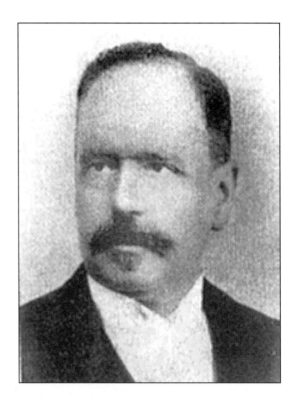

José Eugenio Olavide (1831-1901)

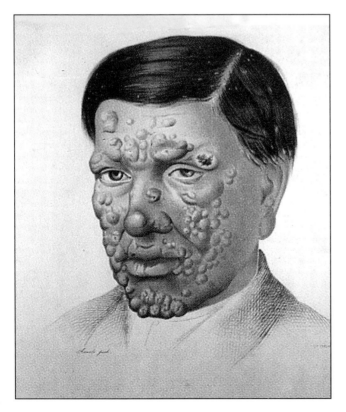

Olavide began his great atlas in 1871 as a small collection of loose-leaf prints, recording his clinical material in support of his dermatologic self-education program. The skill of his artist, Acevedo, and the rich supply of clinical material available soon dictated otherwise, and the project assumed far greater dimensions. Drawings and lithographs in folio size, accompanied by explanatory text, appeared irregularly over a nine-year period, the whole resulting in 1880 in a two volume master work entitled "Dermatologia general y atlas de clinica iconográfica de enfermedades de la piel o dermatosis." The cost exceeded Olavide's limited resources, but the Spanish government came to the rescue with the subsidies needed for completion.

Right: Lepra lepromatosa, chromolithograph from the Olavide atlas, 1880.

In 1870 Olavide turned his attention to the wax and cardboard paste moulage. He employed one Enrique Zofio, a skilled craftsman and pupil of Jules Baretta, to create a collection of moulages for teaching purposes. The collection, beautifully wrought, eventually numbered 1,500 pieces. Unfortunately, the San Juan de Dios Hospital was demolished in 1967, and Zofio's creations were relegated to storage. Steps are under way to rescue them and find a suitable place for their display.

99

Nineteenth Century Tools and Devices

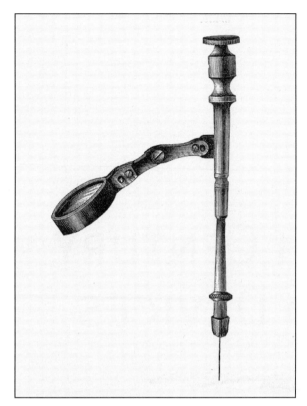

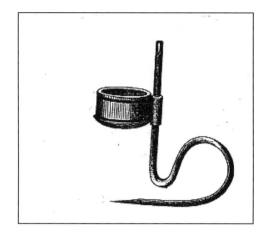

For the presbyopic dermatologist:

Above: scabies mite finder: achromatic magnifying lens attached to a flat sharp needle
Left: achromatic magnifying lens attached to an electrolysis needle.

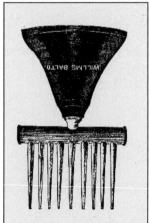

Left: Comb for the application of lotions to the diseased scalp. Handle is hollow and unscrews for filling. Teeth are hollow and perforated at the tip to deliver the medication when run through the hair.
Below: Syringe for the same purpose – medication applied "without making the hair unpleasantly wet. The many patients who have used this method all express themselves as greatly pleased with it."

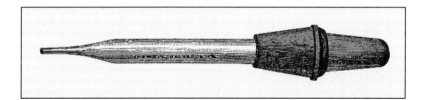

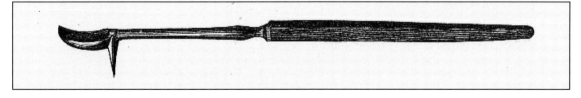

Above: Auspitz Instrument for the treatment of recalcitrant folliculitis barbae:

"The scoops devised by Auspitz of Vienna are of great service. After shaving and applying linen spread with diachylon ointment for several days, the most prominent pustules are opened with the conical point, and then the whole surface is firmly scraped with the scoop so as to remove all pustules, crusts etc. The process is repeated several times a week, the parts being kept covered continually in the intervals with the ointment. In this way brilliant cures are often effected."

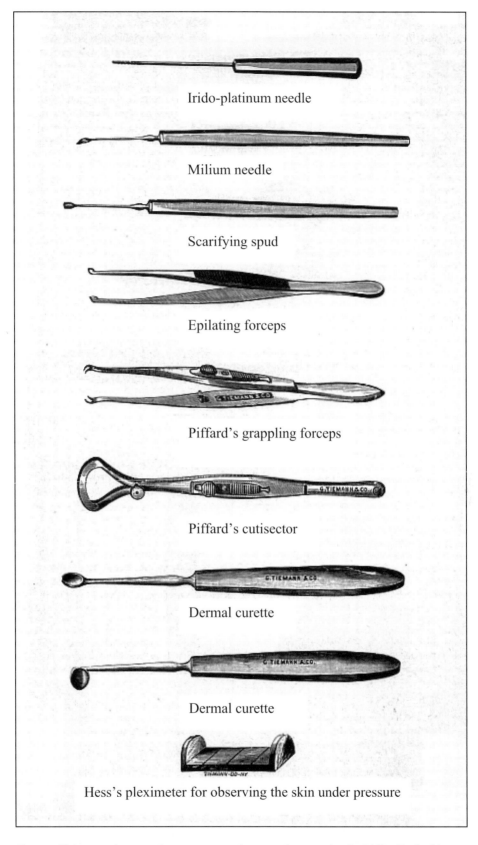

Irido-platinum needle

Milium needle

Scarifying spud

Epilating forceps

Piffard's grappling forceps

Piffard's cutisector

Dermal curette

Dermal curette

Hess's pleximeter for observing the skin under pressure

The scarifying spud was an instrument used to treat lupus vulgaris. Piffard's double-bladed cutisector was designed to cut thin sections of tissue from a lesion for direct microscopic examination. The transparent pleximeter was used mainly to search for the characteristic "apple jelly nodule" of lupus vulgaris.

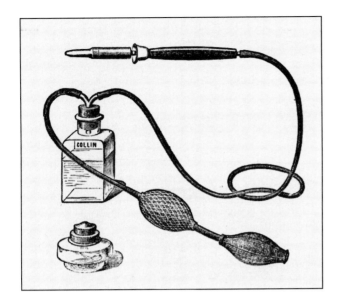

Left: Paquelin's cautery, a benzene fueled heat cautery that was a standard fixture in dermatologic offices well into the early decades of the 20th century. It was displaced by electro-surgical devices.

Below, left: French version of Balmanno Squire's multi-bladed scarification knife for the treatment of lupus vulgaris. Unlikely though it may seem, when this knife was drawn across the lesions to make multiple superficial incisions, and the procedure was repeated at intervals, the lupus often healed, leaving a soft pliant scar.

Below, right: Volkmann's spoons for scraping away lupus vulgaris tissue, and a threaded punch for pulling the centers out of lupus nodules.

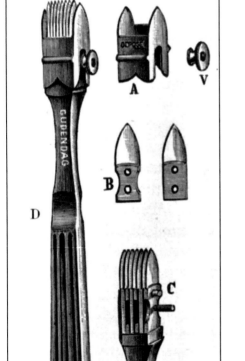

A, manchon ; B, lames ; C, montage des lames ; V, vis servant á fixer les manchons et par suite les lames ; D, instrument complet.

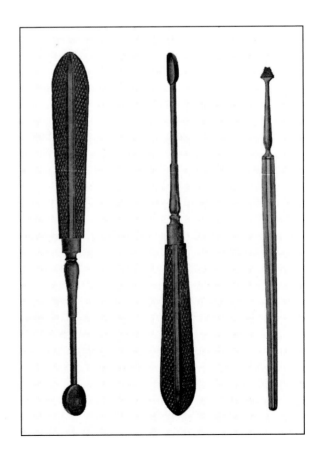

Early Twentieth Century Dermatologists, Events, and Discoveries

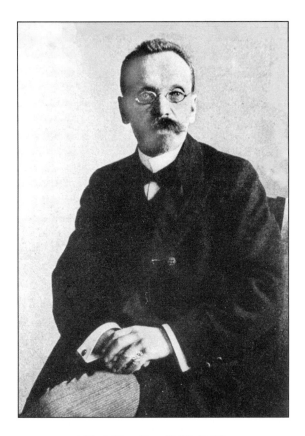

Alfred Blaschko (1858-1922)

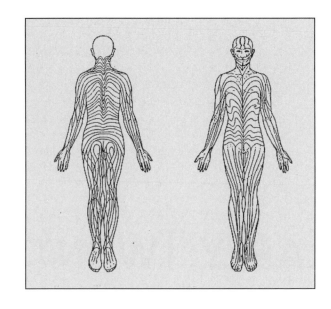

The famous lines as illustrated in Blaschko's classic paper, cited below.

Blaschko A. Die Nervenverteilungen in der Haut in ihrer Beziehung zu den Erkrankungen der Haut. Beilage zu den Verhandlungen der Deutschen Dermatologischen Gesellschaft VII Congress, Breslau. 1901

In 1901, the German dermatologist Alfred Blaschko described "a system of lines on the surface of the human body which linear naevi and dermatoses follow." From his own cases and others in the literature, he outlined on a white plaster statue the paths followed by these linear lesions until the pattern became clear. The statue, a classic Greek "adorant," was later painted green and kept in Blaschko's study. It has long since disappeared. The accuracy of drawings published in his classic paper (above right) can be confirmed almost any day in a busy skin clinic. In the century that has passed since the lines were first described, a good many attempts have been made to identify an anatomic infrastructure to which they correspond. None has been found, but there is evidence that as a result of lyonization, the heterozygous state of some X-linked gene defects may result in mosaic lesion patterns that conform to the mysterious lines.

If it were not for his discovery, Blaschko's name would no doubt be forgotten now, but during his lifetime he was far better known as a political activist at the forefront of many of the liberal causes of the day. He was a founder of the Deutsche Gesellschaft zur Bekämpfung der Geschlechtskrankheiten (1902), the most important society in Germany dedicated to the fight against sexually transmitted diseases (STDs). He was chairman of the organization from 1916 to 1922 - war years and disastrous post-war years in Germany when the incidence of the STDs reached appalling heights.

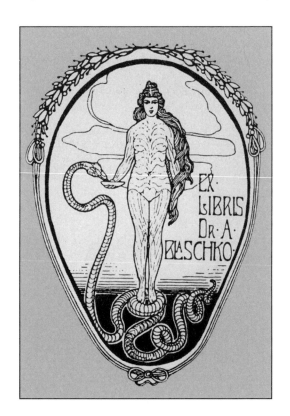

Blaschko's bookplate, into which, with pardonable pride, he worked his lines.

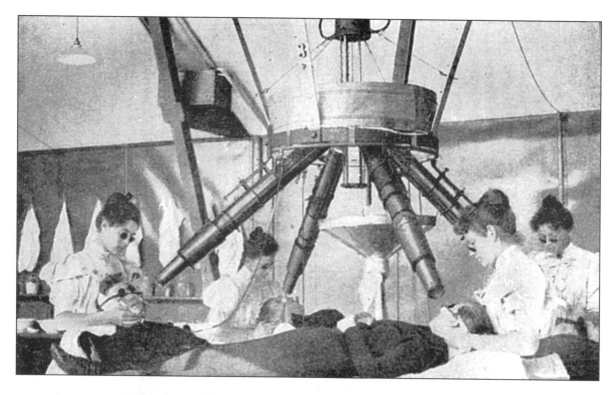

Nurses at work in the famous Finsen Lysinstitute in Copenhagen, ca. 1903. They are compressing lupus vulgaris lesions that are being exposed to ultraviolet rays generated by the carbon arc above.

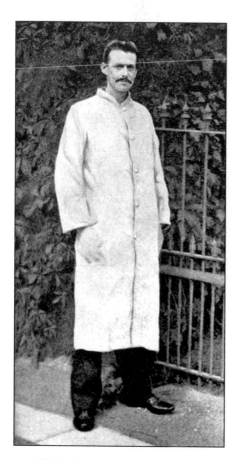

Nils Ryberg Finsen, Danish physician and sometime dermatologist, discovered that mechanical compression of the skin lesions of lupus vulgaris allowed carbon arc or solar generated ultraviolet rays to penetrate deeply enough to kill the tubercle bacilli that cause the disease. In practice many cases responded well. His treatment was regarded as one of the most exciting therapeutic breakthroughs of the time, and in 1903 he was awarded a Nobel prize for his work. Finsen did not enjoy his celebrity status for long. He succumbed the next year to constrictive pericarditis, at the age of 44.

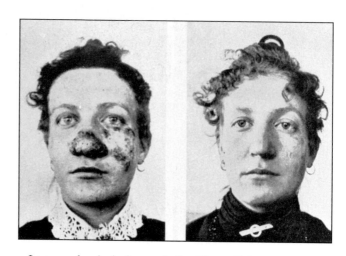

Nils Ryberg Finsen (1860-1904)

Lupus vulgaris, before and after Finsen light treatment.

107

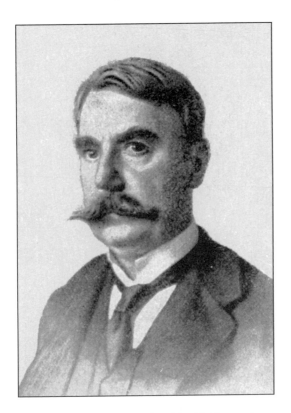

Prof. Charles Tripler (Ca 1849-1906)

Air was first liquefied in the later decades of the 19th century, but its high cost ($3000/ounce) relegated it to the scientific curiosity realm. In 1899 Charles Tripler, a New York inventor, devised a machine to liquefy air at a cost of five cents a quart. Separation of the nitrogen component came a little later. Tripler formed a company to exploit his invention, but the venture became involved in financial difficulties suspicious enough to attract the attention of the local district attorney, and the professor died soon after - alone in a hotel room up in Liberty, NY. The diagnosis was Bright's disease. Archie Campbell White of the Vanderbilt Clinic was the first to use it on skin lesions (1899). He reported his results at an American Medical Association meeting in 1900. Availability problems limited the dermatologic use of liquid nitrogen until after World War II.

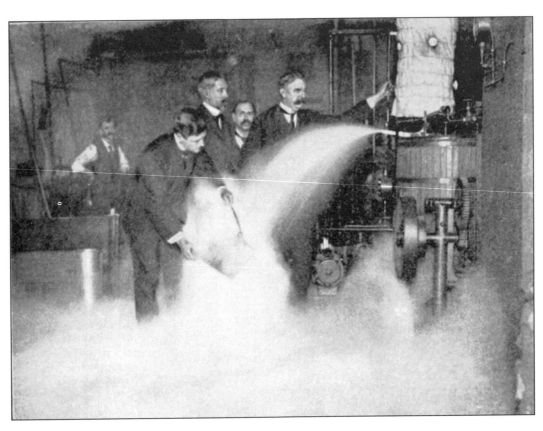

Charles Tripler (arm upraised) demonstrates his new device for the production of liquid air. Photograph from McClure's Magazine (1899)

Wilhelm Conrad Roentgen, German physicist, discovered X-Rays while working with Crookes tubes in Würzburg, Germany, in November 1895. Images such as the early example shown to the right immediately suggested that the rays could be of diagnostic value in many medical situations, and they were put to use for that purpose with "almost wicked speed." Soon afterwards it became evident that the rays were capable of producing hair loss and inflammatory changes in skin. Hairy nevi and cases of ordinary facial hirsutism were depilated. Lupus vulgaris and skin cancers were treated successfully, and within a few years of their discovery Roentgen's rays were turned on many other skin conditions, benign and malignant. With no reliable method available for calibrating machine output and measuring the dose, treatment excesses resulted in severe burns and devastating late sequellae. Nor was it only the patients who suffered. A good many of the physicians and technicians who worked with X-Ray in its early years paid with their lives for their ignorance, enthusiasm, and carelessness. It was not until the 1930s that reasonably reliable methods for calibration were developed.

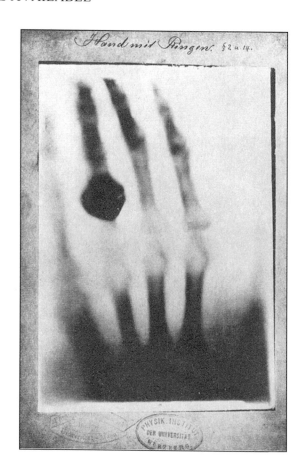

Below: Child with large hairy nevus. Severe radiodermatitis at the site of X-Ray treatment by Leopold Freund (1899)

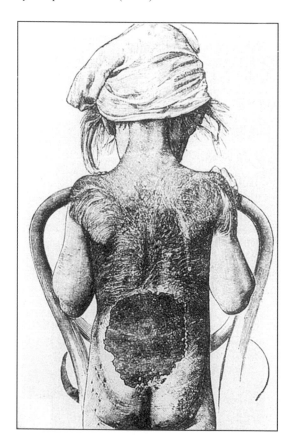

Above: Hand with rings, one of Roentgen's earliest X-Ray images. The subject is believed to have been Frau Roentgen.

The appeal of X-Ray in its heyday is easy to understand; in many intractable conditions - cystic acne vulgaris, lichen planus, and verruca plantaris, for example - it worked better than anything else. As late as 1947, George Miller MacKee and Anthony Cipollaro continued to insist in their famous textbook on the subject that X-Ray is "the most useful and important single agent in the armamentarium of dermatology." The statement accurately described the consensus at the time, and yet by the late 1960s, X-Ray as a treatment for benign skin diseases had all but disappeared. It was the victim to some extent of the Hiroshima syndrome, the often irrational fear shared by many in which radiation in any form, from dental X-Rays to nuclear power plants, is declared anathema. No dose is a safe dose, critics declared. But radiation also succumbed to the advent of improved surgical techniques, powerful antibiotics, topical steroids, and the like.

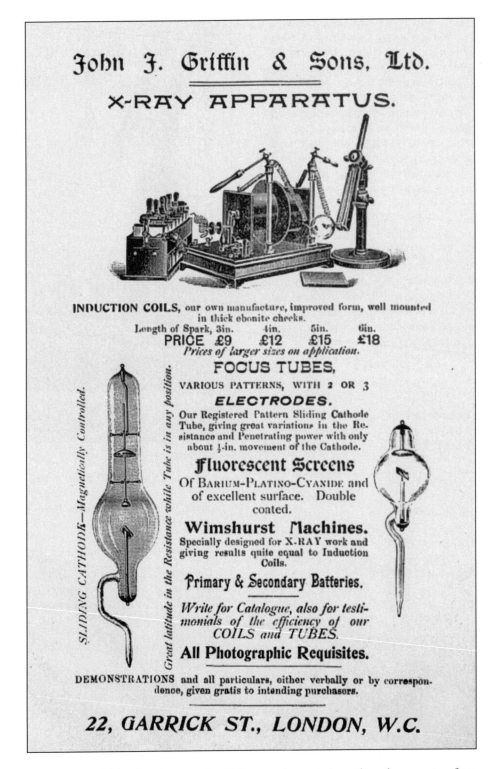

An 1898 British advertisement for X-Ray equipment. Less than three years after Roentgen's discovery a wide variety of machines and parts was available to anyone who could afford the price. Machines did not come as a complete unit. The buyer was expected to select the different components and connect them himself, much as a hi-fi or computer buff assembles a system today. Some machines were powered by induction coils, others by storage batteries or Wimshurst static electricity devices. All were hazardous.

William Allen Pusey, the most influential American dermatologist in the first three decades of the 20th century, was born in Elizabethtown, Kentucky in 1865, received his M.D. from the Medical college of New York University in 1888, and for two years worked with George Elliott at the Skin and Cancer Hospital in New York. As was customary at the time, he devoted another two years to a tour of the skin clinics of Europe and in 1893 settled in Chicago, where he practiced and taught for the rest of his professional life.

It was as an expert in the uses of X-Ray (noted below) that Pusey first gained fame beyond the limits of Chicago, but his talents quickly became evident in other fields, as well. He maintained a life-long interest in syphilology. His essay "Syphilis as a modern problem," published in association with the Panama-Pacific exposition in 1915, is exhaustive and dealt with the clinical and social aspects of the disease in a forthright manner unusual in North America at the time. When America entered World War I in 1917, Pusey was appointed by the Surgeon General to select and head the committee formed to deal with sexually transmitted diseases in the military. The treatment manual he prepared at that time was used throughout the conflict, and continued to be used by many state boards of health well into the 1920s.

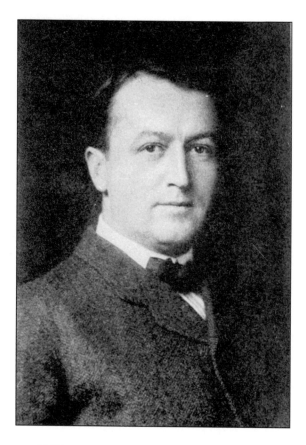

William Allen Pusey, young and ambitious.

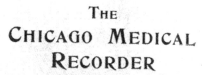

The 1895 publication of Roentgen's remarkable discovery of X-Ray was followed immediately by a period of feverish activity in which investigators around the world applied the new techniques to medical diagnostic problems. With the appearance of the first x-ray burn, it became evident that radiation also exerted profound effects on the skin. It was inevitable that these effects would be investigated and exploited. In 1899 Schiff and Freund in Vienna reported the use of x-ray in the epilation of a large hairy nevus, and that was enough for Pusey. He hurried to the Austrian capital, spent a single evening with Freund, acquired an exact duplicate of the apparatus used by the Viennese physician, and returned at once to Chicago. He hired an electrician to assemble the parts and proceeded to put the machine into action on patients without ever having seen it previously in actual operation. Over the next two years he published a number of reports on his findings, including the first ever uses of X-Ray in the treatment of leukemia and Hodgkin's disease. In February 1902, Pusey presented his "Report of Cases Treated by X-rays" before an SRO meeting of the Chicago Medical Society. From then on and for many years he was the number one authority on X-Ray diagnostic and therapeutic matters in North America, and his 1903 textbook on the subject was accepted as authoritative. The opening of the published report of his Chicago speech is shown to the left.

111

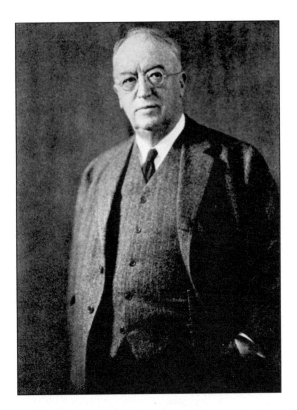

William Allen Pusey, mature and powerful

Pusey was a complete dermatologist. His influential textbook, the title page of which is shown to the left below, appeared in 1907. "Writing it," Pusey's long time associate Herbert Rattner recalled, "was a laborious task to which he gave three or four years. Evenings extending late into the night were spent in the basement of his home, where he had set up an apparatus for making photographs. He himself took nearly all the clinical photographs that were used to illustrate the book, and he personally reviewed all the pertinent literature." Pusey also wrote eminently readable histories of dermatology and syphilis and was the first to use carbon dioxide snow for the destruction of skin lesions.

Above all, Pusey was politically active and a joiner. He held almost every important office in the specialty and went far beyond that. He was elected president of the American Medical Association (the only dermatologist ever to be so honored), when that job was the most prestigious in American medicine.

Success and fame had little effect on Pusey's small town approach to private practice. "The well known country doctor of 7 West Madison St.," one observer called him, and on another occasion a VIP patient, perched precariously on an article of furniture that had seen better days, was heard to exclaim, "By George, Dr. Pusey, you must be a damned good doctor to put patients on a chair like this."

Pusey died quietly at his home in Chicago in 1940, at the age of 74.

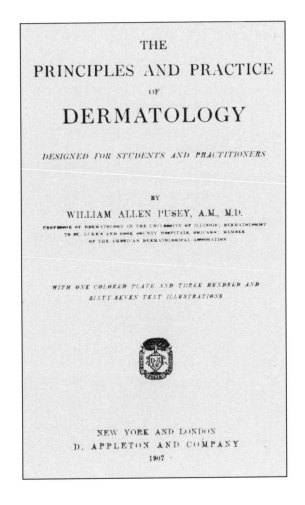

Below: Figure from Pusey's 1903 textbook on X-Ray, showing the primitive type of apparatus he worked with early in his career.

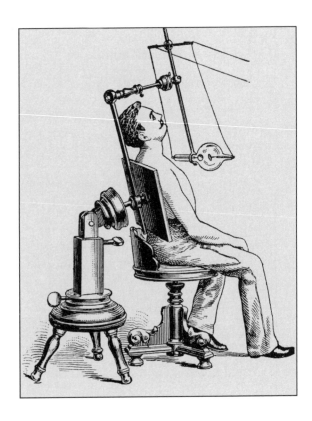

RAYMOND SABOURAUD

Scion of a Parisian medical and artistic family of renown, Raymond Sabouraud received his M.D. from the Paris school, trained in dermatology with Vidal and Besnier at l'Hôpital Saint Louis, and remained associated with that institution throughout his professional life. He also spent an important year early in his career at the Pasteur Institute, where he received a thorough grounding in the techniques of bacteriology.

It was Ernest Besnier who suggested that his pupil investigate the ringworm fungi, the dermatophytes, the literature of which was cluttered with contradictory claims to the point of total disarray. His remarkable work in the field is noted below. In accordance with a grand design set for himself as a young man, Sabouraud labored from 1902 to 1932 to complete a multi-volume work dealing exhaustively with diseases of the scalp. "Les teignes," the third volume of the scalp series (1910), summed up his dermatophyte research and is recognized now as a medical classic.

Sabouraud was a born professor who genuinely enjoyed teaching. His approach to that art was quiet, effective, and charming. He loved the fine arts and was himself a talented sculptor, accomplished enough to produce a number of pieces that were accepted as serious contributions by the artistic critics of the time.

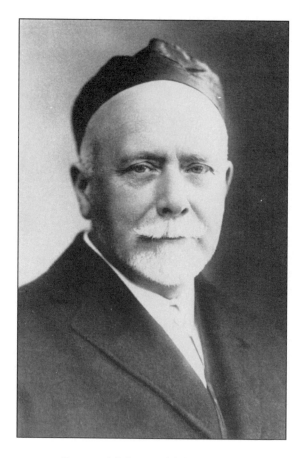

Raymond Sabouraud (1864-1938)

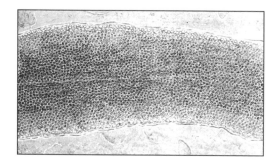

Above: dermatophyte spores within the matrix of the hair shaft (endothrix infection).

Below: spores surrounding the exterior of the hair shaft (ectothrix infection).

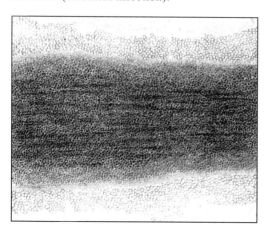

Late in the 19th century, 50 years after the discovery of the first dermatophyte, opinion was sharply divided on the nature of the "trichophytons," as they were commonly called. Is there only one trichophyton, capable of causing all the tineas, or are there many? Sabouraud answered the question by cultivating an impressive variety of colony forms on the dextrose agar culture medium that bears his name and demonstrating his collection to doubters and cynics at international meetings. On clinical and botanical grounds, he divided the dermatophytes into the genera microsporum, epidermophyton, trichophyton, and achorion. The last he later included with the trichophytons. It is a measure of Sabouraud's skill that 100 years later, his classification survives.

The differentiation of the tinea capitis fungi on the basis of the type of invasion of the hair shaft – endothrix or ectothrix – was also an important feature of Sabouraud's work. The figures (shown to the left) illustrating hair invasion types are taken from "Les teignes."

Some of Sabouraud's findings had already been observed and published 50 years earlier by David Gruby, but the work of the Hungarian genius had long since been forgotten. It is to Sabouraud's credit that after exhuming Gruby's reports he acknowledged the older man's work warmly and generously.

113

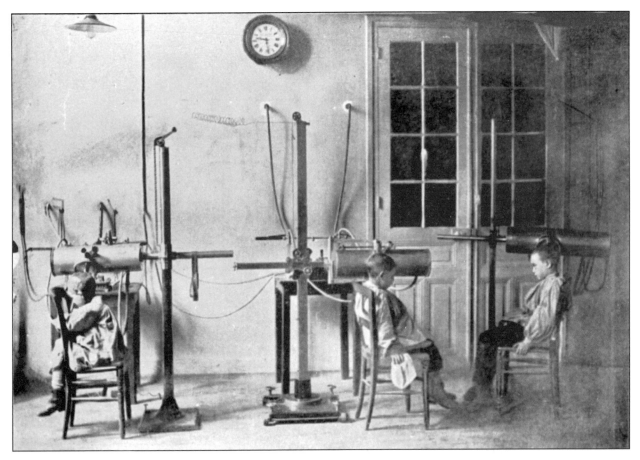

A busy morning in the Sabouraud epilation clinic at l'Hôpital St. Louis

Sabouraud did not reside exclusively in the ivory tower of bench research. He was a busy dermatologic practitioner, a therapeutic activist who concerned himself mainly with diseases of the scalp. He devoted a great deal of attention to the management of tinea capitis. It is estimated that 150,000 children were affected by disease in the Paris of 1900. Dissatisfied with the older topical treatments and the manual epilation approach, Sabouraud was impressed by the preliminary results obtained by the Viennese pioneer radiologist Leopold Freund in the treatment of favus and tinea barbae by X-Ray epilation. The procedure was fraught with danger, and Sabouraud realized that most of the difficulties arose from the inability of therapists to calculate and standardize the energy output of their machines. In 1904 in collaboration with Henri Noiré he developed a measurement technique that utilized disks of paper coated with barium platinocyanide, a substance that turns gradually from green to brown when exposed to X-Ray. Disks included in the treatment field could be matched to a standard brown reference color when the proper dose for epilation had been delivered. Marketed in kit form as the Sabouraud-Noiré radiometer-X the technique remained an important standard for many years. It was replaced eventually by ionization chambers that were far more accurate and easily read. X-Ray epilation continued to be a popular treatment for tinea capitis well into the 1950s, but disappeared abruptly with the advent of griseofulvin in 1959.

Sabouraud's stature in the dermatologic world is well illustrated in this 1908 eyewitness account of a visit to the Paris clinic by a physician from St. Louis, Missouri:

"I went there primarily to see the much-talked-of "bald-headed clinic" of Sabouraud. Everybody has heard of this clinic, where those who have lost their hair come by hundreds, and of the great Sabouraud who pulls a hair (provided there is one remaining) from your head, glances at it, and says "Yes, I can cure you; go into the next room"; to another, "You may be benefited; wait here"; and to a third, "Go and buy a wig; nothing can be done for you." It is said that Sabouraud can tell your moral character, the amount of your yearly income, and what you have eaten for breakfast, by looking at a root of one of your hairs. We will admit that this is perhaps exaggeration, but we want to prove the point that he is a great man, a man every dermatologist in every civilized country has heard of."

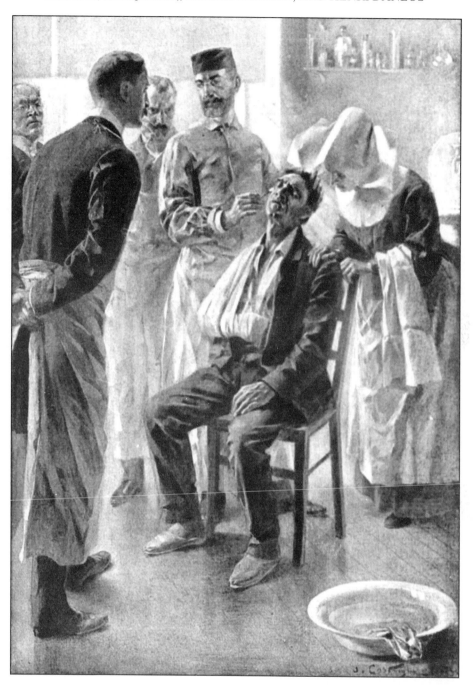

Henri Danlos applying radium to a facial lesion of lupus vulgaris. Paris, circa 1903.

The 1896 discovery by Henri Becquerel that some substances are radioactive and the subsequent isolation of radium by Pierre and Marie Curie were preludes to the development of another form of dermatologic radiotherapy.

On a six hour trip to London in 1901 Becquerel carried in his waistcoat pocket a glass tube containing radium. Ten days later a burn appeared on the skin in the area beneath the pocket. Becquerel consulted Ernest Besnier, who noted the similarity of the lesion to X-Ray burns and suspected that radium might have therapeutic applications. Besnier's associate Henri Danlos began to apply radium in various forms directly to lesions of lupus vulgaris, as shown above. The results were impressive, and radium treatment became popular in many dermatologic centers, especially in the treatment of hemangiomata. Late sequellae followed; popularity declined, and by the late 1950s radium, like X-Ray, had just about disappeared from the dermatologic scene.

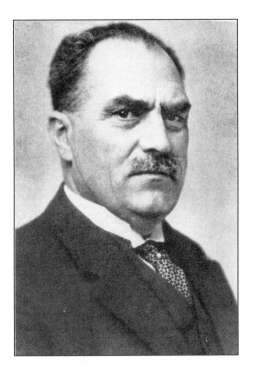

Erich Hoffmann (1868-1959)

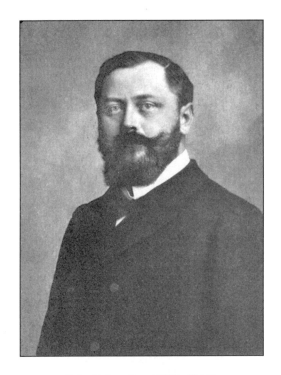

Fritz Schaudinn (1871-1906)

Deeply disturbed by the abysmally high incidence of syphilis in Germany, the government commissioned a research project to be conducted in the dermatologic clinic of Edmund Lesser in Berlin and designed to ferret out the cause of the disease. Dr. Fritz Schaudinn was recalled to Germany from Trieste where he had been conducting animal research on trypanosomiasis. He was chosen because some, including Schaudinn himself, suspected syphilis might be caused by an animal parasite. Erich Hoffmann, a younger member of Lesser's staff, was assigned to the project as a well-trained dermatologist who could be relied upon to recognize a syphilitic lesion when he saw one. Their successful demonstration of *Treponema pallidum* in the lesions of secondary syphilis took place in March, 1905.

The discovery was headline news, but Schaudinn did not enjoy his sudden rise to fame for long. A year later he died from sepsis associated with a rectal abscess. Hoffmann later went on to a distinguished career as chairman of the dermatology department at Bonn. He was a man of principles, the only prominent non-Jewish dermatologist in Germany to protest publicly the unconscionable treatment of his Jewish colleagues during the Nazi era, and in 1934 it cost him his job. He resumed his teaching duties following the conclusion of WWII.

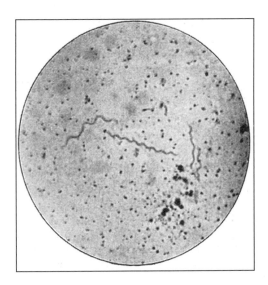

Left: Treponema pallidum. Photograph from the classic 1905 report of Schaudinn and Hoffmann.

Some, soured by the dozens of bacteria erroneously presented over the years as the cause of syphilis, were unimpressed. When Schaudinn first described his discovery at a meeting of the Berlin medical society, the president, Prof. Ernst von Bergmann, cut him short with words he no doubt later regretted. "This," he declared, "terminates this discussion - until the next cause of syphilis is brought to our attention."

To the right: Portion of the first page of the 1905 report in which Schaudinn and Hoffmann described their discovery of *Treponema pallidum* in the lesions of syphilis.

Below: Artist's conception of Schaudinn and Hoffmann at work. Drawing by Karl Krusnyak.

Vorläufiger Bericht über das Vorkommen von Spirochaeten in syphilitischen Krankheitsprodukten und bei Papillomen.

Von

Dr. Fritz Schaudinn,
Regierungsrat

und

Dr. Erich Hoffmann,
Privatdozent.

(Aus dem Protozoen-Laboratorium des Kaiserlichen Gesundheitsamtes und aus der Königlichen Universitätsklinik für Haut- und Geschlechtskrankheiten zu Berlin.)

Auf Veranlassung des Herrn Präsidenten des Kaiserlichen Gesundheitsamtes Dr. Köhler und unter Mitwirkung des Herrn Professor Dr. E. Lesser wurden von uns in Gemeinschaft mit den Herren Dr. Neufeld und Dr. Gonder Untersuchungen über das Vorkommen von Mikroorganismen in syphilitischen Krankheitsprodukten begonnen. Hierbei fand Schaudinn am lebenden Objekt sowie in gefärbten Präparaten Organismen, die zur Gattung Spirochaete gestellt werden müssen, einer Gattung, deren systematische Zugehörigkeit zum Stamm der Protozoen Schaudinn auf Grund seiner Untersuchungen an der Spirochaete ziemanni des Steinkauzes behauptet hat. Die Spirochaeten konnten bisher sowohl an der Oberfläche sezernierender syphilitischer Effloreszenzen als auch in der Tiefe des Gewebes und in den spezifisch erkrankten Leistendrüsen nachgewiesen werden.

Um die baldige Nachprüfung dieser Befunde zu ermöglichen, sollen sie schon jetzt unter Beifügung von zwei Mikrophotogrammen kurz mitgeteilt werden.

Hoffmann himself described the discovery in a conversation with the American dermatologist-syphilologist Charles C. Dennie:

"Schaudinn had a preconceived idea that the cause of syphilis was an animal parasite, and he immediately began to search for this parasite. We scraped the secondary lesions of the syphilitic and collected the serum for microscopic examination. We often worked until the light of the incandescent electric globe was neutralized by the morning rays of the rising sun.

One day we hit the jackpot. All at once Schaudinn let out a yell and said, 'Here it is!' I crowded him away from the microscope and peering into the eyepiece saw a shadowy spiral form slowly turning like a gimlet and at the same time swimming like a fish in slow motion across the microscopic field. We were sure that the microscopic gimlet was the cause of syphilis but we could not prove it at that time."

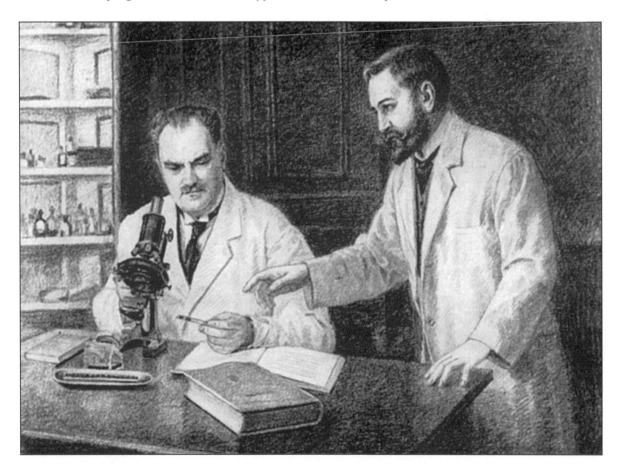

117

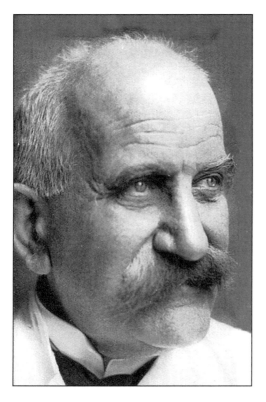

Josef Jadassohn (1863-1936)

Jadassohn J, Lewandoski F. Pachyonychia congenita. Ikon Dermatol 1906;1:29

Below left: pachyonychia congenita, figure from the Jadassohn classic paper referenced above.

Eine eigentümliche Furchung, Erweiterung, und Verdickung der Haut am Hinterkopf. Verhandl Deutsch Dermat Gesell 1906;9:451

Below right: cutis verticis gyrata, figure from the Jadasshohn classic paper referenced above.

Josef Jadassohn, the most complete dermatologist of his time, studied and worked with Neisser in Breslau. He was called to the chair of dermatology in Bern Switzerland at the age of 33, and in 1917 returned to Breslau to succeed Neisser as the chief of that prestigious department. He retired in 1931, and following the Nazi takeover in 1933 moved to Switzerland where he died two years later.

The scope of Jadassohn's work defies summarization. The morphology, immunology, and pathogenesis of cutaneous tuberculosis, dermatophyte infections, leprosy, eczematous eruptions, and sexually transmitted diseases, the characterization of congenital anomalies, all were and studied intently at one time or another by this remarkable man. Clinical and laboratory experiments were joined seamlessly with diagnosis and treatment. Jadassohn was the first to apply objective experimental methods to the study of cutaneous immunology. He was the first to apply patch tests in the study of contact dermatitis, and the first to discriminate clearly between idiosyncrasy in the production of eczematous and drug eruptions. His name will forever be linked to the great "Handbuch" (1927-1937) which he edited and to which he made valuable contributions – 41 volumes, by far the largest work on skin diseases ever published.

Jadassohn's skills as a clinician were also legendary and are reflected in the impressive list of classic descriptions that came from his pen – blue nevus, anetoderma, granulosis rubra nasi, and more, including pachyonychia congenita and cutis verticis gyrata, noted below.

"His integrity, his kindness, his indescribable charm, his delightful sense of humor and his genuine modesty – his character, in short – was a rare addition to his intellectual gifts." Those are the words of Marion Sulzberger, who knew Jadassohn well.

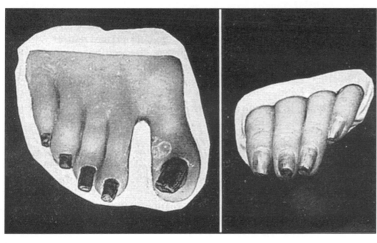

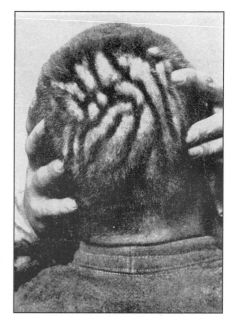

Bruno Bloch, Swiss dermatologist and eminent researcher, received his most significant training under Josef Jadassohn and later became chief of dermatology at Basel. In 1908 he agreed to occupy the newly created chair of dermatology at Zürich, but no suitable facilities existed. To remedy this Bloch became the only dermatologist in history to canvas the local taxpayers personally, door to door, to explain his predicament and solicit their support to build a clinic for him and his staff. Once in place in his grand new clinic he demonstrated convincingly that their money was indeed well spent.

Like many Germanic academics of the day Bloch was a perfectionist and a workaholic to whom the time of day meant nothing. He made notable contributions to mycology, particularly in the study of immunologic responses to dermatophyte infections, and concerned himself with the immunology of contact dermatitis as well. In 1926, he demonstrated his clinical prowess with the classic description of incontinentia pigmenti. His most important discovery, shown below, lay in the field of pigment research.

Bloch's premature death, at the age of 54, resulted tragically from an unrecognized reaction to Allonal, an analgesic then commonly in use, which he took for colds, headaches, and the like.

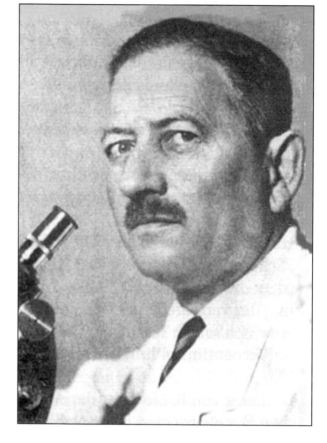

Bruno Bloch (1878-1933)

Bloch B. Chemische Untersuchungen ueber das spezifische pigmentbildende Ferment der Haut, die Dopaoxydase. Ztschr f physiol Chem 1916;98:226-54.

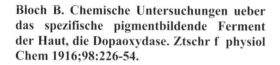

To Bruno Bloch belongs the credit for showing the proper route to follow to solve the mysteries of human cutaneous pigmentation. His classic 1916 study, shown to the left, was the first to establish the presence of an enzyme in human skin. The enzyme, which he called dopa oxidase, catalyzed the transformation of dopa (dihydroxyphenylalanine) into the pigment melanin. Three decades later Thomas Fitzpatrick, Aaron Lerner et al were able to show that dopa oxidase is in fact tyrosinase, and that dopa is itself the product of the interaction of tyrosinase and the amino acid tyrosine, the first step in the formation of melanin.

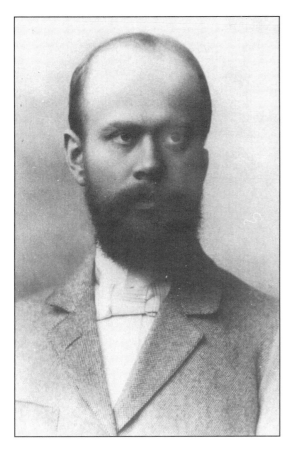

Ernst Kromayer (1862-1933)

Ernst Kromayer, German dermatologist who pioneered in cosmetic surgical procedures, received his M.D. from the university at Halle. In 1899, the Prussian government commissioned him to set up a dermatologic outpatient clinic in that city, and from the beginning Kromayer, a natural born rebel with a taste for conflict, found himself at odds with the local bureaucracy. His attempts to better his position and his clinic were frustrated at every turn by inertia and incompetence. Fed up, he resigned his post in 1904, ripped his enemies in a vitriolic pamphlet that was read with interest throughout the German academic world, and headed for Berlin.

Kromayer was no mere academic troublemaker; he was a multitalented, ambitious, hard-working, innovative physician. Shortly after arrival in the German capital, he acquired an abandoned factory building and turned it into a successful hospital. He also set up a fine private clinic in the vicinity of the Kurfürstendamm, where for years he conducted an enormously remunerative dermatologic practice based to a great extent on his surgical skills.

Well off now, Kromayer became what used to be called a "penthouse warrior;" he embraced the revolutionary tenets of the hard German Left, while living luxuriously in an elegant parkside villa. With the establishment of the Third Reich those credentials and the fact that he was Jewish would most certainly have meant future trouble on the grand scale for Kromayer, but in 1933, the year Hitler came to power, he discovered he was hopelessly ill and escaped it all by committing suicide.

In recognition of Kromayer's contributions to his alma mater, and in celebration of the 100th anniversary of his birth, a bronze plaque (shown to the right below) was cast in 1962 and installed in the library of the Halle clinic.

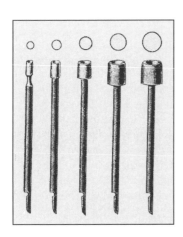

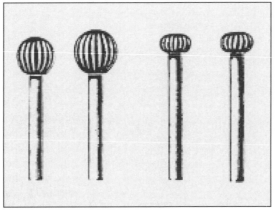

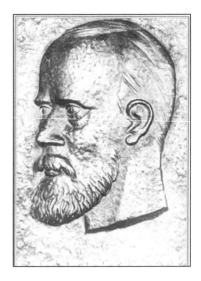

Early in his career Kromayer was interested in dermatopathology and published an impressive monograph on the dermal-epidermal interface, which he called the "parenchymhaut. He is best remembered now for his surgical innovations and for his development of the water-cooled "Kromayer" ultraviolet lamp that could be placed directly against the skin in the treatment of lupus vulgaris and plaque psoriasis. He developed the power driven biopsy punches and the rotary rasps, shown above, and used the latter with great skill in the treatment of scars. The rasps, which remained in use in many clinics into the 1950s, were displaced by the wire brushes developed by Abner Kurtin in the heyday of dermabrasion. Kromayer's influential textbook on the treatment of cosmetic skin problems (Behandlung kosmetischer Hautleiden) appeared in 1913.

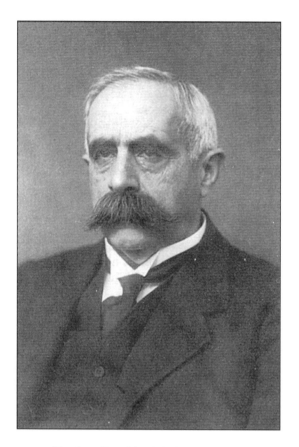

Abraham Buschke (1868-1943)

Below: Title page of Buschke's 1902 treatise on European blastomycosis (cryptococcosis).
Below, right: An entrance to the German concentration camp at Theresienstadt in Czechkoslovakia. Buschke was imprisoned here in 1942 and died of dysentery four months later.

Abraham Buschke, German dermatologist of international repute, received his M.D. in Berlin and his dermatologic training in the clinics of Albert Neiseer (Breslau) and Edmund Lesser (Berlin). He set up a private practice in Berlin, joined the faculty of the university, and in 1904 became chief of dermatology at the enormous Rudolf-Virchow Krankenhaus, in charge of its 400 beds devoted to skin diseases.

Buschke made good use of the rich supply of clinical material available to him. Endowed with a restless, inquiring mind and boundless energy, he published several hundred scientific reports and trained a large number of young dermatologists who expressed their gratitude to the master in many ways in later years.

Among the best known of Buschke's contributions were his studies on cryptococcosis. With Otto Busse, he reported the first case of the disease and later published an impressive monograph on the subject, the title page of which is shown below. He also published the classic descriptions of scleredema adultorum (Buschke's disease, 1902), giant condylomata (the Buschke-Löwenstein tumor, 1925) and, along with his associate Helen Ollendorf-Curth, the assembly of nevoid defects known as the Buschke-Ollendorf syndrome (1928).

Buschke doubted both the efficacy and safety of Ehrlich's salvarsan in the treatment of syphilis, a stand that put him severely at odds with the university power structure and probably cost him the chair of dermatology at Berlin, for which he was being considered.

An observant Jew who was proud of his ethnic heritage, Buschke was relieved of his hospital post by the Nazis in 1933 and relegated to lesser positions. In 1937, he and his wife Erna visited the United States where their children had taken up residence. The children begged their parents to stay, but they insisted on returning to Berlin. In November 1942, both were "transported" to the German concentration camp at Theresienstadt, where Buschke died of dysentery four months later. Erna survived the war and lived out her years with her children in America.

Buschke the man was complex, an introspective workaholic, thoroughly trained as a scientist and yet attracted to mysticism and even astrology. He was an accomplished musician, a violinist who regularly played in chamber music ensembles.

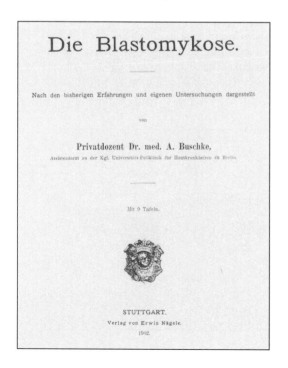

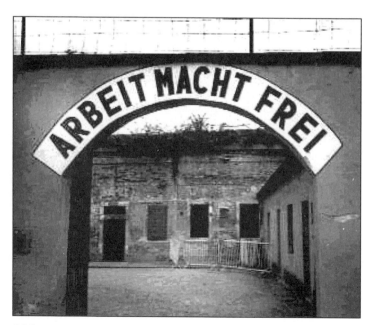

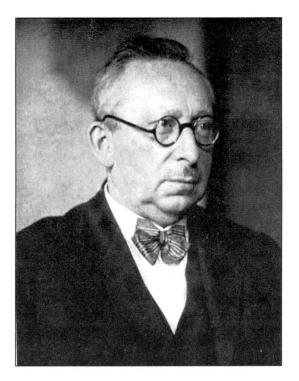

Felix Pinkus (1868-1947)

Felix Pinkus, outstanding Berlin dermatologist, was Jewish and therefore relieved of his official posts in 1933, despite the fact that he had fought for his country in WWI and had been awarded the Iron Cross. He hung on, living dangerously, until 1939 when he emigrated to Norway and later found his way to the United States by a circuitous route that took him through Denmark, Russia, and Japan. He resided the last six years of his life in Monroe MI with his son, Hermann, who was also a distinguished dermatologist. He worked in his son's office and busied himself with the preparation of a new textbook on dermatologic pathology, but died before he could complete it.

Trained by Neisser in Breslau, Pinkus made a name for himself as a histopathologist. His description of lichen nitidus, noted below, is classic, and his voluminous monograph on the anatomy of the skin in the Jadassohn Handbuch was the most comprehensive ever written up to that time.

A modest, friendly man, Pinkus had an artistic side. He loved to sketch and could often be seen at meetings capturing the likeness of the speaker.

Pinkus F. Ueber eine neue knötchenförmige Haut-eruption: Lichen nitidus. Arch f Dermatol Syph 1907;85:11.

Translation of the beginning of the classic Pinkus paper on lichen nitidis cited above: "As early as 1897, during my assistantship at the University of Breslau clinic for skin diseases, I saw a striking skin affection which after a most exact analysis could not be fitted into any known disease picture, and which after an attempt to clarify matters by histological examination, proved to be a new entity in its structure as well. After long and repeatedly futile experiments to determine whether or not it might be related to lichen planes, which is most similar to it, or to one of the known granulomas, I must conclude finally that it is unknown. I have followed it zealously during the succeeding years, and accordingly have gotten a large number of observations together. I believe that I have found the proper place here to report them."

Über eine neue knötchenförmige Haut-eruption: Lichen nitidus.

Von

Felix Pinkus.

(Hiezu Taf. II—IV.)

Bereits während meiner Assistentenzeit an der Breslauer Universitätsklinik für Hautkrankheiten, 1897, ist mir eine Haut-affektion aufgefallen, die bei genauester Analyse in kein bekanntes Krankheitsbild eingeordnet werden konnte und die, beim Versuch, ihr durch histologische Untersuchung näher zu kommen, nicht minder Neuheiten in ihrem Bau enthüllte. Nach langen und immer wiederholten vergeblichen Versuchen, ob sie dem Lichen planus, dem sie am ähnlichsten war, oder einer der bekannten Granulationsgeschwülste anzugliedern wäre, mußte ich sie zum Schluß als unbekannt ansehen. Ich habe sie mit Eifer die ganzen Jahre weiter verfolgt und habe dabei ein recht großes Beobachtungsmaterial angesammelt, für dessen Mitteilung ich hier den würdigsten Platz gefunden zu haben glaube.

Below, right: The classic histologic changes of lichen nitidus are easily recognized in Fig II of the Pinkus report. RW=lesional margin, P=Parakeratosis, Gr=Granuloma with giant cells, R=Round cell infiltration, Schw=sweat gland.

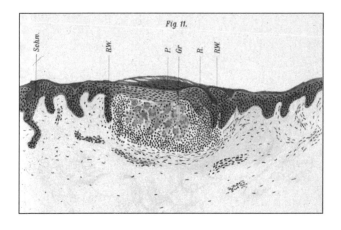

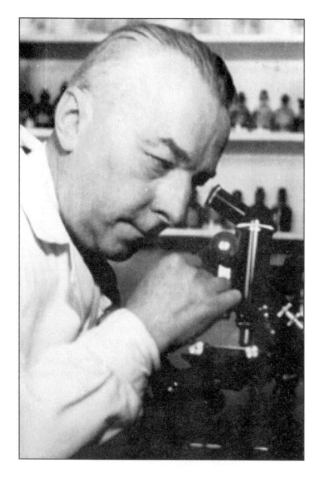

Franjo Kogoj (1894-1983)

Franjo Kogoj, Croatian dermatologist of note, received his M.D. in Prague and his dermatologic training in Zagreb, Brünn/Brno, Breslau, Strassburg, and Paris. He became chairman of the department of dermatology in Zagreb in 1932, successor to Pavel Savnik, and remained in that position until his retirement in 1965.

Kogoj was the author or co-author of more than 200 scientific papers, book chapters, and monographs, which he published in several different languages. Like most educated Europeans, particularly those from the smaller countries, he had mastered the art of slipping easily from one tongue into any of several others, a facility most North Americans find difficult to imagine.

Kogoj was particularly interested in the sexually transmitted diseases and published two textbooks on the subject that were well received. Allergic skin diseases also received his special attention. He is best remembered now for his description of the "spongiform pustule of Kogoj," noted below. It is the hallmark of the acrodermatitis continua of Hallopeau, a condition regarded now by most observers as a variant of pustular psoriasis. Similar pustules occur in Reiter's disease. Kogoj described this histopathologic feature in 1927 while studying in Strassburg with Lucien Pautrier, who was a skilled histopathologist in his own right.

Kogoj was a warm, friendly, cultured man, devoted to classical literature and classical music, especially Mozart.

Below, right: Figure "a" from the Kogoj's classic 1927 spongiform pustule report.

Kogoj F. Un cas de la maladie de Hallopeau. Acta Dermato-Venereol 1927/28;8:1-12

Kogoj's original description reads as follows:

"The most remarkable changes are found in the epithelium. Above the acanthosis just mentioned and beneath the stratum corneum two vesicles are noted containing numerous neutrophils that have migrated across the epithelium in great numbers. No eosinophils can be found in the pustule. The most interesting finding is in the larger pustule. The picture clearly shows that this pustule may be compared to a sponge, the peripheral parts of which possess openings that become enlarged toward the center, and the interior part of which is cavitated."

Kogoj characterized his finding as a "spongiform pustule" in later publications.

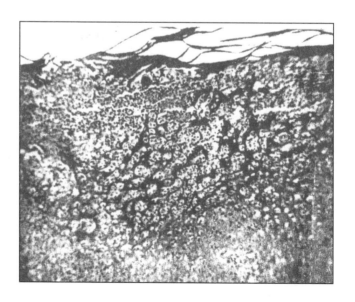

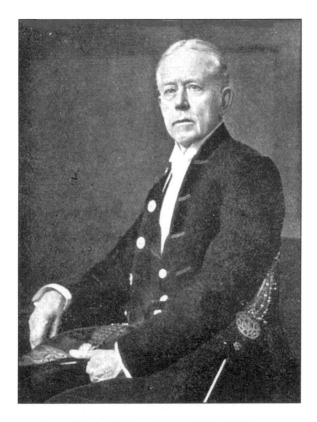

Ernest Graham-Little (1867-1950)

The most distinguished British dermatologist of his generation, Ernest Graham-Little received his training in London and Paris. In 1902 he succeeded Malcolm Morris as the chief of service St. Mary's in London, where he established himself as a diagnostician and therapist second to none. A compulsive attendant at medical meetings, he is reputed to have exhibited more cases at these gatherings than any other dermatologist in England.

Graham-Little's ability to write clear and elegant prose was also celebrated; it is particularly evident in his 1935 retrospect of dermatology in Great Britain, an invaluable historical resource that is a masterly repository of penetrating insights intermixed with personal reminiscences that catches both the spirit and the facts of his subject.

Graham-Little continued in his whirlwind round of dermatologic activities until circa 1930, when he redirected his life. Elected to Parliament in 1924, he now immersed himself in politics and all but abandoned dermatology. He abhorred the Socialistic tendencies of Britain at the time and became a fierce opponent of the National Health Service. A genial, kindly man with a good sense of humor in his circle of friends and medical colleagues, he was quite the opposite in political life. He died after a lingering illness in 1950 at the age of 83.

Below: Arthur Whitfield (1868-1947)

A graduate of King's College in London, Arthur Whitfield spent three years in the dermatology clinics in Vienna and Berlin. In 1896 he returned to England, where he served for some time as an assistant to Thomas Colcott Fox at Westminster Hospital. In 1906 he became Professor of Dermatology at his alma mater, which position he held until his retirement in 1927.

A member of the generation that succeeded England's "big five," Whitfield absorbed the clinical expertise that characterized the work of the older group and added to it an abiding interest in the basic sciences acquired in his years on the Continent. He was particularly fond of bacteriology and mycology, and it is for his work in the latter field that he is best remembered. In 1906 he published an influential report in which he demonstrated convincingly the causative role of fungi in tinea pedis. He followed it up with the introduction of the benzoic acid-salicylic acid ointment that is associated with his name. Cheap, effective, and long a standard topical treatment for tinea pedis and other forms of ringworm, Whitfield's ointment has now been superseded by more modern fungicides.

Whitfield, perpetually young in outlook and curious, was a vigorous and forthright contributor to discussions at meetings. He passed away in 1947 at the age of 79.

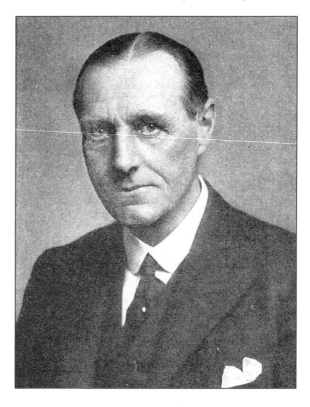

Henry W. Stelwagon, highly respected Philadelphia dermatologist and author, received his medical degree from the University of Pennsylvania and spent two years abroad in the skin clinics of Vienna and Berlin. He taught at his alma mater and at Jefferson Medical College, and assumed the chair of dermatology at the latter institution in 1904.

Successful in practice, scholarly, and as well read as any dermatologist of his day, Stelwagon wrote constantly, contributing chapters to encyclopedic medical works, original papers on clinical subjects, student manuals, and the like, and he translated the popular German atlas of Franz Mracek, adding to it a number of plates of his own. His fine 1902 textbook, "Diseases of the Skin." is noted below.

"[Stelwagon] was indeed a gentle man," his long time friend Milton Hartzell wrote, and he added that he had never heard Stelwagon say an unkind word to or about anyone. In the late afternoon of October 18, 1919, after the close of office hours, Stelwagon was found dead, seated in his office chair. The diagnosis was coronary occlusion.

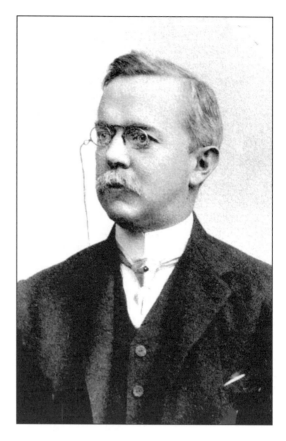

Henry W. Stelwagon (1855-1919)

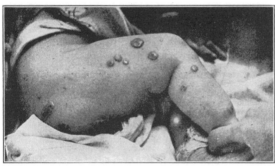

DERMATITIS MEDICAMENTOSA.   425

undergo epitheliomatous degeneration (referred to under psoriasis and epithelioma), and in a few instances death has finally resulted.

Belladonna—Atropin.—Not infrequent, especially in children ; scarlatinous type most usual ; patchy erythematous areas or flushings occasional. The eruptions are, as a rule, upon suspending the drug, of short duration. Exceptionally erythema and gangrene of scrotum have been observed. Itching is sometimes troublesome.

Bromin Compounds.[1]—Quite common. An acne-like papulopustular and pustular, about the regions of the face and shoulders and back most frequently ; although the lesions are usually discrete, several or more may tend to group and become in places confluent, forming a sluggish, conglomerate patch studded with pustular points, and bearing slight resemblance to a superficial carbuncle. The eruption may be in some instances more or less generally distributed.

FIG. 104.—Dermatitis medicamentosa in a young child, from the ingestion of *potassium bromid*; the lesions of a pustulopapillomatous character, and of somewhat general distribution, but most numerous and marked on the face and lower extremities (courtesy of Dr. G. T. Jackson).

Occasionally erythematous, vesicular, papular, urticarial, furuncular, and carbuncular eruptions are observed to follow its administration. Exceptionally an eruption somewhat similar to erythema nodosum is encountered. Bullous development is rarely observed.

[1] Crustaceous and papillomatous eruptions : Jackson (2 cases (1 child)), *Jour. Cutan. Dis.*, 1895, p. 462 ; Elliot (2 cases—infants), *Trans. Amer. Derm. Assoc. for 1895 ;* Panichi, *Giorn. ital.*, 1897, fasc. 5, p. 559—abs. in *Annales*, 1898, p. 395 ; Malherbe (vegetative and ulcerative), *La Presse médicale*, May 24, 1899, p. 243 ; Hallopeau et Trastour (suppurating plaques), *Annales*, 1900, p. 883 ; Feulard, " Bromisme Cutané," *ibid*, 1891, p. 531 ; Pini (Bromoderma nodosum fungoides), *Archiv*, vol. lii., 1900, p. 161, with 4 plates—3 histologic—and some literature references ; Colcott Fox, *Brit. Jour. Derm.*, 1892, p. 287 ; see also paper by Van Harlingen, *loc. cit.;* Hall (confluent pustular, child, with illustration), *Quarterly Med. Jour.*, Nov., 1902, p. 138 ; Myers, *Jour. Cutan. Dis.*, 1904, p. 231 (with illustration) ; Hallopeau and Vielliard (gangrenous), *Annales*, 1904, p. 442 ; Parkes Weber (granuloma-like or mycotic type case demonstration), *Brit. Jour. Derm.*, 1905, p. 63. Pasini, " Sur la pathogenie des eruptions bromiques (with review and bibliography), *Annales*, 1906, p. 1 (papulopustular, discrete, and confluent).

It is as the author of an outstanding and innovative dermatologic textbook that Stelwagon really shines. Henry Radcliffe Crocker's "Diseases of the skin" (1888), with its concentration on the written word and the intense and intimate personal involvement of the author with all of the problems discussed in his pages, stands as the last and finest of the nineteenth century's magisterial treatises in English. In sharp contrast, Henry Stelwagon's 1902 textbook of the same name, with its plethora of photographs, elaborate documentation, and visible effort at personal detachment, represents the new wave, the first great twentieth century textbook on the subject. All the new features are present in the typical page from the 5th edition of the work (1907), shown to the left. Stelwagon's text served as a model later for many successful American efforts – textbooks by Richard Sutton and by Oliver Ormsby, for example – until the middle of the twentieth century when the complexity and sheer volume of material available on skin diseases rendered textbook authorship by one or two individuals impractical.

John Templeton Bowen, another proper Bostonian and Harvard graduate, became in 1907 the first Edward Wigglesworth professor of dermatology at his alma mater. He learned his dermatology in three years of study abroad in the clinics of Vienna, Berlin, and Munich. Bowen was a shy retiring man who shunned the spotlight, found lecturing an unbearably stressful experience, and wrote and published only when he was convinced he had something important to say. On at least two occasions such was the case. In 1889 he published a pioneering study of the epitrichium (periderm), and in 1912 the account of the "precancerous dermatosis" noted below.

Histopathology was Bowen's forte, although he was also a fine clinician. He never married, and in later life became something of a recluse. He died in 1940 at the age of 83.

Below right: Figure 1 from Bowen's classic report: Lesion on the left buttock of his first patient. Below left: Figures 2 and 3. L.P. shows "proliferation of the rete, vacuolization and abnormal cornification of cells, dilatation of vessels of the corium with cell masses surrounding them." H. P. shows "peculiar 'clumping' of nuclei and kariokinesis."

It was no less than Jean Darier who suggested that the condition be called "Bowen's disease." Most workers in the field consider the entity to be a form of squamous cell carcinoma in situ.

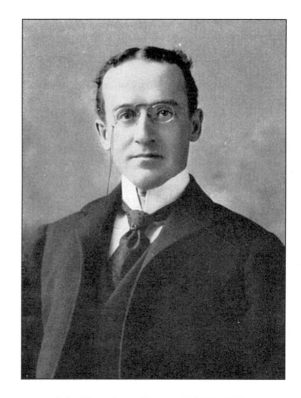

John Templeton Bowen (1857-1940)

Bowen JT. Precancerous dermatoses: a study of two cases of chronic atypical epithelial proliferation. J Cutan Dis 1912;30:241-255

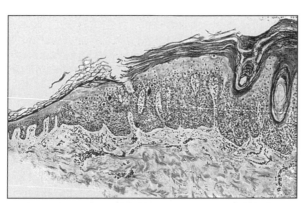

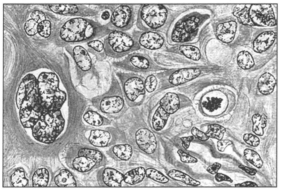

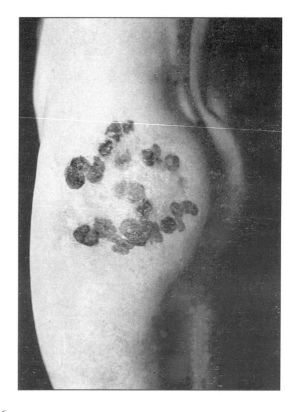

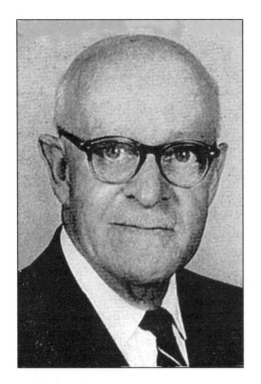

Udo J. Wile (1882-1965)

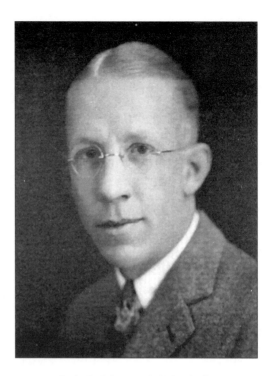

Lyle B. Kingery (1892-1972)

Below: Berkefeld filtering apparatus used by Wile and Kingery in their 1919 experiments.

Wile UJ, Kingery LB. Etiology of common warts. JAMA 1919;83:970-973

Wile UJ, Kingery LB. Etiology of molluscum contagiosum. J Cutan Dis 1919;37:431-44

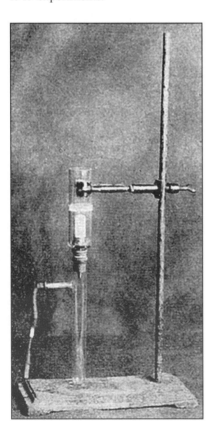

Johns Hopkins graduate and Unna trained, Udo Wile practiced and taught in New York City until 1910, when he became the chief of dermatology at the University of Michigan. Under his leadership the Michigan department rose to prominence on the international scene. Wile's interests lay largely in skin diseases of infectious origin., particularly syphilis. He was acknowledged everywhere as an authority on the latter disease second to none.

Wile's associate, Lyle B. Kingery, also did postgraduate work in Europe before completing residency training at Michigan. He later became chief of dermatology at the University of Oregon.

In 1919 Wile and Kingery collaborated in a series of experiments (referenced above) to determine whether common warts and the lesions of molluscum contagiosum might be caused by a filterable virus. They curetted tissue from clinically typical lesions, added normal saline, ground the material in a mortar and pestle, and rendered it bacteria-free by passing it through a Berkefeld filter. They inoculated themselves and volunteers with the filtrates and observed the appearance of clinically typical lesions at the sites of inoculation. Diagnoses were confirmed by biopsy – QED. The numerous reports in the older literature on bacterial causes for the two diseases were shown to be wrong.

We have it from reliable sources that the junior author of the Wile-Kingery experiments did the lion's share of the work, an arrangement not unheard of even now.

Kingery's son Frederick (Ted) is himself a prominent Oregonian dermatologist.

German born, William H. Goeckerman arrived in the United States with his parents when he was 10 months old. He grew up in Milwaukee and received his M.D. from the Wisconsin College of Physicians and Surgeons, and his dermatologic training with John Stokes at the Mayo Clinic. He remained at the Mayo Clinic for 15 years, during which time he made significant contributions to the study of lupus erythematosus, the psychic factors in dermatologic diseases, and the famous "Goeckerman treatment" for psoriasis, noted below.

In 1932 Goeckerman left the Mayo clinic and moved to Los Angeles, California, where he opened a private practice. He joined the faculty of the University of Southern California and resumed his clinical investigational work, including studies on the effects of estrogens on acne vulgaris.

Goeckerman was an introspective, well read, cultured man, with a love of the classics. Horace, Virgil, and Montaigne were among his favorites.. He died in 1954 at his home in Whittier, California after a long illness.

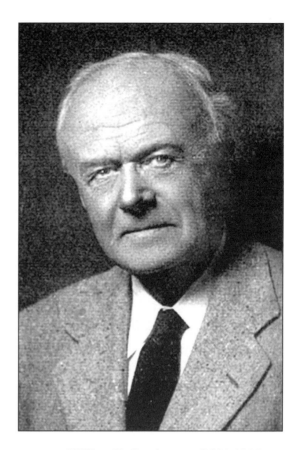

William H. Goeckerman (1884-1954)

Goeckerman WH. The treatment of psoriasis. Northwest Med 1925;24:229-231

Cited above is Goeckerman's classic 1925 paper on the tar plus ultraviolet light (UVL) anti-psoriatic treatment that bears his name. The report begins with a mini-review of the literature, a depressing litany of therapeutic failures from the past; it goes on to describe the new technique in considerable detail. Crude coal tar ointment was applied to the patches and left in place for 24 hours. Excess ointment was then removed with olive oil and the lesions exposed to UVL generated by a quartz lamp and delivered daily (later at longer intervals) in gradually increasing doses. Goeckerman's experience is described in the report as a "reasonably large series of cases," and he assured his readers that "it should be possible to remove all patches of psoriasis in from three to four weeks."

Despite the fact that the paper was published in a journal with a relatively limited circulation, the procedure caught on and soon became standard. It continues in widespread use today, and many thousands of psoriasis sufferers have benefited and continue to benefit from the discovery.

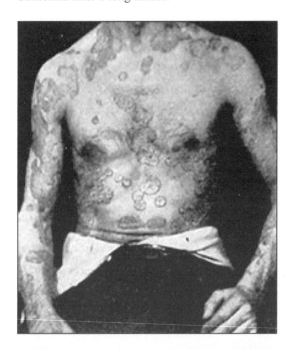

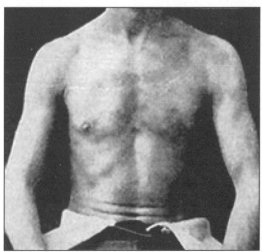

Left, top: Figure 1 from Goeckerman's classic paper. Case of psoriasis before treatment.
Left, bottom: Figure 2. Same case nineteen days after treatment. Dark patches are the result of residual pigmentation.

The quartz mercury vapor lamp was the most popular source of ultraviolet rays for the treatment of skin diseases in the first half of the twentieth century. The spectrum emitted was mainly UVB. Two types were common. The "Kromayer" type was water cooled; the lamp head enclosed in its casing was placed against the area to be treated, often with compression. Only a small area at a time could be treated. The Kromayer was usually used to treat lupus vulgaris (a la Finsen) or psoriatic plaques. More popular were the air cooled types, which could cover wide areas. These lamps were used to treat a long list of diseases – acne vulgaris, pityriasis rosea, psoriasis, alopecia areata, eczematous eruptions, ringworm – just about everything but sun burn. The development of the efficient longwave UVL emitters, used now with such success in the PUVA treatment of psoriasis, did not take place until the 1970s.

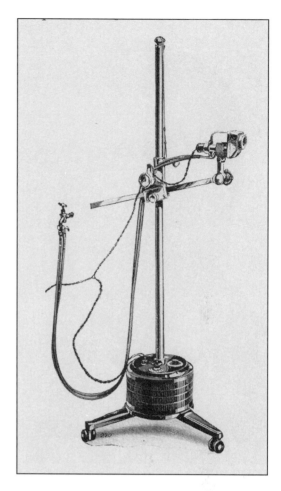

"Kromayer" type, water cooled quartz mercury vapor lamp.

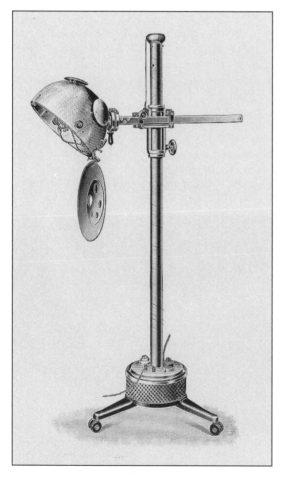

The Emesay-Hanovia quartz mercury vapor lamp. "Percy Hall" model.

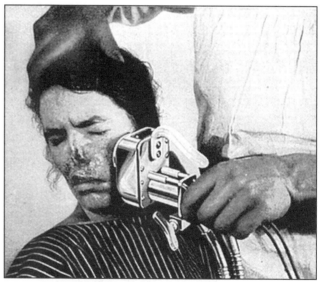

"Kromayer" lamp in the treatment of lupus vulgaris of the face. The area under treatment is being compressed.

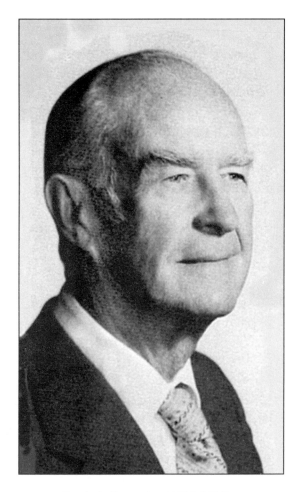

Louis A. Brunsting (1900-1980)

Louis A. Brunsting, American dermatologist known for his clinical acumen, received his M.D. from the University of Michigan and his dermatologic training at the Mayo Graduate School of Medicine. In 1930, he was appointed to the staff of the Mayo Clinic, and became Chief of the Section of Dermatology in 1953, which position he held until his retirement in 1962.

Situated in the Mayo Clinic, Brunsting was confronted regularly with the serious, the recalcitrant, and the unusual in the catalogue of skin diseases. He was adept at spotting common threads that linked odd cases together even when years separated their initial appearances before him. He is best remembered now for his classic 1930 account of pyoderma gangrenosum, noted below. He collected five cases over a three-year period, and his meticulous description of the lesions bears the unmistakable stamp of the born and practiced morphologist. His name is also associated with the uncommon localized form of bullous pemphigoid often called "Brunsting-Perry disease," which he described in collaboration with his associate Harold O. Perry. Brunsting published illuminating reports on scleroderma, lupus erythematosus, and porphyria, as well.

In 1965, Brunsting bid goodbye to the inclemencies of the north and moved to Tucson, Arizona where he engaged in private practice. He retired again in 1976, and settled finally in San Diego, California, where he died in 1980.

Brunsting LA, Goeckerman WH, O'Leary PA. Pyoderma (ecthyma) gangrenosum: clinical and experimental observations in five cases occurring in adults. Arch Dermatol Syphilol 1930;22:655-80

Right: Case 4 from Brunsting's classic paper cited above, a 32 year old farmer who had had recurrent cutaneous ulcers for five years and ulcerative colitis for nine:
"Lower portion of right leg during a later period of exacerbation. There are active ulcerations on the leg and a verrucous area on the dorsum of the foot."

Four of the five patients reported also had chronic ulcerative colitis; the fifth had chronic empyema. Staphylococci and hemolytic streptococci were found in the lesions "with consistent regularity."

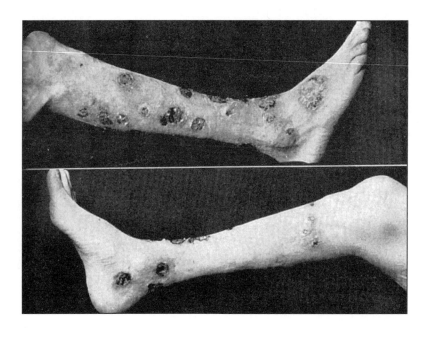

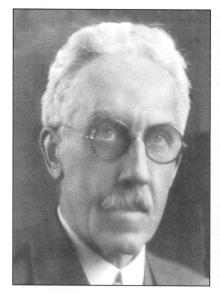
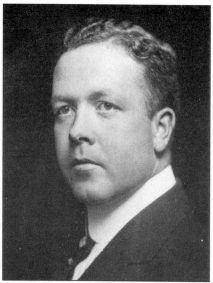
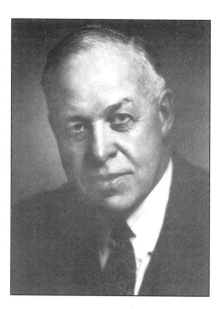

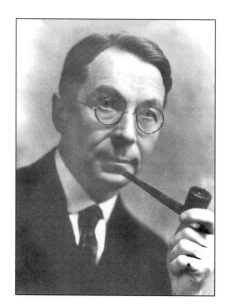

Above, left: George Gordon Campbell (1863-1932) of Montreal, QC. He taught at McGill University. Campbell wrote the first Canadian dermatologic textbook, "Common diseases of the skin" (1920).

Above, center: Omar Matthew Wilson (1880-1933) of Ottawa, Ontario. He worked and taught at the Ottawa Civic Hospital.

Above, right: Emerson James Trow Sr. (1886-1958) of Toronto, Ontario. He taught at the University of Toronto.

Left: William Reginald Jaffray (1887-1950) of Hamilton, Ontario. Formerly a bacteriologist, he practiced dermatology in Hamilton.

After attending a meeting of the Ontario Medical Association in London, Ontario, these four men, in the words of William Jaffray, "got together over a bottle of Old Parr and dreamed up the Society." The date was May 1924, and the "Society" is now the Canadian Dermatology Association (CDA), although it began its existence more modestly as the Interurban Dermatological Society. The organization met for the first time in Montreal in 1926. In addition to the four original "dreamers," the list of founders includes David King-Smith and Hamet A. Dixon of Toronto, and Philip Burnett and John Frederick Burgess of Montreal.

Old Parr is a deluxe Scotch whiskey, aged in oak for 12 years.

Emerson J. Trow received his dermatologic training at the Skin and Cancer Hospital in New York, but the majority of the others trained in England and had friends in the British Association of Dermatology and Syphilology. It seemed natural, therefore, for the fledgling organization to set up a working relationship with the British group, an arrangement soon completed, and for the next twenty years the Association was known as the British Association of Dermatology and Syphilology (Canadian Branch). By 1946 the specialty had grown strong enough in Canada to wish to stand on its own. The name was changed again – to the Canadian Dermatological Association - although the members were careful to maintain close ties with their British colleagues. The final change in the name to The Canadian Dermatology Association took place in 1987.

Since World War II, the CDA has met annually in dermatologic centers across the whole of the country and has been a significant force in raising the standards of the specialty in Canada to the present levels of unquestioned excellence. The organization now has 543 members, concerns itself with undergraduate and postgraduate teaching, publishes the Journal of Cutaneous Medicine and Surgery, and sponsors the Canadian Dermatology Foundation (CDF). The CDF has an endowment fund of more than two million dollars, which it disperses to underwrite dermatologic research in Canada.

131

Barney David Usher, the first Canadian dermatologist to have his name eponymically attached to a disease, was born in Montreal, received his M.D. from McGill University, and his dermatologic training under Pusey and Senear at the University of Illinois. In 1926, in collaboration with Francis Senear, Usher published the classic report on pemphigus erythematodes, commonly called the Senear-Usher syndrome. From the beginning, the condition has presented taxonomic difficulties. The consensus is that the condition is a special form of pemphigus foliaceus, with features in some instances of lupus erythematosus.

Back in Montreal, Usher entered into private practice, joined the faculty at McGill, and taught at the Montreal General Hospital for more than 50 years. He was one of the first in Canada to attempt investigative work along with his clinical practice. He published studies on sweating, on the pathogenesis of eczematous diseases, and on the incidence of emotional disturbances in various dermatoses.

While recovering from a heart attack circa 1975, Usher was urged by his friend Roy Forsey to write his autobiography. The result was a sober, terse, and remarkably frank document that summarizes the development of the specialty in eastern Canada, warts and all, and is essential reading for anyone researching the subject. Usher remained active to the end. He was preparing for his usual Friday morning teaching session when he suffered his final heart attack and died at the age of 79.

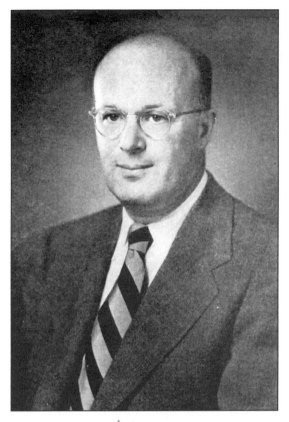

Barney Usher (1899- 1978)

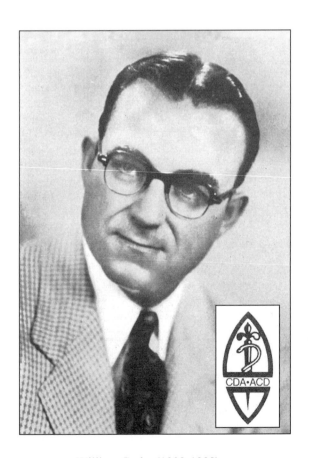

William Garbe (1908-1998)

William Garbe, well known Canadian dermatologist, received his M.D. from the University of Toronto, spent a year in dermatology in the New York Postgraduate Medical School, and two years (1934-36) in the private offices of Fred Wise and Marion Sulzberger. In collaboration with Sulberger he published the classic 1936 account of exudative discoid and lichenoid chronic dermatosis ("oid-oid disease"), often called Sulzberger-Garbe disease. The status of the condition as a disease *sui generis* has been challenged repeatedly, but more than 100 cases have been reported under the name.

Garbe returned to Toronto, opened a private practice, and became chief of the dermatology service at the Mount Sinai Hospital. He is well and justly remembered now for his superb work in setting up and securing funds for the Canadian Dermatology Foundation, the chief source of revenue available to underwrite Canadian dermatologic research. He pursued colleagues, patients, friends, accountants, lawyers, and bankers with the relentless zeal of the truly committed until he had amassed a sizeable sum. He was unanimously elected first president of the Foundation, a position he held for the first five years of its existence.

Garbe also organized a competition among art students to develop a logo for the Canadian Dermatological Association. The winning design, superimposed on Garbe's portait to the left, now adorns the CDA masthead.

132

Professor and chief of service at l'Hôpital St. Louis from 1928 until his retirement in 1951, Henri Gougerot was the best known French dermatologist of his generation. Early in his career he became interested in mycology and made a name for himself as an expert on sporotrichosis. The disease was first described in 1898 by the American physician Benjamin Schenck, but the full picture of sporotrichosis and the nature of its causative organism were worked out by Gougerot in association with the mycologist de Beurmann in a series of studies that culminated in a classic report published in 1912.

In 1914 WWI erupted and Gougerot accepted a commission in the French army, served throughout the conflict, and was awarded the Croix de Guerre. Back at St. Louis his interests expanded exponentially and his publications eventually covered nearly the whole field of dermatology. He was much admired as a teacher. His textbooks on dermatology and on syphilology, large well illustrated practical compendiums, were best sellers that remained in print for more than thirty years,

Gougerot's name is associated with the Gougerot-Carteaud syndrome (confluent and reticulate papillomatosis), the Gougerot-Houwer-Sjörgren's syndrome, the Gougerot-Ruiter syndrome, and the pigmented purpuric lichenoid dermatoses of Gougerot and Blum, all of which he described.

Distinguished and elegant, he was gentle, open, and affectionate towards the many who journeyed to Paris from all parts of the world to learn from him.

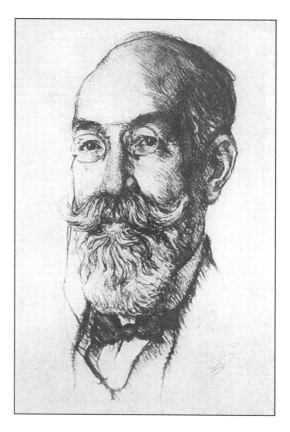

Henri Gougerot (1881-1955)

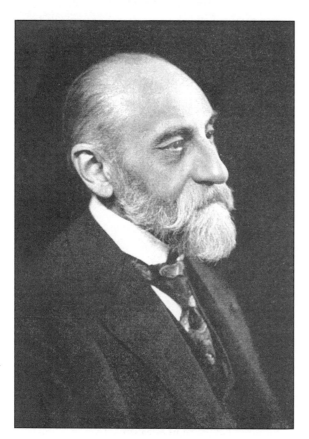

Edouard Jeanselme (1858-1935)

Edouard Jeanselme, prominent French dermatologist at l'Hôpital St. Louis in the early decades of the 20th century, was best known as an expert on tropical dermatology. A pupil of Hallopeau, he became interested in leprosy early in his career and was one of the first to establish the usefulness of nasal smears as a reliable diagnostic test for the disease.

In 1899, at the request of the French government, Jeanselme embarked on a two year tour of Indochina, parts of China, Siam, and the Dutch Indies (Indonesia) to catalogue the diseases of those areas, a task he carried out assiduously. Back in France he lectured and wrote extensively on his findings. His publications on the juxta-articular nodes of leprosy, the study of which he began in Indochina, are classic. He was also influential in the establishment of the Pavillion de Malte at St. Louis, a structure devoted to the study and treatment of leprosy.

Jeanselme was also one of the foremost experts on syphilis of his time. He headed up the major French societies in the battle against sexually transmitted diseases, and greatly expanded the hours and facilities devoted to the subject at St. Louis. He was passionately involved in every aspect of what was then called venereology - treatment, laboratory diagnostic techniques, prevention, legislation, and more. In 1931 he wrote a superb history of syphilis that can be a most rewarding place to look when historical research stalls.

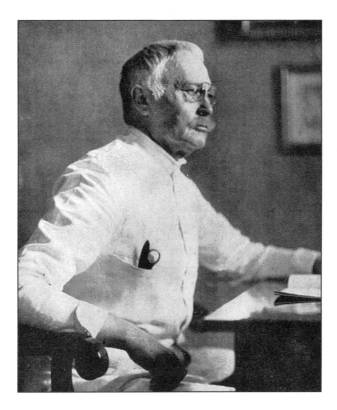

Carl Rasch (1861-1938)

A pupil of Besnier, Carl Rasch occupied the chair of dermatology at Copenhagen from 1906 to 1931. He was, in the words of Svend Lomholt, "the founder of scientific and systematic dermatology" in Denmark. Acknowledged everywhere as Denmark's finest morphologist, he was particularly interested in eczematous eruptions and was one of the first to validate the clinical synthesis that we call atopic dermatitis and he called "Besnier's prurigo" in honor of his teacher who had introduced the concept at the end of the 19th century.

Rasch wrote the first and for many years the only dermatologic textbook in the Danish language, and in 1899 he founded the Danish Society of Dermatology. He was also one of the founders of the Northern Dermatological Association.

A man of high literary culture who also loved art, Rasch had the largest collection of copper plate prints in Denmark. He willed the proceeds from the sale of his collection to the Dermatological Society to be used, among other things, as travel stipends for young Danish dermatologists.

Edvard Ehlers, much traveled Danish dermatologist who trained in Berlin, Breslau, Vienna, and Paris, practiced in Copenhagen and from 1911 to 1932 directed the special service of the Kommunehospitalet in that city.

Ehlers was best known in his own time for his work on leprosy. He initiated the first international congress on that disease (1897) and studied all aspects of it on the scene in Norway, Iceland, the Balkans, and the Caribbean. Intensely interested in syphilis as well, he published valuable studies on the history and epidemiology of the disease, worked tirelessly for the abolition of prostitution, and was active in the establishment of special Welander homes for the care of children suffering from "lues congenita."

Ehlers is remembered today largely for his 1901 description of the collagen disorder known as the Ehlers-Danlos syndrome, which has subsequently turned out to be far more complex than its describer ever imagined. He shares the credit for the initial characterization of the syndrome with the French dermatologist Henri Danlos (1855-1912), and that is not surprising. Ehlers was an ardent Francophile; he spoke the language perfectly, visited Paris often, and was as much at home in Parisian dermatologic circles as his own. The French were extremely grateful for the care he gave French prisoners of war during the murderous influenza epidemic of 1918.

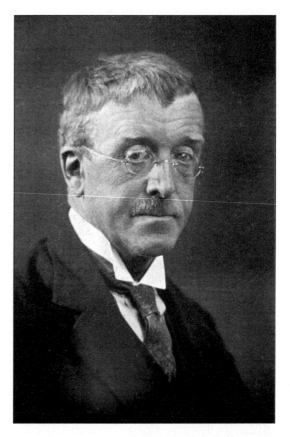

Edvard Ehlers (1862-1937)

Holger Haxthausen, Danish dermatologist and eminent clinical investigator, succeeded Carl Rasch as chairman of the department of dermatology in Copenhagen.

Early in his career Haxausen was interested in light and its effects on the skin. He published an influential monograph on the subject and improved and simplified the Finsen light treatment of lupus vulgaris by suggesting the introduction of the heat absorbing Jena-blau Uviol glass in the light path. He is best remembered now for his research on allergic contact dermatitis (ACD), which subject he took up in earnest at the age of 50. From 1942 through 1951 he published a series of remarkable studies that complemented and extended the work of other ACD investigators, notably Chase and Landsteiner, and were key works in the establishment of ACD as a form of delayed or cell mediated hypersensitivity. His ingenious reciprocal mini-graft transplantations in identical twins, one sensitized, the other not, did away with the widely held belief that ACD antibodies are fixed in the skin. Other studies identified and emphasized the importance of regional nodes, lymphocytes, and hapten binding in the pathogenesis of disease.

Haxthausen was something of a "loner" in scientific endeavors. His many experimental trials were "performed in 'splendid isolation,' as if he was shy," wrote a colleague who knew him well. "He never wore his heart on his sleeve," another noted. Be that as it may, his laboratory at the State Hospital in Copenhagen was a Mecca for dermatologists from everywhere, and the professor welcomed them all.

Haxthausen was also a talented musician, an athlete, and prominent promoter of physical fitness.

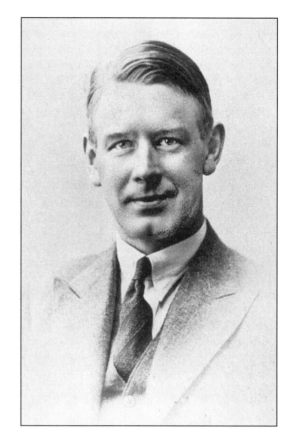

Holger Haxthausen (1892-1959)

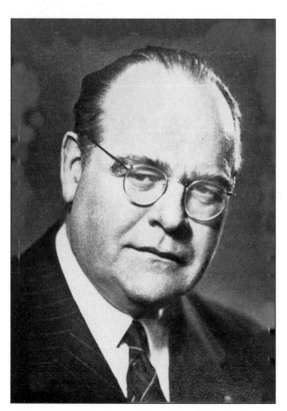

Svend Lomholt (1888-1949)

Svend Lomholt, dynamic, idealistic Danish dermatologist and expert on lupus vulgaris, received his M.D. from the University of Copenhagen and his dermatologic training under Ehlers and Rasch. In 1932, he became Senior Physician at the Finsen Institute and in 1939, Professor of Dermatology at his alma mater.

As a young man Lomholt engaged in basic research on the fate and distribution of mercury, bismuth, and gold in patiends treated for syphilis and other diseases. His best known achievements came later during his tenure at the Finsen Institute, where he completely redesigned the Finsen lamp, vastly improving its efficiency, introduced Dowling's calciferol treatment of lupus vularis at the Institute, and succeeded in bringing the pervasive Danish lupus problem under control once and for all.

Lomholt was also an outstanding teacher. By the time of his death in 1949, fully half the physicians in Copenhagen had first been introduced to the world of skin diseases by him. Multilingual and internationally known, he was the perfect choice to carry out the duties of Secretary General of the highly successful 1930 International Congress of Dermatology, held in Copenhagen that year.

A devoutly religious man, Lomholt published works on educational problems, marriage, sexual mores, and prostitution; he injected himself fearlessly into politics, vehemently protested perceived judicial injustices, and willingly engaged in the polemics generated by his deeply held convictions.

Niels Danbolt, leader of Norwegian dermatology for 35 years, received both his M.D. and his dermatologic training at the University of Oslo. From 1936 to 1971, he was Professor of Dermatology and Venereology at the Rikshospitalet in that city.

Danbolt was a dermatologist of the old school, who used his mastery of morphology to make his diagnoses, confirmed them with simple laboratory tests, and treated the patients with a formulary rooted firmly in the trials and errors of long experience. The best known of his contributions is his classic description of acrodermatitis enteropathica, noted below. He was also responsible for the popularization of the intradermal "Kveim test," developed in 1941 by his assistant Ansgar Kveim. The test is still useful to support a diagnosis of sarcoidosis, although preparation and administration of the antigen and interpretation of the results require special knowledge and care.

In his formal portrait, shown to the right, Danbolt looks a bit forbidding, but he was in fact a charming, friendly man. His lectures were sparkling, combining clinical expertise with edifying asides on ethics, humanity, and loyalty. He was constantly in demand as a speaker and toastmaster for banquets and special occasions and never failed to instruct and entertain.

Danbolt died in Oslo in 1984 at the age of 83. "Nobody," wrote one of his students, "who had the privilege of being his pupil, colleague, patient, or friend will ever forget him."

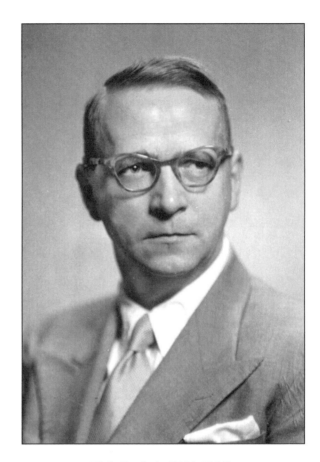

Niels Danbolt (1900-1984)

Danbolt N, Closs K. Akrodermatitis enteropathica. Acta Dermato-venerologica 1942;17:513-

Left: Acrodermatitis enteropathica, Figure 1 from Danbolt's classic report, cited above.

Written during the Nazi occupation of Norway in World War II, Danbolt's report is in German, as required by the censors. Danbolt's co-author, Karl Closs, was a biochemist. The summary in English, appended by the authors, read as follows:

"The disease is characterized by a pustular dermatitis which is frequently familial and appears in early childhood, often when the child is weaned. The dermatitis is preferentially located around the natural openings of the body and on the protruding parts of the head, trunk, and extremities (acrodermatitis). The terminal phalanges of the fingers are swollen up, and there is pustulous paronychia and atrophy of the nails. Furthermore, there is total alopecia, photophobia and blepharitis, and sometimes affections of the mucous membranes of the oral cavity (papillomata of the tongue). The course of the disease is rather chronic with recurring exacerbations, during which there is diarrhea with foamy, stinking pale yellowish-grey motions."

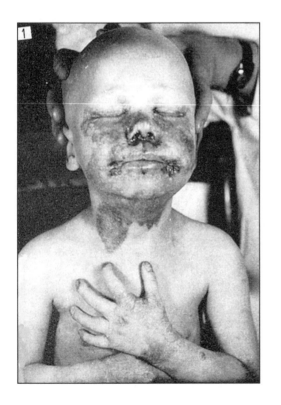

Louis Nékám, Vienna and Paris trained Professor of Dermatology in Budapest, was a multilingual world traveler who was well acquainted with virtually all the prominent dermatologists of the Western World. He was the ideal choice to preside over the International Congress of Dermatology held in Budapest in 1935, and he never had a tougher job. The Great Depression was at its height, Europe was once more seething with unrest, and World War II was imminent. Hitler had come to power, and Germany was putting the pressure on to prevent or limit meeting attendance by Jewish dermatologists and even such non-Jewish trouble makers as the fiercely independent Erich Hoffmann. All this Nékám handled with aplomb. The meeting went off with no major explosions, and the historical volume "De Dermatologia et Dermatologis," and the atlas "Corpus Iconum Morborum Cutaneorum" put together by Nékám to commemorate the event are dermatologic treasures.

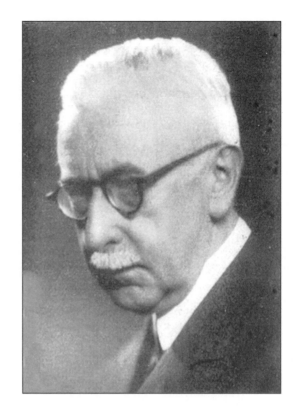

Louis Nékám (1868-1957)

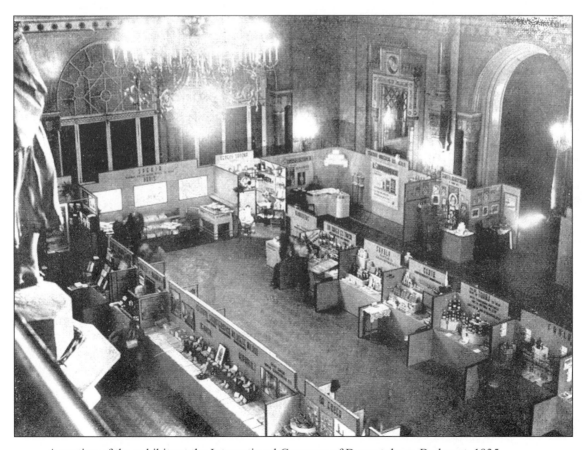

A portion of the exhibits at the International Congress of Dermatology, Budapest, 1935

137

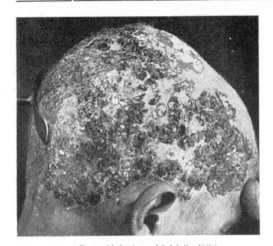

1224. Favus (Achorion schönleini). *Nékám.*

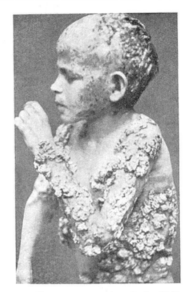

1225. Favus cutaneus et intestinalis. *Nobl.*

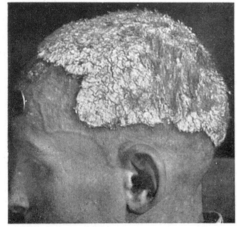

1226. Favus (Achorion schönleini). *Nékám.*

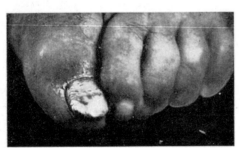

1227. Favus hallucis (Achorion quinckeanum). *Nékám.*

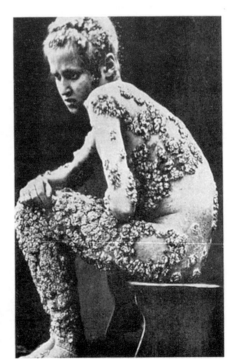

1228. Favus universalis. *Lailler.* (Phot. Méheux.)

A typical page from the magnificent atlas, "Corpus Iconum Morborum Cutaneorum," put together by the noted Hungarian dermatologist Louis Nékam in conjunction with the International Congress of Dermatology held in Budapest in 1935. It contains four thousand five hundred and fifty six photographs, all but two hundred or so in black and white, and is the most riveting, bizarre, and engrossing collection ever assembled of the evils the cutaneous flesh is heir to. It was the final fling for black and white photography in its losing battle with the newly developed Kodachrome, but demonstrates clearly the power of the monochromatic image to force the observer to concentrate profitably on patterns and configurations when freed from the distractions of color.

Mid-Twentieth Century Dermatologists, Events, and Discoveries

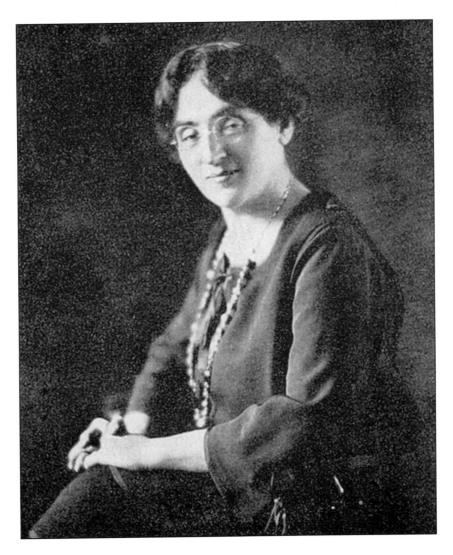

Rose Hirschler (1875-1940)

Rose Hirschler, America's first woman dermatologist and the first woman in the world to chair a dermatology department, was born in Butler, Indiana in 1875. Her route to the chairmanship was unusual. Certified as a masseuse by the Royal University of Uppsala in Sweden in 1896, she received her M.D. three years later at Women's Medical College (WMC) in Philadelphia, studied dermatology briefly in Berlin, and spent some time with Unna in Hamburg in 1904. From 1899 to 1919 Hirschler practiced general medicine intermixed with dermatology, and during this time worked closely with the noted Philadelphia dermatologist Jay Frank Schamberg. She was appointed professor and chair of the dermatology department at WMC in 1936, and held this position until her death, from chronic lymphatic leukemia, in 1940.

Hirschler's publications deal with skin cancer, hydroa puerorum, and the treatment of syphilis. She was particularly interested in X-Ray therapy; she organized the radiology department at WMC and was the first woman to recommend the rays for the treatment of acne vulgaris.

Hirschler was the second woman to be certified by the American Board of Dermatology, and the only woman among the founders of the American Academy of Dermatology. In recognition of her many accomplishments the Women's Dermatologic Society in 1992 created the Rose Hirschler award to be given annually to individuals who have enhanced the role of women in the specialty.

George Miller MacKee, long time Professor of Dermatology at Columbia University College of Physicians and Surgeons and Director of the New York Skin and Cancer Unit, received his dermatologic training under John A. Fordyce at New York University and Bellevue Hospital Medical College. Throughout his professional life he was a dermatologic perpetual motion machine. In addition to the endless duties associated with his teaching positions, he found time to author highly regarded textbooks on general and pediatric dermatology. MacKee was also regarded world wide as an authority on the therapeutic uses of X-ray. He devised dose measurement techniques that were standard for many years, and his textbook on X-ray and radium, coauthored in its later editions by Anthony Cipollaro, was constantly in the hands of residents until radiation all but disappeared from the dermatologic scene in the early 1960s.

As important as any of MacKee's contributions was his essential role in organizing and launching the Society for Investigative Dermatology (SID). He was the first president of that organization, and in his 1938 inaugural address not only laid out the goals of the Society with clarity, but also warned that a failure to keep up with the times through organizations such as the SID would result in gradual dismemberment of the specialty and its final demise.

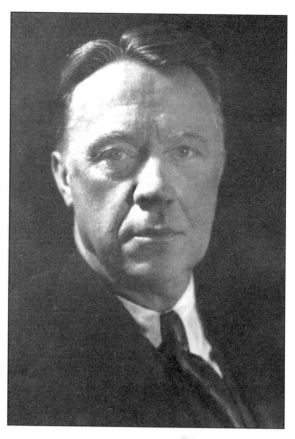

George Miller MacKee (1878-1955)

Founding Members of the Society for Investigative Dermatology:

S. William Becker	Samuel M. Peck
J. Gardner Hopkins	Sigmund Pollitzer
Joseph V. Klauder	John H. Stokes
George M. MacKee	Marion B. Sulzberger
Hamilton Montgomery	

IN WITNESS WHEREOF, the undersigned have made, subscribed and acknowledged this certificate this 14ᵗʰ day of April, 1937.

Marion B. Sulzberger

Gardner Hopkins

[signature]

John H. Stokes

J. [signature]

♦ 3799-60-6

The Society for Investigative Dermatology was born into a hostile world. Many of the dermatologic elite felt threatened by the young Turks who created the organization and presided at its delivery. For one thing, some of the most prominent among the new breed – Marion Sulzberger, William Becker, and Samuel Peck – chose to train in Europe, an educational decision the old guard considered both unnecessary and a demeaning relic of the past. Xenophobia, resentment of the new immigrants who were enthusiastic supporters of the venture, also played a significant role. But a sturdy cadre of unassailably American dermatologists with the highest of credentials put their reputations on the line in support, and the "SID" came into being at an organizational meeting held at the Hotel Dennis in Atlantic City, June 10, 1937. Less than a year later the Society could point with pride to a membership of 435. The names of the founding members and the signatures appended to the certificate of incorporation that put the legal finishing touches on the organization are shown to the left.

From the beginning, the officers and directors of the newly formed Society for Investigative Dermatology had seen the need for a journal that could concentrate in one place reports on the sort of research activities the Society hoped to encourage. Such a publication, they declared, "would demonstrate that dermatology has emerged from a state of purely morphologic, static, and dead description and classification," and "would further demonstrate that dermatology is a living, integral part of modern medicine …" As might be expected, many older dermatologists, clinicians of distinction, concluded that these and similar statements were pejorative and denigrated the activities to which they had devoted their lives. The hostility generated in this way between the clinically and research minded lasted for some time and surfaces occasionally even now.

The new publication was called the Journal of Investigative Dermatology (JID). In its early years, it was financially unstable; reports of the publishing committee chaired by M.B. Sulzberger are filled with fiscal forebodings. But all that changed, and who would deny that the JID has accomplished over the years exactly what its founders had in mind?

The title page of the first issue of the journal (1938) is shown to the right.

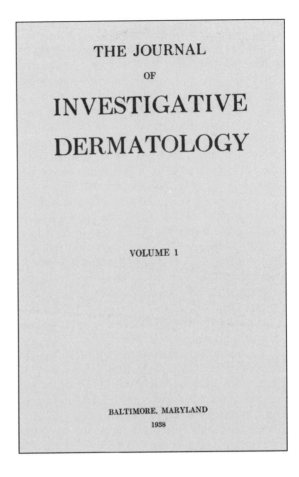

THE JOURNAL
OF
INVESTIGATIVE
DERMATOLOGY

VOLUME 1

BALTIMORE, MARYLAND
1938

Below: Naomi Kanof (1912-1988)

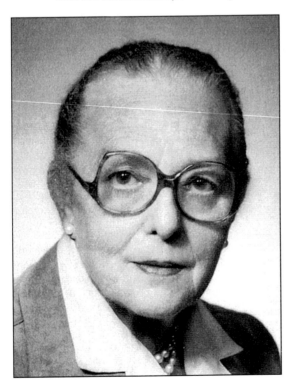

Daughter of Russian immigrant parents, Naomi Kanof was born in Brooklyn, NY. She received her dermatologic training at the Skin and Cancer Unit, now a part of New York University. In 1938 she opened an office in Washington DC and joined the faculty of Georgetown University, where she rose to the ranks to become Professor of Medicine in Dermatology. When her friend Marion B. Sulzberger withdrew as executive editor of the Journal of Investigative Dermatology in 1949, Kanof was chosen as his successor. She held that demanding position until her retirement in 1967, coping with great success with the ideological storms that erupted over the direction the journal was to take in those years of constant change.

Kanof also took on the onerous task of correcting, adding, and deleting terms for two editions of Stedman's Medical Dictionary, a job only a born and dedicated editor would accept or could handle.

Among the many honors she received in her lifetime for her contributions to the specialty was the Gold Medal, the most prestigious award of the American Academy of Dermatology. Kanof was the first woman to be so honored.

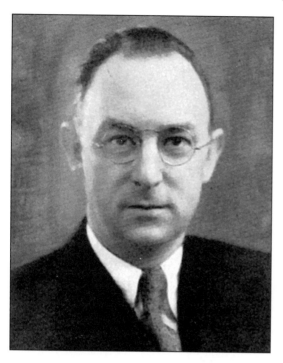

Earl D. Osborne (1895-1960)

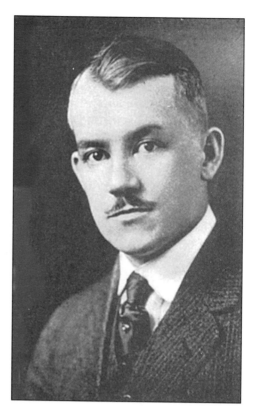

Harold N. Cole (1884 -1966)

June 10, 1937 found Earl Osborne of Buffalo, NY and Harold Cole of Cleveland, OH lunching at the Traymore Hotel in Atlantic City, NJ and engaged in an earnest conversation of considerable significance to dermatology. They were brainstorming, formulating plans for a national organization, an academy open to all qualified dermatologists and devoted to setting and maintaining the highest standards for the specialty through continuing education. Others had entertained similar ideas, but these two men had the inner drive, the know-how, and the connections essential to an organizational task of this pitch and moment. They agreed to present their ideas the next day at the dermatological section of the American Medical Association then in session, Paul O'Leary of Rochester, MN, presiding. O'Leary appointed a committee to consider the matter; the committee, the true founders of the organization (shown to the right), set up the first meeting, an organizational session that convened at the Statler hotel in Detroit, MI, January 14, 1938. Some 300 dermatologists attended. A program consisting of sections on syphilis, immunology, histopathology, and mycology was cobbled together and presented in St. Louis, MO later in the year. The American Academy of Dermatology was off and running.

The survival of the Academy during its infancy owes much to its first secretary, Earl Osborne. "The chief thing I remember during the first few years," wrote Joseph Hathaway of Honolulu, " was the tremendous time and energy that was given by Earl Osborne, and I do not think anyone contributed more to the success of the organization."

Founders of the Amerian Academy of Dermatology, 1938:
Harold N. Cole, M.D., Cleveland
Harry R. Foerster, M.D., Milwaukee
Howard Fox, M.D., New York
C. Guy Lane, M.D., Boston
George M. MacKee, M.D., New York
Howard Morrow, M.D., San Francisco
Paul O'Leary, M.D., Rochester
Oliver S. Ormsby, M.D., Chicago
Earl D. Osborne, M.D., Buffalo
William Allen Pusey, M.D., Chicago
Elmore B. Tauber, M.D., Cincinnati
H. J. Templeton, M.D., Oakland
Martin T. Van Studdiford, M.D., New Orleans
Fred S. Weidman, M.D., Philadelphia
Richard S. Weiss, M.D., St. Louis
Udo J. Wile, M.D., Ann Arbor
Fred Wise, M.D., New York

The first officers of the AAD were Howard Fox, President; Paul O'Leary, vice president; Earl Osborne, secretary; and Clyde Cummer, treasurer.

"The crucial idea of excising the cancerous site layer by layer and systematically examining the undersurface of each excised layer under the microscope by means of frozen sections is so logical that it is surprising that it was not thought of a century ago."

Those are the 1978 words of Frederick E. Mohs. He is a surgeon, not a dermatologist, but "the Mohs technique" has been embraced so enthusiastically by the surgically inclined among us for the treatment of certain types of skin cancer that it seems unnatural not to claim him as one of our own. A University of Wisconsin Medical School graduate, he served as a Bowman Cancer Research Fellow for three years and rose through the ranks to become Clinical Professor of Surgery at his alma mater.

In 1941, Mohs published a landmark paper in the Archives of Surgery describing a method he had developed in which cancerous tissue fixed in situ by the application of zinc chloride was excised a layer at a time and examined under the microscope. The process was repeated until no further evidence of the cancer could be found. In 1953, he discovered that the process could be speeded up by substituting frozen sections for zinc chloride fixation, and the latter was abandoned.

Immensely successful in practice, Mohs has attracted and trained many in the art of microscopically controlled surgery, and the procedure has long since secured a permanent place in anti-cancer therapy. Indeed, no cancer treatment center today can afford to be without services of a "Mohs surgeon," and over the years large numbers of skin cancer patients dismissed as hopelessly inoperable have been rescued by the application of the Wisconsin surgeon's ingenious approach.

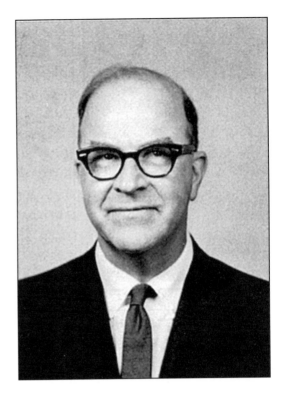

Frederic E. Mohs

Mohs FE. Chemosurgery: a microscopically controlled method of cancer excision. Arch Surg 1941;42:279-95

Below: Figure 1 from the Mohs landmark paper referenced above. In this example four excisions were required to reach a completely cancer-free zone.

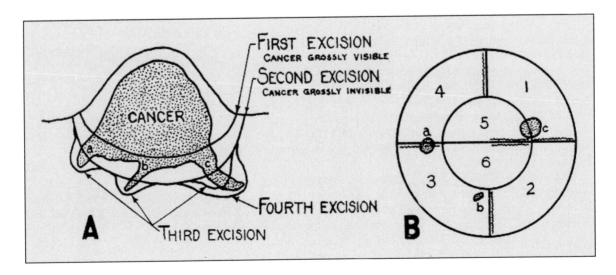

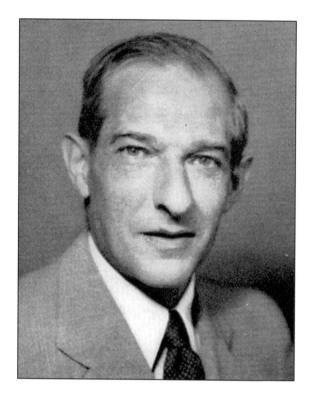

Stephen Rothman (1894-1963)

Rothman S, Rubin J. Sunburn and para-aminobenzoic acid. J Invest Dermatol 1942;5:445-57.

Rothman and Rubin were the first to recognize and demonstrate the effectiveness of PABA as a sunscreen. Their classic paper, referenced above, appeared in 1942. They showed that the substance absorbed the "sunburn rays," ultraviolet circa 300 mμ:. "By incorporating 10 to 15% para-aminobenzoic acid into ointment bases," they stated, "an extremely effective preparation against sunburn was obtained." However, it was not until the 1963 in depth study of topical agents that prevent sunburn by Madhukar Pathak, Thomas Fitzpatrick, and Edgar Frenk, showing the superiority of PABA, that the study and marketing of sunscreens really took off. The fair skinned among us have benefited greatly ever since.

Right: Figure from the 1942 report of Rothman and Rubin. The caption reads: Molar extinction coefficients of p-aminobenzoic acid and acetyl-p-aminobenzoic acid.

A native of Budapest, trained in both physiology and dermatology, Stephen Rothman held professorial positions in Hungary and Germany before emigrating to the United States in 1938. He joined the faculty of the University of Chicago and became the Chair of the Section of Dermatology at that institution in 1942, serving with great distinction until his retirement in 1959. His reputation as an authority on dermatologic research was unexcelled. Among his best known contributions are his investigations on sun screens, the iron pigment of red hair, the pharmaco-dynamics of axon reflex sweating, the biochemistry and pathophysiology of the lipid-aqueous surface film of human skin , and the endocrine control of sebaceous glands. His encyclopedic knowledge of the world basic research literature on cutaneous matters amazed his colleagues and students and fitted him admirably to pull it all together in his 1954 masterpiece, "Physiology and biochemistry of the skin," a book treasured and in active use in every dermatologic center at the time.

Rothman also enjoyed a reputation as a teacher of the first rank. He did not reside exclusively in the ivory tower, and therein lay the secret of his success. He was a fine clinician with experience on the firing line of practice and was able to combine those skills with his basic knowledge of the way the skin reacts to provide the sort illuminating insights that have always delighted students.

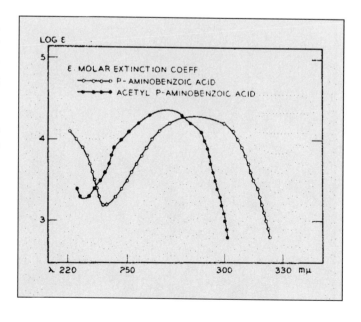

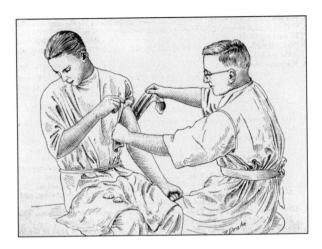

One of a series of line drawings in "Modern Clinical Syphilology" illustrating simple clinical techniques. The patients depicted are non-descript, but the star is easily identified.

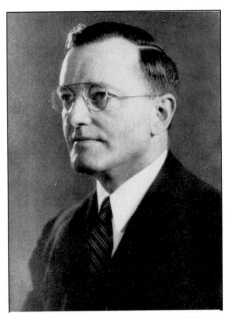

John Hinchman Stokes (1885-1961)

After training with Udo Wile at Michigan and William Allen Pusey in Chicago, John Hinchman Stokes (above, right) organized the Section on Dermatology at the Mayo Clinic (1916), and in 1924 took over the Chair of Dermatology and Syphilology at the University of Pennsylvania, which post he occupied with great distinction until his retirement in 1945.

Stokes was an eloquent lecturer, a master clinician, and a prolific writer with a keen ear for the well turned phrase. Like many of the renowned physicians of that era he was a martinet on the job and abundantly supplied with amour propre. His finest work was "Modern Clinical Syphilology," particularly the massive third edition (1945), which the residents at Penn affectionately called the "green monster." Joseph Earle Moore, a syphilologist of equal fame, pronounced it "the best text of its kind in any language."

Below: Stokes and his associates and residents, 1935. Sitting, L to R: Herman Beerman, Vaughn Garner, Stokes, Donald Pillsbury, Allen King. Standing: Carmen Thomas, Lamar Callaway, Norman Ingraham, Thomas Sternberg, Bertram Shaffer, Leonard Anderson, George Fonde.

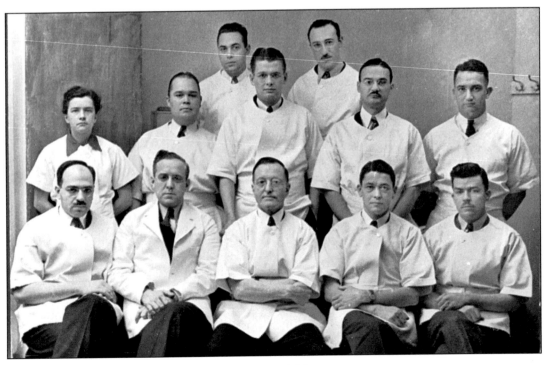

146

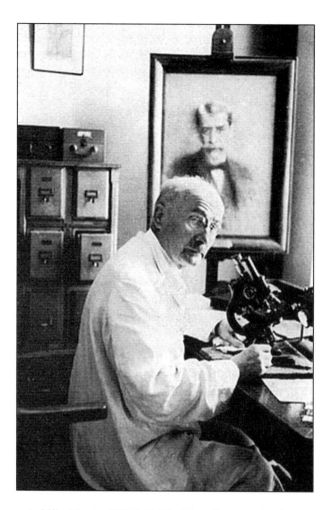

Achille Civatte (1877-1956). Note the portrait of Civatte's mentor, Jean Darier, on the easel behind the desk.

Achille Civatte, distinguished French dermatologist and favorite pupil of Louis Brocq at l'Hôpital St. Louis, also studied in the skin clinics of England, Germany, and Austria. He was associated with Jean Darier early in his career and remained at St. Louis throughout his professional life.

Ever the scholar, Civatte worked quietly and patiently to master all aspects of dermatology. He was the author of the valuable chapter on the physiology of the skin in the mid-twentieth century Bible of French dermatology, the "Nouvelle pratique dermatologique," and he demonstrated his clinical acumen in his classic description of the distinctive photosensitity reaction known ever since as "the poikiloderma of Civatte."

Dermatopathology was Civatte's first love, a passion that originated no doubt in his early association with Darier, who was also a past master of that art. Recognized later as an expert in his own right, Civatte and the huge collection of microscope slides over which he presided (Musée d'Histologie) attracted students from all over the world. His name continues to be associated with the colloid bodies (Civatte bodies) commonly observed in lichenoid reactions of the skin, particularly lichen planus, and his research on the histopathology of the bullous diseases was of great importance. Working under difficult circumstances in Nazi-occupied Paris, he published the 1943 classic report, noted below, in which he identified acantholysis (loss of cohesion between keratinocytes) as the hallmark of true pemphigus in its various presentations, and for the first time separated pemphigus from all the other bullous diseases on grounds other than clinical.

Civatte the man was reserved and somewhat austere in aspect, but a sincere and loyal friend to those who got to know him. He was a lover and connoisseur of literature, painting, and classical music.

Diagnostic histopathologique de la dermatite polymorphe douloureuse ou maladie de Duhring-Brocq. Ann Dermatol Syph 1943;3:1-17

Right: Figure 8 from the classic Civatte report on bullous diseases cited above.

"Pemphigus vegetans. Floor of a bulla at the edge of a vegetation: Malpighian cells at the cleavage line. Their connecting filaments have completely disappeared (total acantholysis). The cells have become detached and exist now as opaque bodies that are somewhat reminiscent of the "grains" of the dyskeratoses. They accumulate to form a sort of epidermal sediment or are suspended in the purulent melieu that fills the lower portion of the bulla. These purulent accumulations are made up almost entirely of polynuclear neutrophils. – No eosinophils in this case."

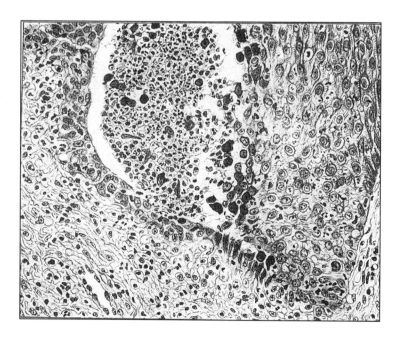

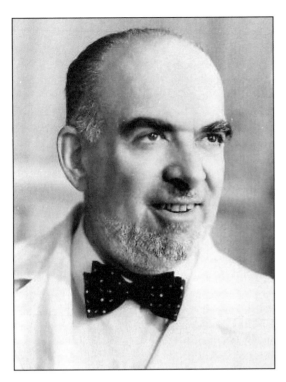

Robert Degos (1904-1987)

Degos R, Delort J, Tricot R. Dermatite papulo-squameuse atrophiante. Bull Soc Fr Dermatol Syph 1942;49:148-50, 281

In 1942, Degos presented before the Société Française de Dermatologie a case he believed to represent something new. He brought along a newly minted wax moulage to demonstrate the patient's lesions. His classic report on the case is cited above.

The patient was a 49-year old plumber who had suffered repeated outbreaks of a skin eruption for several months. The lesions, which were mostly on the trunk, began as pale pink papules that soon became umbilicated. Central areas were white, depressed, and covered by non-adherent scale. Lesional biopsies examined by Achille Civatte reinforced the contention that the disease process was something new. "The contrast between the marked epidermal lesions," he wrote, "and the absence of infiltrate in the dermis, with vascular changes leading up to thrombosis, make these sections unique." Seven months after the onset of the eruption the patient experienced an acute attack of abdominal pain. A laparotomy was performed, and numerous small yellowish spots were observed on the small bowel, but no perforation. The patient died six days later.

By 1979, Degos was able to point to more than 70 cases in the literature. Involvement of the central nervous system and numerous viscera had been added to the disease catalogue. The cause remains unknown, and treatment is ineffective.

Robert Degos, the most prominent figure in French dermatology following WWII, studied dermatology with Albert Touraine and Gaston Milian, and joined Gougerot's department at l'Hôpital St. Louis. He took care of the service of Arnault Tzanck, pro temp, while the latter, who was Jewish, spent the war years in exile in Chile. In 1951, Degos succeeded Gougerot as a department head..

It is as a superlative clinician that Degos is best remembered. A student, Stéphane Belaïch, recalled fondly his performances on Friday morning rounds. "It was then that he showed his qualities as a brilliant clinician and made each session a truly masterly lesson. We all remember his dazzling, intelligent, almost mischievous eyes when he encountered a difficult diagnostic problem and found a solution."

Degos' publications number more than 1,000 and include an extremely popular "Précis de dermatologie" that passed through eight editions. With Civatte and Belaïch he also published an encyclopedic loose-leaf work, updated yearly, that exerted great influence both in France and in the Latin countries that look to Paris for dermatologic authority.

Degos' name is associated with malignant atrophic papulosis, the frequently fatal skin-bowel syndrome noted below, which he first described in 1942. In 1954, independently of G.B. Dowling, Degos also described the inherited pigmentary disturbance commonly called Dowling-Degos disease (reticular pigmented anomaly of the flexures).

Charming, witty, and articulate, Degos had an instinct for the ironic and was willing and able to make his points forcefully in the rough and tumble of clinical debate.

Below: Figure from the classic Degos report on malignant atrophic papulosis, showing lesions on the patient's chest. It is a wax moulage.

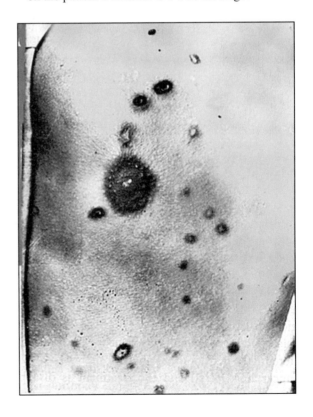

ERICH URBACH AND NECROBIOSIS LIPOIDICA DIABETICORUM

A native of Prague, Erich Urbach received his medical and dermatologic training at the University of Vienna, joined the faculty of his alma mater, and rose to the rank of associate professor. He served as a lieutenant in the Austrian army in World War I and was twice decorated for valor. But Urbach was Jewish and past patriotic services carried no weight with the Nazis when they took over Austria. In 1938, Urbach emigrated to the United States, where under the sponsorship of John Stokes he became associated with the University of Pennsylvania. He was a vigorous teacher and a skilled and inventive clinician whose bottomless bag of therapeutic tricks continually impressed the resident staff.

Already well-known in Europe for his numerous publications, including the classic descriptions of necrobiosis lipoidica (noted below) and lipoid proteinosis, he nevertheless insisted on taking the American Board of Dermatology examination. He passed successfully, but the stress associated with the experience cost him his life. He died of a massive coronary attack shortly after taking the exam.

Urbach's son Frederick, who emigrated with his father from Austria, is also a well-known dermatologist, whose work on photobiology and global warming is of considerable importance. He went on to become chairman of the department of dermatology at Temple University.

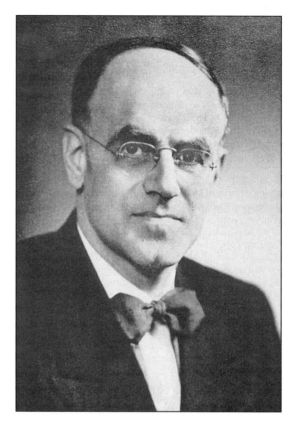

Erich Urbach (1895-1946)

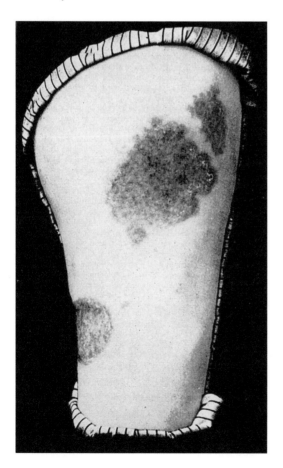

Urbach E. Eine neue diabetische Stoffwechseldermatose: Nekrobiosis lipoidica diabeticorum. Arch f Dermatol Syph 1932;166:273-85

Left: Necrobiosis lipoidica diabeticorum, figure from Erich Urbach's classic paper, referenced above. The original is in color. The clinical and histopathologic characteristics of the "new" disease were laid out with such precision in this report that it became, even for beginners, a diagnosis easily made.

Urbach had a life-long interest in the skin diseases associated with metabolic and nutritional problems. He published several books on the subject, the last of which, "Skin diseases, nutrition, and metabolism," appeared just before his untimely death (1946). Allergic diseases were also of particular interest to him, and works on hayfever, asthma, and allergic skin diseases are also well represented in his bibliography.

Oscar Gans received his dermatologic training from Paul Gerson Unna at the Dermatologikum in Hamburg. In his early years he worked at the university clinic in Heidelberg, where he engaged among other things in research on cutaneous respiration and pH, mineral residues in skin ash, and sulfur assimilation, but his real interest lay in cutaneous histopathology. With the publication of his remarkable textbook on the subject (described below), he was called in 1930 to take over the chair at Frankfurt. But Gans was Jewish, and despite the fact that he had fought for his country in World War I and was a fervent German patriot, he was removed from his post by the Nazis in 1933 and replaced by a nonentity. He emigrated to India, where he spent the war years doing research on leprosy.

Gans was one of the few Jewish dermatologists to return to Germany after the war. He resumed his duties at Frankfurt in 1949 and was, with his colleague Albert Marchionini, a figure of great importance in rebuilding German dermatology during the post war years.

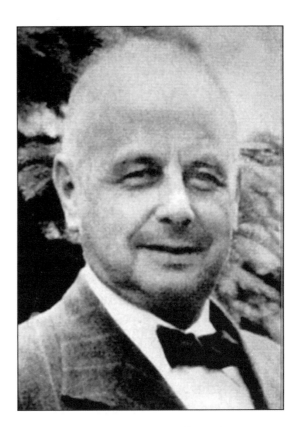

Oscar Gans (1888-1983)

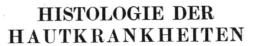

The years of study with Unna prepared Gans admirably for his later role as the Mr. Histopathology of the European dermatologic world. During this period he internalized completely the Hamburg master's famous dictum, "Evaluate the histological manifestation with a clinically trained eye, and the clinical manifestation with an eye trained at the microscope." Intensive research along these lines culminated in the master work, "Histologie der Hautkrankheiten" (1925-1928), the title page of which is shown to the left. This work, with its penetrating insights and beautiful illustrations, became the Bible of cutaneous histopathology in Europe and was influential in North America as well.

Otto Braun-Falco, who knew Gans well, described him as "a personality marked by a pleasant simplicity in speech and movement, by friendliness and kindness, an exquisite knowledge of our field, and a deep and thorough education, with a tendency toward humorous statements and Rhenish Gemütlichkeit, especially during the occasional late meeting over apple wine." Braun-Falco also remembered Gans for "his willingness to help and the complete absence of any form of vanity or self-aggrandizement."

Leo Ritter von Zumbusch trained with Kaposi and Riehl in Vienna. He took over the chair in dermatology in Munich in 1915 and over the next three decades transformed his clinic into one of the finest dermatologic centers in Europe. His name is still connected with his 1907 description of pustular psoriasis, and in 1925 he coauthored (with Gustav Riehl) one of our favorite books, a fine atlas of diseases of the skin featuring color photographs taken from life, not from wax moulages, images that are really superb despite the limitations of color photographic processes as they existed at the time.

In recognition of his outstanding contributions to the University of Munich, von Zumbusch was elected rector of the school. Munich in those days was Hitler's main base of operations. Von Zumbusch knew him, and after reading "Mein Kampf" concluded that the Führer was a lunatic. He said so, and got on badly after that. Sarcastic replies to arrogant Nazi petty Beamters who attempted to tell him how to run the university's business resulted in his removal as rector in 1933. He hung on as chief of dermatology until replaced in 1935, and during that time resisted Nazi interference in departmental affairs in any way he could, short of losing a great deal more than his job. He died in 1940, shortly after the beginning of World War II.

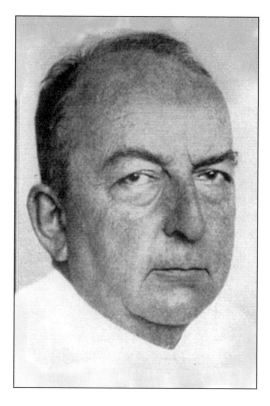

Leo von Zumbusch (1874-1940)

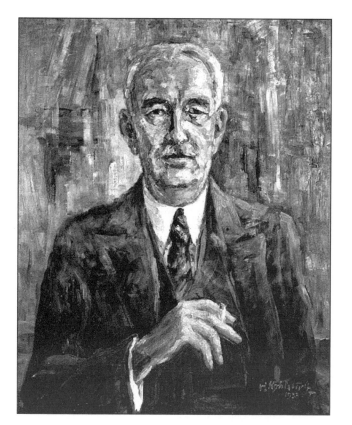

Heinrich Gottron (1890-1974)

Heinrich Gottron was the most charismatic dermatologic figure in post-World War II Germany, and perhaps also Europe's most talented morphologist. His clinic at Tübingen became the Mecca for the young and ambitious, many of whom have themselves gone on to positions of significance and prestige. Gottron's name is associated with papillomatosis cutis carcinoides, erythrokeratodermia congenitalis, acrogeria, scleromyxedema, all of which he described, and of course with "Gottron's papules," the distinctive violaceous lesions over the knuckle prominences that have enabled clinicians everywhere to make a presumptive diagnosis of dermatomyositis at the bedside.

During his lifetime Gottron received a great many of the medical honors his homeland has to offer, but to some in Germany and many in other countries, his Nazi-tainted past detracts from his reputation and diminishes his appeal.

Alfred Marchionini, prominent German dermatologist whose home base prior to World War II was Freiburg, found his career permanently on hold when he would have no truck with the Nazi party, and it was discovered that his wife's grandmother was Jewish. He emigrated to Turkey in 1938, where he took over the chair in the dermatology department in Ankara. He spent the war years in research on diseases common in his new location. After the war he was able to return to Germany with a clear conscience and his scientific reputation intact, which placed him in perfect position to lead in the daunting task of restoring respectability to German dermatology and starting it out on the road to parity with the rest of the Western World.

After a brief stay in Hamburg, Marchionini took over the chair in Munich (1950). Under his leadership Munich became a teaching and research center second to none in Germany, turning out a remarkable number of students destined to become heads of departments in dermatologic centers all over Deutschland.

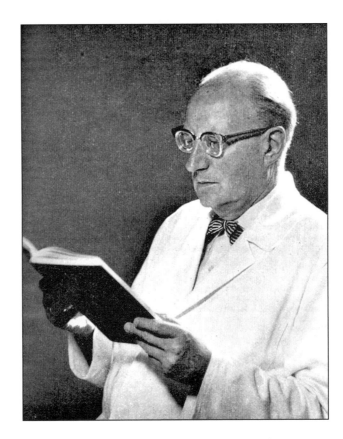

Alfred Marchionini (1899-1965)

Title page of the first issue of Marchionini's new journal, *Der Hautarzt*

Already well known in his Freiburg years for his concept of the "acid mantle" protective layer of human skin (1929), Marchionini also concerned himself in earlier years with dermatologic ethnology and the influence of climate on skin diseases. On his return to Germany he was responsible for the editing and publication of the numerous supplementary volumes of the exquisitely detailed "Jadassohn Handbuch," long the cornerstone of Teutonic dermatology. He also saw the need for a new journal designed to call to the attention of German-speaking dermatologists the many practical and scientific advances then being made worldwide, particularly in North America. His creation made its debut in 1950 as *Der Hautarzt* (The Skin Physician), and it soon established itself as the most important dermatologic journal in the German language.

Marchionini was a warm man with a keen sense of humor. He encouraged his students to travel, observe, and put to use the new things learned, as he himself had done. He was a key figure in the revival of the true scientific spirit that had all but disappeared during the disastrous years of the Third Reich.

Otto Braun-Falco, outstanding, widely acclaimed figure in the post-World War II rejuvenation of German dermatology, received his M.D. from the Johannes Gutenberg University in Mainz and his dermatologic training under Egon Keining in the same city. In 1967 he became professor and chairman of the department of dermatology at Ludwig Maximillian University in Munich. Braun-Falco acknowledges the salutary influence on his career, and on that entire generation of young German dermatologists, exerted by Oskar Gans, who had returned from wartime exile to take over as chief of the university skin clinic at nearby Frankfurt/Main.

Scarcely any area of dermatology has escaped the notice of Braun-Falco. His research activities include the investigation of the structure and function of normal and diseased skin using histochemical and electron microscope modalities. Psoriasis, skin allergies, and disturbances of hair growth received his attention, along with cutaneous lymphomata and malignant melanoma. He was deeply involved in the development of dermatoscopy for the evaluation of pigmented skin lesions and was among the first in Europe to put the laser to use in the treatment of a variety of cutaneous disturbances. He has had an abiding interest in all aspects of the AIDS epidemic, including the early detection of the disease by dermatologic observation. His textbook of dermatology, noted below, is the most popular and widely read dermatologic work in the German language.

Hiking, modern art, and botany rank high among Braun-Falco's non-medical interests.

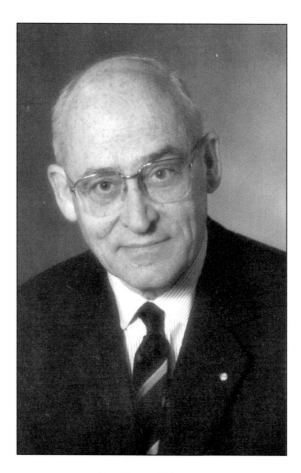

Otto Braun-Falco

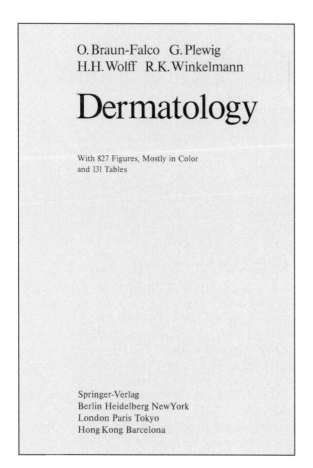

O. Braun-Falco   G. Plewig
H. H. Wolff   R. K. Winkelmann

Dermatology

With 827 Figures, Mostly in Color
and 131 Tables

Springer-Verlag
Berlin Heidelberg New York
London Paris Tokyo
Hong Kong Barcelona

Left: Title page of the 1991 English-language edition of the popular textbook of Braun-Falco and colleagues.

The first two editions in German (1960 and 1969) were written by Keining and Braun--Falco. Follwing the death of Keining (1971), Braun-Falco, with his assistants of Gerd Plewig and Helmut Wolff, thoroughly revised the text. The secret of the popularity of the work lay in the ability of the authors to introduce the newer research-based concepts of pathogenesis in palatable form and combine them with succinct disease descriptions and a clear exposition of both classic and modern methods of topical and systemic treatment. The value of the text was further enhanced by the inclusion of more than 800 color photographs. The English version of 1991 followed the same general pattern.

The expansion of the specialty in recent times to include many surgical procedures designed to improve appearance rather than treat disease, and the addition to dermatology of concerns that were once the province of cosmetology has placed new burdens on authors and editors of textbooks. Attempts to adjust to these new realities are evident in the most recent Braun-Falco works. Prospective authors may wish to examine his approach.

Klaus Wolff, key figure in the revival of Austrian dermatology in the aftermath of World War II, received his M.D. from the University of Vienna, and his dermatologic training at the same institution. He did postgraduate work in the United States at the National Institutes of Health and at the Mayo Clinic. He returned to Vienna in 1966, rejoined the faculty of the university, and in 1981 became chairman of the department of dermatology.

Equally interested in clinical and investigational dermatology, he has made a great many valuable contributions to both. His research activities include investigations on the cellular chemistry of the Langerhans cell, melanosome kinetics, insights into the concept of the skin as an immune organ, and antigen mapping in bullous diseases. An important example of the latter – the ultrastructural location of pemphigus autoantibodies - is noted below.

On the clinical side, Wolff was the first to treat pemphigus successfully with azathioprine. In his department, he put together the most sophisticated European center of its time for the retinoid-PUVA photochemotherapy of psoriasis. Melanoma research also claimed his attention, and he played an important role in the development of epiluminescence microscopy (dermatoscopy) for the evaluation of pigmented skin lesions.

Wolff is an energetic man of purpose who commits himself wholeheartedly to any task he undertakes. He is a devotee of modern and contemporary art and literature.

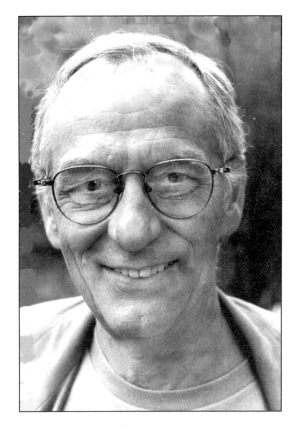

Klaus Wolff

Wolff K, Schreiner E. Ultrastructural localization of pemphigus autoantibodies within the epidermis. Nature 1971;229:59-61

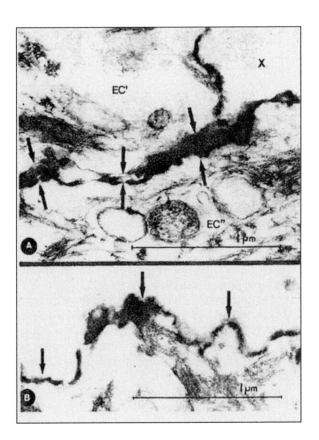

Left: Figure 2 from the landmark report cited above. A. Ultrastructural localization of the antibody-peroxidase conjugate. The electron dense reaction product is confined to the intercellular space (arrows) between two adjacent epidermal cells (EC.'EC"). It is also seen coating the cell surface in the area where the intercellular space is distended (x). B. Immunoglobulins (arrows) coating the surface of an acantholytic cell.

The classic 1964 report of Ernst Beutner and Robert Jordon had established the presence of autoantibodies in the area, but the resolution of immunofluorescent microscopy was insufficient to establish whether they are deposited in the intercellular space proper, on or in cytomembranes, or in the peripheral cytoplasm of epidermal cells.

"Our observations," Wolff and Schreiner concluded," show that the autoantibodies of pemphigus are deposited in and confined to the intercellular spaces of the epidermis."

Thomas B. Fitzpatrick, a household name in American dermatology, received his training in the specialty at the Mayo Clinic, set up and served as chairman of the department of dermatology at the University of Oregon (1952), and later became the chief at Harvard. From the earliest years of his professional life to the present he has been involved in nearly every aspect of melanin research and in the effects and uses of ultraviolet light. Shown below is his landmark publication on the chemistry of human melanogenesis. His talents are not confined to the laboratory. He identified and described the white leaf-shaped macule recognized now by clinicians world-wide as the earliest sign of tuberous sclerosis. Working with Wallace H. Clark and Martin C. Mihm, he also helped establish the clinical criteria for early detection of malignant melanoma.

Fitzpatrick's zeal for teaching and research is communicable. Of the 114 residents trained by him, 44 have chosen careers in academic dermatology. His name is also familiar everywhere as the originator of "Fitzpatrick's dermatology in general medicine," the most successful American magisterial textbook on skin diseases of our time, edited now by Irwin M. Freedberg.

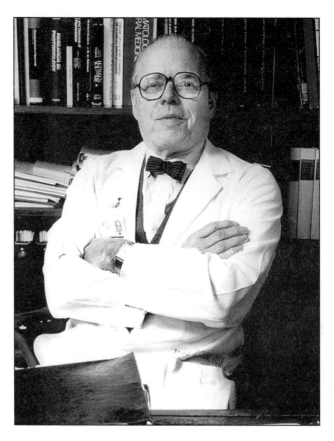

Thomas B. Fitzpatrick

Fitzpatrick TB, Becker SW Jr., Lerner AB, Montgomery H. Tyrosinase in human skin: demonstration of its presence and of its role in human melanin formation. Science 1950;112:223-5.

This report established for the first time that the enzyme tyrosinase does exist in human skin, although in an inactive or partially inhibited form. It also demonstrated that the enzyme identified by Bruno Bloch as dopa oxidase in his pioneering study three decades earlier is in fact tyrosinase, and that dopa (dihydroxyphenylalanine) is itself the product of the interaction of tyrosinase and the amino acid tyrosine, the first step in the formation of melanin. With these facts in hand researchers since have been able to pin point the location of the problem in many diseases characterized by disturbances in pigmentation.

Below, left: Figure 2a from the 1950 report of Fitzpatrick et al: Pigmented dendritic melanoblasts in human skin which has been exposed in vivo to ultraviolet light and incubated in tyrosine phosphate buffer.

Below, right: Figure 1 from the same paper: Enzymatic oxidation of tyrosine to melanin by mammalian tyrosinase.

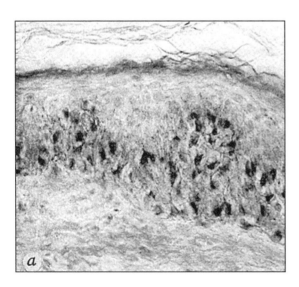

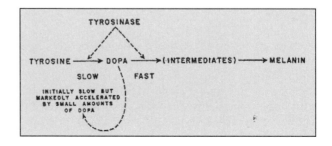

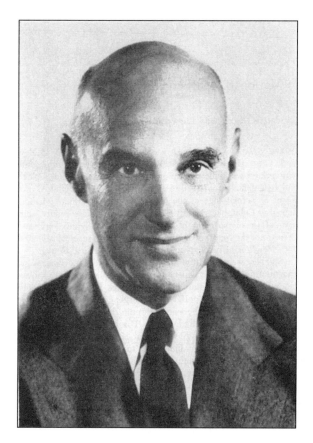

Marion B. Sulzberger (1895 -1984)

Sulzberger MB, Witten VH, Yaffe SN. Cortisone acetate administered orally in dermatologic therapy. AMA Arch Dermatol Syphilol 1951;64:573-9

Marion B. Sulzberger, easily America's best known dermatologist in the 1950s, 60s, and 70s, was born in New York City and received his medical degree in Zürich, Switzerland. He received his dermatologic training with Bloch in Zürich and with Jadassohn in Germany. Returning to New York, he entered private practice with Fred Wise, began to teach at the New York Skin and Cancer Unit, and in 1947 succeeded George Miller MacKee as director of the New York Post-Graduate Medical School and Hospital.

Sulzberger made his name first in basic research. While still abroad he succeeded in demonstrating the phenomenon of specific immunologic tolerance and clarified the role of the skin in initiating hypersensitivity. After returning to New York he joined forces with Fred Wise to introduce the epicutaneous patch test to the United States. He popularized Lewis Webb Hill's term atopic dermatitis and furnished a description of that disease that would be difficult to improve upon. He contributed to our knowledge of heat stroke and pointed out the importance of shearing forces in the production of decubitus ulcers. With Victor Witten, he published the earliest studies on the dermatologic use of corticosteroids, as noted below and on the following page. A veteran of World War I, he willingly interrupted his career to serve as the chief of dermatology in the U.S. Navy throughout World War II.

Sulzberger's clinical and communicative skills were legendary. Patients loved him; his practice and his fees grew apace, and his clientele included the ultra-rich and famous from all over the world. Having held every important dermatologic office, chaired virtually every significant committee, and received all possible honors at home and abroad, he retired from his practice and teaching duties in 1961 and moved to California, where he closed out his active years as director of research at the Letterman Army Institute of Research in San Francisco.

Among the principal purposes for which we administered cortisone orally were the following: (1) to get the patient "over the hump" of the acute phase of a dermatoses, e.g., atopic dermatitis, dermatitis herpetiformis, nummular eczema, distinctive exudative discoid, and lichenoid chronic dermatosis of Sulzberger and Garbe; (2) to give relief from the annoying, incapacitating, or dangerous symptoms and lesions of an acute or chronic dermatoses, such as penicillin urticaria or multiform drug eruptions, even though the condition was one which could be predicted to be "self limited;" (3) to afford relief while a dermatoses, such as severe pruritus ani or vulvar or generalized pruritus, was being investigated further; (4) to get a dermatoses "under control" so that other forms of therapy could be used effectively; (5) as a purely temporary measure of practical usefulness; for example, to make a patient able to travel and thus move to a section of the country where persons with similar dermatoses are known to do well (e.g., in cases of atopic dermatitis, distinctive exudative discoid, and lichenoid chronic dermatoses); (6) to help a patient meet an "emergency," such as a wedding or a debut party, where he must look and feel well "at all costs;" (7) to produce and maintain remissions in diseases in which the eventual prognosis is very poor (as in pemphigus vulgaris or sub acute and acute disseminated lupus erythematosus) by means of continued administration of the lowest effective doses.

This is an excerpt from the first report (cited above) of the systemic use of a corticosteroid to treat dermatologic conditions. Cortisone acetate was administered by mouth in starting doses of 100 to 200 mg a day and gradually decreased. Thirty-two patients were treated, and as might be expected from the multiplicity of indications listed in the excerpt, they suffered from a variety of conditions. The majority of the dermatoses were eczematous, the most common diagnosis being atopic dermatitis. Side effects were covered in some detail, but considering the tremendous implications for the future of dermatologic therapy evident in the dramatic improvement in most of the diseases treated, the tenor of the paper is surprisingly low key.

Victor H. Witten, who collaborated in these the earliest reports of the dermatologic uses of the corticosteroids, was for many years associated in practice with Sulzberger at 999 Fifth Ave. in New York, and is himself an accomplished dermatologist. In addition to his work on steroids, he published studies on the use of radioisotopes to measure skin penetration and on the gonadal radiation dose received by patients undergoing X-ray treatment for acne vulgaris.

Now retired and living in Florida, Witten also made a truly outstanding contribution to the study of dermatologic history. Over a period of forty years, beginning in 1959, he conducted and recorded interviews with more than 200 dermatologists, including many of the most prominent members of the specialty, preserving for all time their personal reminiscences. He has now donated his collection, 240 audiotapes, 30 videotapes, and 4000 pages of transcripts, to the National Library of Medicine, where they are available for study.

Witten, who from his long association knew Sulzberger better than anyone else, took on and carried out admirably the difficult task of editing and filling in the gaps in Sulzberger's autobiography, the manuscript of which was unfinished and in disarray when the author died in 1983.

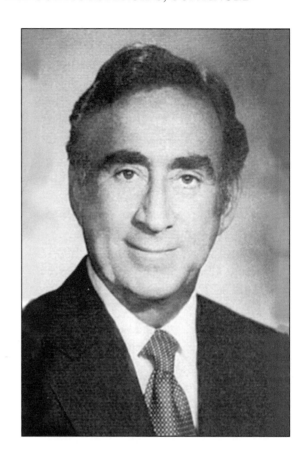

Victor H. Witten

Sulzberger MB, Witten VH. The effect of topically applied Compound F in selected dermatoses. J Invest Dermatol 1952;19:101-2

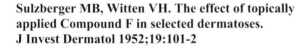

TABLE I

Comparison Between Areas Treated with Compound F Ointment and Those Treated with Control Ointment

CASE	AGE	SEX	DIAGNOSIS	COMPOUND F TREATED AREAS AS COMPARED TO CONTROL SITE		
				Much better	Slightly better	No better
1. (S. M.)	2	M	Atopic dermatitis		X	
2. (H. W.)	16	M	Atopic dermatitis		X	
3. (M. S.)	28	M	Atopic dermatitis		X	
4. (H. S.)	48	F	Atopic dermatitis			X
5. (C. W.)	35	F	Atopic dermatitis		X	
6. (G. H.)	19	F	Atopic dermatitis		X	
7. (E. M.)	35	F	Atopic dermatitis (?)	X		
8. (J. L.)	18	M	Atopic dermatitis (?)			X
9. (N. J.)	15	F	Psoriasis			X
10. (I. M.)	50	M	Psoriasis			X
11. (W. S.)	52	F	Chronic discoid lupus erythematosus			X
12. (M. F.)	36	F	Chronic discoid lupus erythematosus			No control No improvement (?)
13. (L. G.)	56	F	Chronic discoid lupus erythematosus			No control No improvement
14. (J. F.)	30	F	Chronic discoid lupus erythematosus			No control No improvement
15. (W. H.)	46	F	Widespread discoid or subacute lupus erythematosus		X	
16. (A. K.)	34	M	Exudative discoid and lichenoid chronic dermatosis			X
17. (E. S.)	41	M	Pemphigus vulgaris			No control No improvement
18. (C. L.)	20	F	Alopecia areata			No control No improvement
19. (W. K.)	46	M	Alopecia areata			No control No improvement

The earliest topical preparations containing cortisone acetate, both ointments and lotions, were completely ineffective, a great and unexpected disappointment to the world of dermatology. When Merck and Co. made the more biologically active "Compound F" (*hydro*cortisone acetate) available for study, Sulzberger and Witten incorporated it in an ointment base (25 mg/g of base) and put it to use. The results, summarized in the table to the left that appeared in the classic report cited above, were hardly earth-shaking either. But they were enough to start the ball rolling, and in the end topical steroids virtually displaced all other topical modalities, particularly in the treatment of eczematous eruptions and psoriasis. Improvements in these preparations and the marketing of them in pre-packaged form contributed greatly to the demise of compounding, the arcane art topical ingredient mixing that required years to master and manifested itself in the lovingly complex and lengthy prescriptions written by dermatologists in earlier times.

Donald M. Pillsbury was graduated M.D. from the University of Nebraska and and trained in dermatology under John Stokes at the University of Pennsylvania (Penn). He became chairman of the dermatology department at Penn in 1946.

From the beginning, Pillsbury was interested in the basic sciences. He had received special training in biochemistry and was convinced that the survival of our specialty depended on unraveling the secrets of clinical disease through basic research. Early in his career, he investigated cutaneous carbohydrates, water metabolism, and the normal and abnormal bacterial flora of human skin. World War II put a halt to these activities. Colonel Pillsbury served throughout the war as Senior Consultant in Dermatology for the European Theater of Operations.

Much decorated and honored for his military service, Pillsbury returned to Philadelphia to take over the chair at Penn. Under his leadership, the department expanded rapidly. With its numerous faculty and 23 residents, it was at the time the largest in North America, and it turned out a most impressive number of individuals destined for positions of leadership in dermatologic departments worldwide. Pillsbury presided over the diverse, talented, noisy, and often-quarrelsome inhabitants of his fiefdom with a preternatural composure that had to be experienced to be believed. He pushed no one and yet extracted from all the best they had to offer.

The spirit and the accomplishments of the Penn department are all on display in the grand textbook "Dermatology," completed in 1956 by Pillsbury, Walter Shelley, and Albert Kligman. Arriving at a time when the standard textbooks in English had failed to keep up with the new developments in basic science and continued to give space to theories and treatments woefully obsolete, "Dermatology" was like a breath of fresh air. It was the most successful magisterial work of its day.

Recipient of almost every honor dermatology had to offer, Pillsbury died in 1980, at the age of 78.

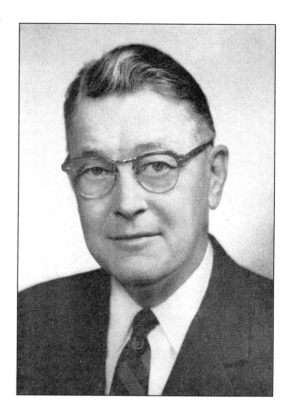

Donald M. Pillsbury (1902-1980)

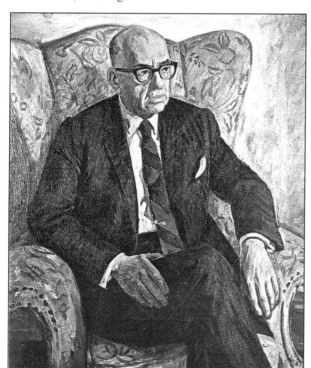

Herman Beerman (1901-1995)
Portrait by Roswell Weidner

Herman Beerman, highly respected American dermatologist, syphilologist, and histopathologist, received both his M.D. and dermatologic training at the University of Pennsylvania. He joined the faculty of his alma mater, rose through the ranks, and became Professor and Chairman of the Graduate School of Medicine in 1949, and Professor of Dermatology at the medical school proper in 1956.

His primary interest lay in the study of syphilis, reflecting the influence of John Stokes, whom he much admired. His knowledge of the voluminous literature on syphilis was simply incredible, and over the years he published scores of reports on virtually every aspect of the disease. He was also recognized worldwide as a superior histopathologist, particularly skilled in the diagnosis of cutaneous neoplasms.

Beerman was the ultimate organization man. He is best remembered now for his long service as secretary and treasurer of the Society for Investigative Dermatology in its early years, during which time he steered that often-wayward vessel away from the rocks of fiscal irresponsibility and the shoals of unnecessary divisiveness. Countless other dermatologic organizations, committees, convocations, and the like in the ever-busy world of American dermatology benefited greatly from his steady hand and prudent counsel, as well.

Warm and friendly, with a sly sense of humor, Beerman was an inspiring teacher, a devoted family man, a connoisseur of art, a bibliophile of note, and an expert on Sherlock Holmes.

158

Aaron Bunsen Lerner, American dermatologist and the universally acknowledged Dean of pigmentation research, received his M.D. and Ph.D. degrees from the University of Minnesota. He spent productive years at the universities of Michigan and Oregon, the latter in association with Thomas Fitzpatrick, and from 1958 to his retirement was Professor and Chairman of the Department of Dermatology at Yale.

At the University of Michigan, Lerner pioneered in the use of psoralens in vitiligo treatment, studied the effects of melanocyte stimulating hormone (MSH), and investigated benoquin depigmentation. He also assisted in the landmark Fitzpatrick study that established the presence of tyrosinase in human skin.

At Oregon, Fitzpatrick and Lerner joined forces in investigating and finally isolating MSH. They succeeded in changing the older term melanoblast to melanocyte.

At Yale, among other things, Lerner isolated and determined the structure of melatonin (noted below), worked out the sequencing in the formation of MSH and ACTH, studied eye color, looked for answers to the knotty problem of the relationship of vitiligo and melanoma, and concerned himself with the pathogenesis of acanthosis nigricans.

His 60 years in pigmentation research have convinced Lerner that the next 60 years will see cures for vitiligo, melanoma, and other pigmentary disorders, and people will be able to change the color of their skin at will.

In a recent communication Lerner, now 80 years old, reflected that he never saw himself as a mentor and did not even realize he had become one until two or three years ago. The rest of us in dermatology realized it much earlier than that.

Below: Figure from the 1959 paper of Lerner et al, showing the structure of melatonin, N-acetyl-5-methoxytryptamine.

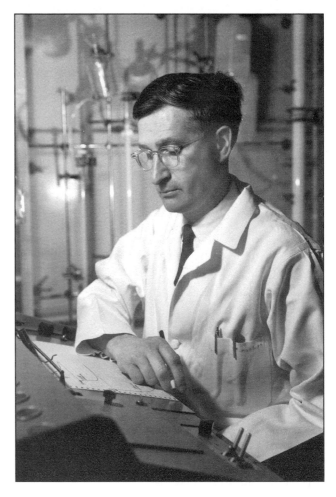

Aaron Bunsen Lerner

Lerner AB, Case JD, Takahashi Y, Lee TH, Mori W. Isolation of melatonin, the pineal gland factor that lightens melanocytes. J Am Chem Soc 1958;80:2587

Lerner AB, Case JD, Heinzelman RV, Structure of melatonin. J Am Chem Soc 1959;81:6084-85

In the two landmark papers cited above Lerner and his associates isolated melatonin from bovine pineal glands, named it, and determined its molecular structure. The work took four years to complete and involved the use of 250,000 pineal glands. In Lerner's own words, "It took the mystery out of the pineal gland and reset the course of research on biologic rhythms." Melatonin has proven useful in the management of insomnia, jet lag, and other sleep disorders, and is being actively investigated in a wide variety of other venues – seasonal affective disorders, bipolar affective disorders, animal breeding, and much more.

159

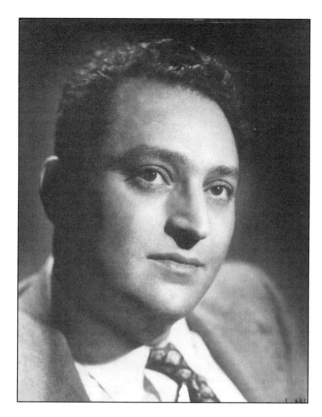

Abner Kurtin (1911-1955)

In 1953, Abner Kurtin, young New York City dermatologist, suddenly found himself the center of attention in the world of dermatologic surgery He had revived, modified, and improved the operative technique called surgical planing or dermabrasion, designed 50 years earlier by the German dermatologist Ernst Kromayer to improve the appearance of unsightly scars. Kurtin, who was one of the first physicians to enter the German concentration camp at Dachau during his army service in World War II, was led to experiment with dermabrasion in an effort to remove the hated identification numbers tattooed on the arms of the inmates by their Nazi captors.

After the war, he completed his dermatologic training at the Skin and Cancer Hospital in New York and entered private practice, where he spent five years perfecting his dermabrasion technique. With the publication of his results (noted below), the procedure skyrocketed in popularity, reaching its peak in the mid 1960s. Since then, dermabrasion has undergone an erratic but pronounced decrease in popularity, due principally to an exaggeration in the media of untoward results and the development of laser resurfacing methods that require less skill and are more easily taught.

Kurtin died young, of coronary artery disease in 1955 at the age of 43. He was appointed chief of dermatology at Albert Einstein College of Medicine shortly before his death. His son Stephen is a well-known New York dermatologist.

Kurtin A. Corrective surgical planing of skin. Arch Dermatol 1953;68:389-97

This report of 273 patients, most of them with facial acne scarring that had been dermabraded with satisfactory results, was received with great interest by surgically inclined dermatologists throughout North America and to a lesser extent in Europe. The procedure, as perfected by Kurtin, represented a considerable improvement over the earlier efforts of Kromayer. Kurtin introduced the rotary driven wire brush, which in combination with ethyl chloride as a refrigerant anesthetic transformed dermabrasion in trained hands into a safe and effective procedure that can be performed on an outpatient basis. His instruments are shown to the right.

Many improvements in the instruments, anesthesia, and control and care of the surgical field have been made over the years, but dermabrasion continues to lose ground. John Yarborough of New Orleans, one of America's finest masters of the technique, estimates that at present no more than 5% of dermatologists continue to dermabrade.

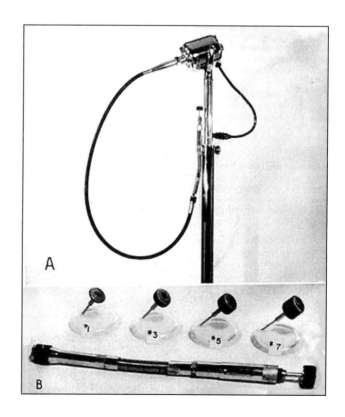

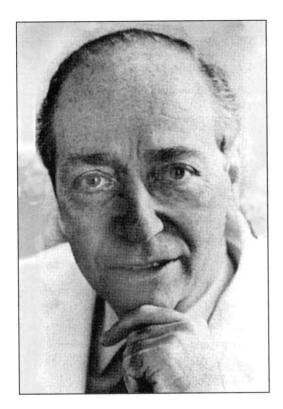

Rudolf Baer (1910-1997)

Rudolf Baer, internationally acclaimed, German-born, American dermatologist, studied medicine in several German schools, but was forced by anti-Jewish licensure regulations introduced by the Nazis to move to Switzerland to complete his course work. He received his M.D. from the University of Basel in 1934 and in the same year emigrated to the United States. In New York City he took his dermatologic training at the Montefiore Hospital and the New York Skin and Cancer Unit, where he met and was greatly influenced by Marion Sulzberger. He joined Sulzberger in practice in 1940, but spent the war years at Cornell doing basic research on insect repellants and on ointments designed to prevent the vesicant effects of poison gas. He rejoined Sulzberger after the war, but struck out on his own in 1947, joined the faculty of the NY Skin and Cancer Unit (SCU) as a clinician-investigator, and remained with that institution for the rest of his life. In 1961 he became chairman of the dermatology department at New York University (NYU), which by that time had united with the SCU and the Post-Graduate Medical School and Hospital with which the SCU had been affiliated. Under Baer's leadership the department expanded remarkably both in size and in influence, and Baer's ability in his new position to keep one foot in both the clinical and investigative worlds was responsible to a great extent for the salutary influence he exerted on the future course of American dermatology.

Early in his career, working with Sulzberger, Baer made valuable contributions to the study of contact dermatitis, establishing the fact that the antigenicity of certain simple chemicals is a function of their ability to combine with proteins. He also published helpful observations on dermatophyte epidemiology, photosensitivity, and atopic dermatitis. Later he joined Inga Silberberg-Sinakin, Jeannette Thorbecke, and others in establishing firmly the importance of the Langerhans cell in the antigen presentation phase of contact dermatitis.

The credibility that accrued from all these studies enabled Baer to promote effectively within his own department, and by example elsewhere, his mission to strike a better balance in American dermatology between clinical and research activities. He played an active role in the formative years of the Society for Investigative Dermatology, even to the point of translating articles from German publications to include in the Society's journal when, as sometimes happened in the earliest days, the cupboard was bare. He was delighted to discover that German research methods hybridized well with the thriving, largely clinical dermatologic infrastructures he found in the United States, and that the informality and willingness of Americans to work together facilitated the process. His successes along these lines made him the logical choice to head what was perhaps the most significant project in post-World War II American dermatology, the preparation of the 1969 *National Program for Dermatology* report, which provided guidelines followed profitably by the specialty ever since.

A quiet, serious, and yet friendly man, Baer was incapacitated by a stroke late in life, and succumbed to its effects in 1997 in his 87th year.

Below: The New York Skin and Cancer Hospital, Second Avenue and 19th St., home base of Rudy Baer in his early years.

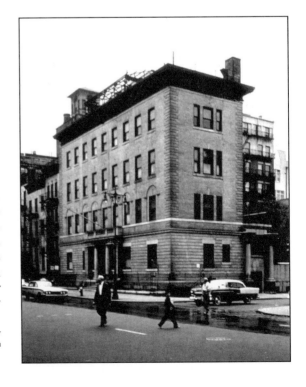

Walter F. Lever, German-American dermatologist and expert dermtopathologist, received his M.D. from the University of Leipzig and emigrated to the United States in 1935. He trained in dermatology under C. Guy Lane at the Massachuetts General Hospital, following which he spent two years as a research fellow with John Talbot at the same institution and received further training in pathology with Tracy B. Mallory at the Boston City Hospital. In 1944, he joined the faculty at Harvard, and in 1959 was appointed to the chair of dermatology at Tufts University School of Medicine.

From the beginning, Lever was interested in all aspects of the bullous diseases, particularly pemphigus, and he made outstanding contributions to the study of these entities throughout his career. His success in separating bullous pemphigoid from pemphigus and the other blistering diseases is noted below. Lever was also greatly interested in the appendage tumors of the skin, and in 1968 published an influential in depth monograph on the subject in collaboration with his friend Ken Hashimoto, who often joined him in bullous disease research as well.

While still at Harvard, Lever instituted a course in dermatopathology for the resident physicians, and because there was at the time no suitable textbook available in English, he wrote one – "Histopathology of the Skin," first edition 1949. The work was an instant success, has passed through many editions, has been translated into all major languages, and continues in print to this day.

In 1983, Lever returned to Germany to be with his second wife, Gundula Schaumberg-Lever, an accomplished electron microscopist, who had accepted a research post in Berlin.

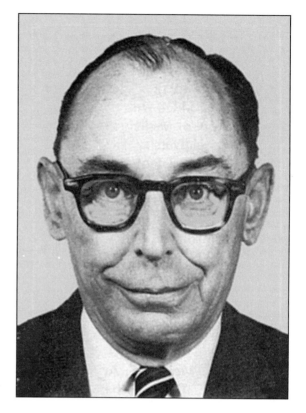

Walter F. Lever (1909-1992)

Lever WF. Pemphigus. Medicine 1953;32:1-124

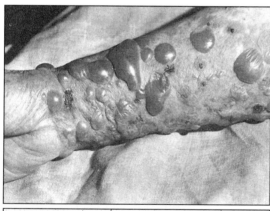

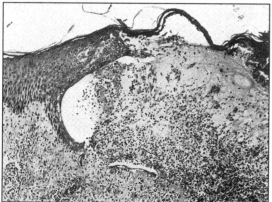

Left: Figures 20 and 50 from Lever's classic 1953 paper on pemphigus in which he separated bullous pemphigoid from pemphigus and named the disease.

Figure 20: Bullous pemphigoid. The flexor surfaces of the arms are the most commonly involved areas.

Figure 50: Bullous pemphigoid. Part of a completely subepidermal bulla. The malpighian cells in the central portion of the roof of the bulla have disintegrated, leaving only the horny layer qs cover.

The renowned French dermatologist Achille Civatte was the first to identify acantholysis as the characteristic histopathologic feature of true pemphigus (1943), but he believed that the disease we now call bullous pemphigoid (BP) is a form of dermatitis herpetifomis. A controversy of sorts arose between the Civatte and Lever camps over the validity of Lever's contention that BP is a completely separate entity. The controversy persisted until the 1970s when jejunal biopsies and immunofluoresence studies established once and for all that Lever's position is correct.

162

Hermann Pinkus, son of the renowned Felix Pinkus, avoided the pitfalls that so often await sons and daughters who attempt to follow in the footsteps of a famous parent and made it on his own. He received his M.D. in Berlin and his dermatologic training with Jadassohn in Breslau. He later began to teach in Breslau. A practicing Christian, with a Jewish father and a non-Jewish mother, Pinkus was removed from his post by the Nazis in 1934. Shortly thereafter, he emigrated to the United States where he arrived without job or money, but not without friends. Marion Sulzberger came to the rescue and secured for him a position at the University of Michigan in tissue culture research. He later completed a fellowship in pathology at Wayne County General Hospital, joined the dermatologic faculty at Wayne State University, and in 1960 took over the chair of dermatology at that institution.

It is as an expert in dermatohistopathology that Pinkus is best remembered, and his many original contributions to the field gained him worldwide recognition. Along with other superior histopathologists, he had the ability to visualize the cellular constituents of his tissue sections in three dimensions and in motion, but he possessed an additional gift less common - a central nervous system with an unusual capacity for data storage and instant recall. This gift is well illustrated in his classic description of alopecia mucinosa, noted below. Once a year for six years, on the average, Pinkus noted among the thousands of slides submitted to him for examination an accumulation of mucinous material in hair follicles and sebaceous glands in biopsies taken from patients suffering from localized hair loss. By case number three, links had already been established in his mind, and by case number six he was ready to publish.

By nature soft-spoken, quiet, modest, and subdued, Pinkus was nevertheless able to maintain his positions in dermatologic controversies with the tenacity and self-assurance that revealed the strength of the inner man.

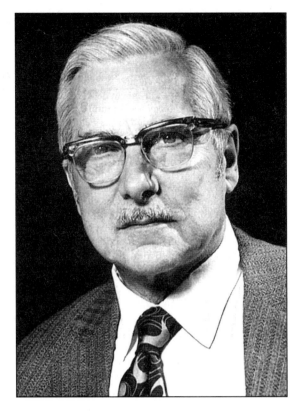

Hermann Pinkus (1905-1985)

Pinkus H. Alopecia mucinosa. Inflammatory plaques with alopecia characterized by root sheath mucinosis. AMA Arch Dermatol 1957;76:419

Figure 3 from the classic Pinkus paper on alopecia mucinosa cited above.

"Low-power photographs of sections from Cases 1-4, stained with hematoxylin and eosin. A (Case 1), note that not all follicles are affected. "X" marks area of inflammatory infiltrate around free mucin in the corium. B (Case 2), sebaceous gland and middle portion of root sheath affected. Lower part of follicle fairly normal with growing hair ("X"). C (Case 3), edema of outer root sheath and cysts. D (Case 4), edematous follicles resemble nests of basal-cell epithelioma."

This "new" entity, described so well by Pinkus, is now accepted as genuine and is commonly divided into three types - a primary acute variety usually seen in young people, a chronic variety that occurs in older individuals, and a type secondary to various benign and malignant diseases.

The pathogenesis remains obscure but, as Pinkus noted, the histologic picture is characteristic

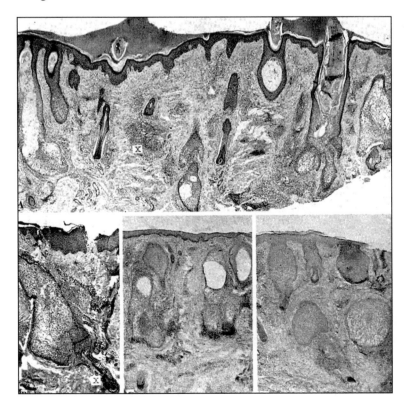

Norman Orentreich, New York dermatologist, is the universally acknowledged father of modern hair transplantation. He received his training in dermatology at the New York University School of Medicine, Skin and Cancer Unit in New York City, and is currently clinical professor of dermatology at NYU.

While studying vitiligo in the early 1950s, Orentreich observed that hair-bearing punch grafts taken from lesions and transplanted to hairless skin on the same patient continued to grow hair in a normal fashion. It occurred to him that this procedure might be useful in the treatment of various alopecias, particularly male pattern baldness (MPB), which usually provides an abundant supply of transplantable hair on the sides and back of the head. And so it was. When he had successfully transplanted hair in 65 cases, 59 of them MPB, he wrote them up carefully and sent the report off to a well-known dermatologic journal. It was rejected out of hand –"can't be done" was the rejection message. Ultimately published by the NY Academy of Sciences, the procedure described caught on immediately. From the beginning, Orentreich has shared his expertise willingly with colleagues worldwide, and hair transplantation, modified and improved by the efforts of many, has become standard in dermatologic offices everywhere.

Orentreich has greatly expanded his horizons. His Orentreich Foundation for the Advancement of Science has concerned itself with the problems of aging, hair loss, cancer, hormonal replacement therapy, Alzheimer's disease, and more. Still active, Orentreich has been joined in practice by his son David and daughter Catherine.

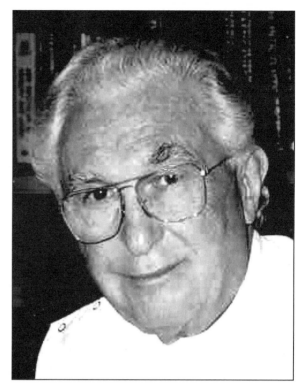

Norman Orentreich

Orentreich N. Autografts in alopecias and other dermatological conditions. Ann NY Acad Sciences 1959;83:463-79

Below: Figure 7 from the report cited above: A patient with alopecia prematura. (a) grafts at various stages following transplantation. Grafts 1 and 7 show crusts one week after grafting. Grafts 2, 5, and 6 show healing one month later. Grafts 3 and 4 show hair growth 6 months later: (b) hair growing on the patient's left frontal scalp.

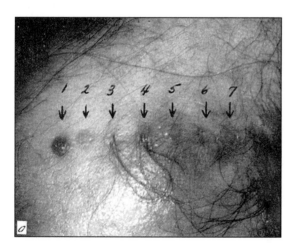

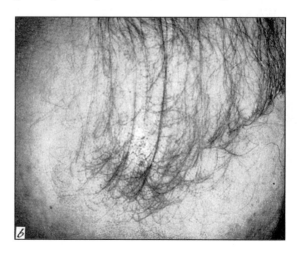

Geoffrey Barrow Dowling, preeminent and revered British dermatologist was born in South Africa. He was received his M.D. from Guy's Hospital in London and his dermatologic training at the same institution. In 1926 he was appointed Consulting Physician to the Department of Skin Diseases at St. John's Hospital for Diseases of the Skin, and in 1933 accepted the position of Consulting Physician to the Department of Dermatology at St. Thomas's Hospital.

Dowling is recognized as the most influential figure in the renaissance of British dermatology in the post-World War I period. He was a superb clinician, endowed with a formidable and sometimes devastating talent for separating the real from the imaginary in clinical investigations. Early in his career, with J.H.H. Macleod, he confirmed the role of pityrosporon ovale in the pathogenesis of seborrheic dermatitis, and in 1938 described the genodermatosis now known as the reticulated pigmented anomaly of the flexures (Dowling-Degos disease). His most famous contribution was the introduction of calciferol in the treatment of lupus vulgaris (1945). Long since superceded by newer anti-tuberculosis medications, it was nevertheless a welcome and highly successful alternative to the Finsen light.

Affectionately known as "Daddy Dowling" by his students and juniors, he was perhaps best known in his day for the extremely popular informal journal and traveling club he established in 1948 to promote knowledge and friendship among the younger dermatologists. The organization is now known as the Dowling Club.

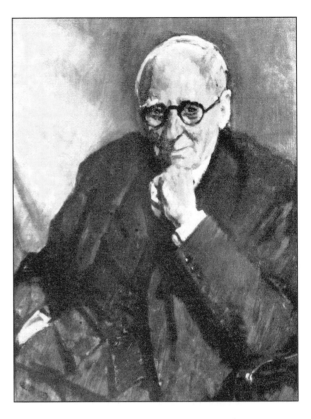

Geoffrey B. Dowling (1891-1976)

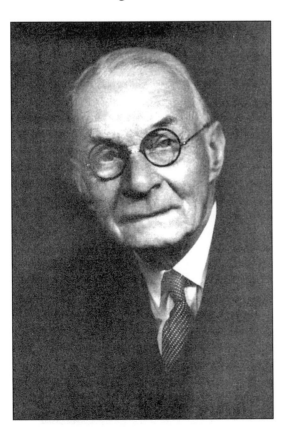

Archibald Gray (1880-1967)

Archibald Gray, distinguished British dermatologist and organizational mavin, received his dermatologic training under Josef Jadassohn in Switzerland. In 1909, he succeeded Radcliffe-Crocker as Physician for Diseases of the Skin at the University College Hospital, and over the years greatly expanded the unit's dermatologic facilities.

Gray was a fine clinician, particularly interested in pediatric dermatology. In addition to his primary appointment, he was associated for years with the Goldie Leigh Hospital, which specialized in the treatment of childhood skin diseases. Sclerema neonatorum and tinea capitis were among Gray's favorite topics for study.

Organization was Gray's true forte. Scarcely any significant British dermatologic society, committee, or task force escaped his attention. The dermatologic sections of the Ministry of Health, Royal Air Force, Royal Society of Medicine, and the Institute of Dermatology all benefited from his ministrations, and he served as President of the highly successful 10th International Congress of Dermatology held in London in 1952.

Gray is especially identified with the British Association of Dermatologists (BAD). It was he who suggested the formation of the organization in 1919, the purpose being in part to control and support the *British Journal of Dermatology*, which he edited from 1916 to 1929. Dermatologic historians owe him a debt of gratitude. As treasurer of the BAD, he convinced the association in 1957 to make a generous donation to the Royal College of Physicians toward the construction of its new building in Regent's Park. He made the donation contingent on the establishment of "the Willan Room" on the premises to house the BAD's fine oil portrait of Robert Willan, along with manuscripts and other objects of historical interest. It is well worth a visit.

Alan Lyell, esteemed Scottish dermatologist, received his medical degree from Cambridge in 1942. As a medical officer in the British Army, he was wounded in the Normandy invasion in June of that year. Following the war, he received his dermatologic training with C.H. Whittle at Addenbrooke's hospital, Cambridge. He later joined G.H. Percival at the Edinburgh Royal Infirmary, spent some time as Consultant Dermatologist at the Royal Infirmary in Aberdeen, and in 1962 was appointed in charge of the Skin Department of the Glasgow Royal Infirmary, which position he held until his retirement in 1980.

Lyell's interests are wide-ranging. He has made valuable contributions to the study of warts, cutaneous bacteriology, artifactual skin diseases, and delusions of parasitosis. He is also a student of dermatologic history. His accounts of Daniel Turner, Alexander Ogston, and Joseph Lister are both scholarly and eminently readable.

Lyell is best known for his classic description of toxic epidermal necrolysis (TEN), the opening paragraph of which is shown below. The four cases described by Lyell resembled the condition characterized by Ritter von Rittershain in 1878 as dermatitis exfoliativa neonatorum (Ritter's disease). A period of confusion followed during which Lyell and other investigators attempted to differentiate between the two conditions on the basis of histopathology and cause. It has been established beyond doubt that they are different. Ritter's disease, now known as the staphylococcal scalded skin syndrome (SSSS), is caused by toxigenic strains of *Staphylococcus aureus*, while TEN is a cytotoxic immune reaction, usually caused by drugs.

Although long retired, Lyell still keeps an eye on the relevant literature. He believes the name TEN should be abandoned, along with "Stevens Johnson syndrome" and erythema multiforme bullosum, and that all should be united under the term "exanthematic necrolysis."

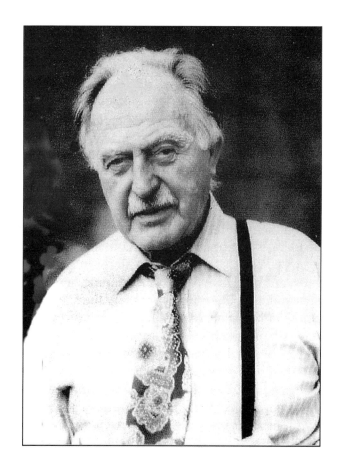

Alan Lyell

Lyell A. Toxic epidermal necrolysis: an eruption resembling scalding of the skin. Br J Dermatol 1956;68:355-61

TOXIC EPIDERMAL NECROLYSIS: AN ERUPTION RESEMBLING SCALDING OF THE SKIN.

ALAN LYELL.

Assistant Physician to the Skin Department, Royal Infirmary, Aberdeen.

THE purpose of this paper is to describe the course of events in four cases of a toxic eruption which closely resembles scalding in its clinical appearance and in the sensations to which it gives rise in the patient. It is probable that this type of reaction is not uncommon and that it has been classified as a toxic eruption, toxic erythema with blistering, or something similar. But the features of the reaction are so definite and they concern the epidermis so intimately—to the exclusion of the dermis—that I believe it to be useful and important to recognize this sequence of events as a distinct syndrome in which some circulating toxin specifically damages the epidermis and results in its necrosis.

Left: The opening paragraph of Lyell's classic 1956 description of toxic epidermal necrolysis, cited above.

166

Arthur James Rook, the best-known and most influential British dermatologist in the latter half of the 20th century, received his M.D. at St. Thomas' Hospital in 1942, served in the Royal Air Force throughout the war years, and returned to St. Thomas where he trained in dermatology under G.B. Dowling. He received additional training in Paris and briefly in the United States. In 1961, he became senior dermatologist at Addenbrooke's Hospital, where he remained until retirement in 1977.

Rook was a clinician of surpassing skill and great experience who sought to improve his clinical performance through the insights provided by the many new discoveries in basic medical science that appeared in rapid sequence in the post-World War II years. He expressed these views in a steady stream of publications on subjects that interested him, bullous diseases, tropical dermatology, entomology, and many more. In addition to the universally admired "Textbook of Dermatology" noted below, Rook co-authored the successful monographs "Botanical Dermatology" and "Diseases of the Hair."

An insatiable reader with a highly retentive memory, he was ideally suited to the many editorial tasks he accepted over the years. Particularly important was his tenure as editor of the *British Journal of Dermatology*, during which he used his position with great effect in his lifelong mission to maintain in British dermatology standards worthy of its glorious past.

In his later years, Rook turned his attention to dermatologic history and brought to the subject the same analytical skills and devotion to accuracy that characterized his work in every venue.

Rook received every dermatologic honor his country had to bestow and numerous foreign marks of recognition as well, and yet he remained at all times a modest, likeable, soft-spoken man. He faced with great courage the Parkinson's disease that clouded the last 20 years of his life; he succumbed to its complications in 1991.

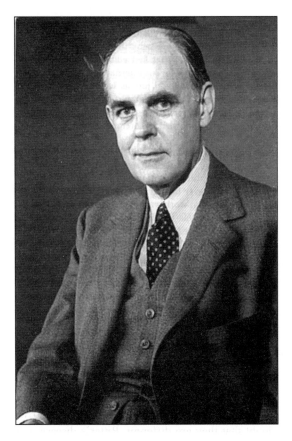

Arthur James Rook (1918-1991)

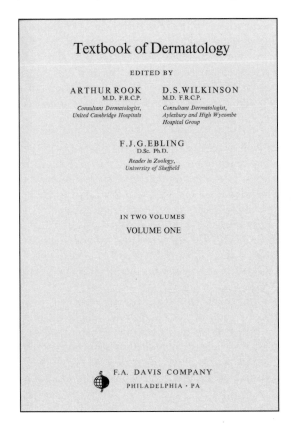

The best known of Rook's productions is the "Rook Book" of 1968, the magisterial textbook widely read everywhere and consulted routinely by North American dermatologists as an eminently reliable source for the European slant on things. The title page of the first edition is shown to the left. Rook's good friend and co-editor, Darrell S. Wilkinson, described the inception of the work in these words:

"In the late 1950s, while at Addenbrooke's Hospital, Cambridge, AJR initially began preparing a textbook on Paediatric Dermatology. However, he soon realised that this covered almost all dermatology and that a full textbook of dermatology was really called for - the first in Gt. Britain for some 25 years. His inauguration of the `Seminars on Progress of the- Biological Sciences in Relation of Dermatology' (published 1960, 1964) also led him to recognise the importance of not only expanding dermatological knowledge but of extending it to include biological aspects and a broader scientific outlook. This was emphasised by his inclusion, as co-editor, and contributor, of the (then) Reader in Zoology, John Ebling, whose breadth of knowledge and critical skills Arthur much admired and who was the perfect epitome of the `non-specialist reader'. I myself made up the triumvirate. We spent many hours together on the floor of his house, going through Chapter after Chapter. The Book could not have come about without Arthur's wide knowledge, enthusiasm and diplomacy in dealing with his contributors!"

Darrell S. Wilkinson, astute English clinical dermatologist and editor and author of note, received his M.D. from St. Thomas' Hospital. Following service in the Royal Navy in World War II, he returned to St. Thomas for dermatiologic training, and later accepted an appointment as Consultant Dermatologist for the Aylesbury and High Wycombe Area. In 1965 he became Consultant Dermatologist for the Wycombe Area Health Authority, which position he held until retirement in 1983.

In 1956, Wilkinson joined with Ian B. Sneddon in the classic description of subcorneal pustular dermatosis, that puzzling entity, the cause and the nosologic position of which continue to generate discussion.

"The summer of 1960 was not notable for its sunshine and cases of photodermatitis were uncommon, at any rate in Buckinghamshire." That is the opening sentence of another important report by Wilkinson. It appeared in the *British Journal of Dermatology* of 1961. He went on to say that in November of that year he was suddenly confronted by a flood of such cases, 53 in all, 29 among workers in a single factory. He soon spotted the thread that linked them all – contact with a pair of germicidal soaps, the active ingredient of which was tetrachlorsalicylanilide. Patch tests confirmed his suspicions that the germicidal ingredient was the cause, and his paper on the subject is a model of proper clinical research reportage, succinct, well argued, and consequential. The soaps are no longer marketed.

In the late 1960s Arthur Rook, impressed no doubt by Wilkinson's keen clinical eye, writing talents, and willingness to sacrifice time and energy for the cause, invited his friend aboard as a co-author and co-editor of the famous "Rook Book" of 1968. Fully retired now and the recipient of many honors, Wilkinson is justly proud of his contributions to that important work. He also takes pride in the main business of his life, the establishment and maintenance of a first class dermatologic center in an area of England where none had existed before.

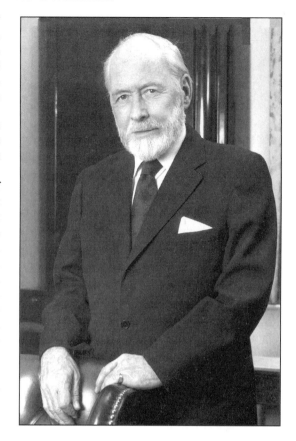

Darrell S. Wilkinson

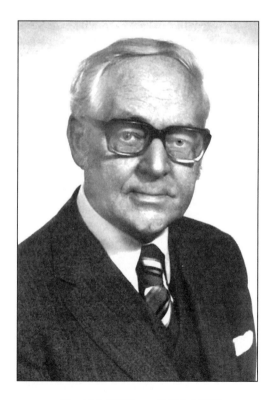

David I. Williams (1913-1995)

David I. Williams, individualistic English dermatologist associated with therapeutic innovation, qualified in medicine at King's College Hospital and received his dermatologic training under Sydney Thompson at the same institution. He spent the World War II years in the R.A.M.C. as an adviser in venereology and a consultant in dermatology and was deeply involved in the secret development of BAL as an antidote to the deadly poison gas, Lewisite. Following the War, he joined the dermatologic staff at King's and remained with that institution until his retirement in 1978.

As a Medical Advisor to the Glaxo Pharmaceutical Company, Williams began working with griseofulvin as early as 1955. In the Fall of 1958, he began studies on the oral administration of the drug to patients with *Trichophyton rubrum* infections. In November that year, he was dismayed to learn that Harvey Blank in Miami had obtained a supply and was about to steal his thunder at the upcoming meeting of the American Academy of Dermatology (AAD). He pushed all the buttons, waved the Union Jack, badgered the editor of *The Lancet*, and succeeded in having his own findings on the use of what he called "this terribly, terribly British drug" appear in print December 6, 1958 - just six days before Harvey Blank delivered his paper at the AAD.

Williams was a captivating speaker, who laced his presentations with irreverent anecdotes and one-liners to the perpetual delight of the audience. He once opened a presentation on his wartime experiences as a venereologist with these words: "I originally intended to entitle this speech 'Prostitutes I have known,' but my wife objected - and quite rightly so." He loved rugby football, was an opera devotee, and played the clarinet at a professional level.

Harvey Blank, much honored American dermatologist, has succeeded throughout his career in combining clinical and investigational skills. He received his dermatologic training at the University of Pennsylvania and at the age of 37 became chairman of the dermatology department at the University of Miami.

From the beginning virus infections of the skin fascinated Blank. His studies of the cytologic smears ("Tzanck" smears) useful in the diagnosis of these infections are particularly valuable, and his interest and expertise resulted in 1955 in a highly esteemed textbook, "Viral and rickettsial diseases of the skin, eye, and mucous membranes of man."

Electron microscopy, basic histologic technique, and the diseases papular urticaria, and juvenile xanthogranuloma - all are subjects that have attracted his attention with beneficial results, and he has also been greatly interested in the cutaneous fungous diseases. His landmark paper on the treatment of dermatophyte infections with griseofulvin is noted below.

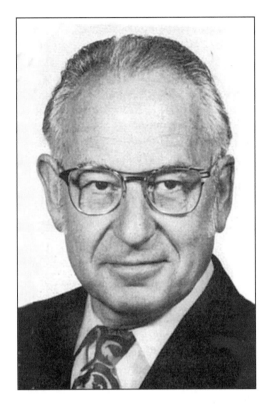

Harvey Blank

Blank H, Roth FJ, Bruce WW, Engel MF, Smith JG, Zaias N. Treatment of dermatomycoses with orally administered griseofulvin. Arch Dermatol 1959;78:259-66

The paper cited above, describing the successful use in humans of a systemically administered antibiotic in the treatment of dermatophyte infections, was for dermatology the number one therapeutic news story of the year. Blank's announcement of his preliminary results at the 1958 American Academy of Dermatology meeting at the Palmer House in Chicago generated unprecedented interest and excitement.

Meanwhile, working independently with griseofulvin in Britain, David I. Williams anticipated Blank's announcement and succeeded in having a preliminary report published in *The Lancet* the very week of the AAD meeting. Therefore, in the matter of precedence, it was essentially a dead heat between the written and the spoken word.

Below: Figure 1 from the Blank report: *T. rubrum* infection of leg. A, before, and B, after three weeks of oral griseofulvin, 5 gm per day. The patient had deep granulomatous lesions elsewhere.

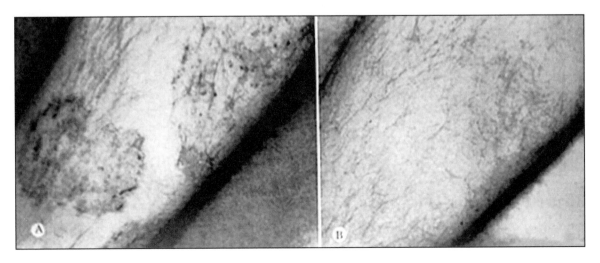

Clayton E. Wheeler Jr., prominent American research dermatologist, received his M.D. from the University of Wisconsin and his dermatologic training at the University of Michigan. In 1962 he joined the faculty of the University of North Carolina and became chairman of the department of dermatology at that institution in 1973, which position he held until his retirement in 1987.

Wheeler is best known for his interest in viral diseases affecting the skin. Early in his career he made valuable contributions to our knowledge of milker's nodules and orf, but soon concentrated his research on infections caused by the herpes simplex virus (HSV), which he studied intently both in the clinic and at the laboratory bench. An intriguing example of his basic HSV research is noted below.

Boarded in internal medicine as well as dermatology, Wheeler has also emerged as an articulate and much-published authority on the cutaneous manifestations of internal disease.

In the 1970s, Wheeler joined with Robert A. Briggaman, later his successor to the chair at North Carolina, in research on the structure of the dermal-epidermal junction at the molecular level. The results of this research have generated intense interest and further investigations worldwide of great value in the study of the many diseases that affect that complex interface.

Wheeler is most proud of his success in elevating his department to its present position in the first rank of excellence. He did so by training and assiduously recruiting faculty and providing a collegial and functional environment in which they could freely develop and express their talents. Prospective department heads can profit from his example.

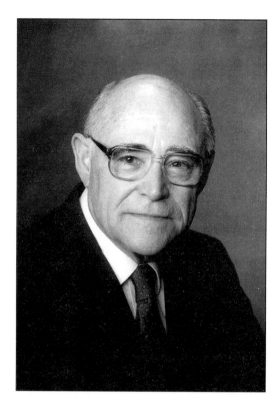

Clayton E. Wheeler, Jr.

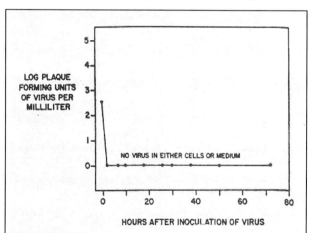

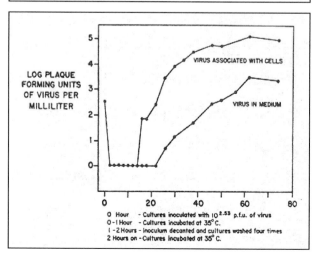

Wheeler CE Jr, Canby CM. Effect of temperature on the growth curves of herpes simplex in tissue culture. J Immunol 1959;83:392-6

It has been known for many years that recurrent herpes simplex infections can be precipitated by febrile illnesses and therapeutic hot boxes. In the well-executed study cited above, Wheeler and his co-worker Charles M. Canby set out to determine whether temperature has a direct effect on the growth of the herpes simplex virus in tissue culture. They inoculated a stock virus strain into cultures of HeLa cells nourished in HSMS medium and maintained the cultures at different temperatures, 25 to 40 °C. At intervals, sample cultures were titrated for virus content. At 25 °C no new virus was detectable in either cells or cell-free medium. Growth increased with each unit rise in temperature; it was optimal at 35 °C and persisted to a significant degree at 40 °C. Figures from the report showing the growth curves at 25 and 35 °C are shown to the left. The investigators concluded that temperature has a profound effect on the ability of the virus to prosper in tissue culture. Do these results provide a plausible explanation for the recurrence of "fever blisters" in febrile patients? Perhaps they do.

170

John S. Strauss, well-known American dermatologist, received his M.D. from Yale and his dermatologic training at the University of Pennsylvania. He joined the faculty of Boston University Medical School in 1961, and in 1978 became chairman of the dermatology department at the University of Iowa, which position he held until his retirement in 1998.

Early in his career, Strauss became interested in the sebaceous gland, its structure, function and diseases. In association with Peter E. Pochi, with whom he often collaborated, Strauss was able to measure the amount and rate of secretion of sebum by the glands in a given area by weighing the output collected on cigarette papers held in place against the skin for varying lengths of time. This clever clinical experiment from 1961 is noted below.

It is as an expert on acne vulgaris and related conditions that Strauss is best known. He has in fact made acne his personal property, publishing numerous cogent reports on every aspect of the disease and sharing his thoughts and expertise on countless occasions with audiences at home and abroad.

Away from the laboratory and clinic, Strauss enjoys sailing and swimming.

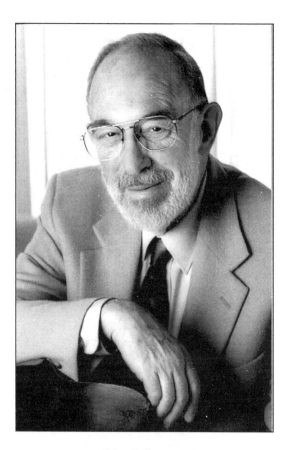

John S. Strauss

Strauss JS, Pochi PE. The quantitative gravimetric determination of sebum production. J Invest Dermatol 1961;37:293-8

Previous attempts to measure human sebaceous gland output failed to furnish reliable data on amount and rate of secretion, information essential to an understanding of the diseases affecting that gland. Using their new technique, the authors were able to demonstrate increased sebum production following administration of methyl testosterone and decreased production following ethynyl estradiol. The report is remarkable for its demonstration that ingenuity and simple tools can combine to produce accurate date useful in a variety of clinical and research situations.

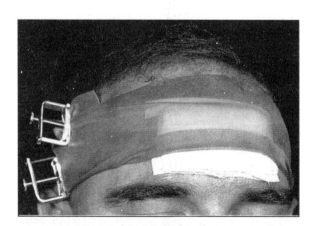

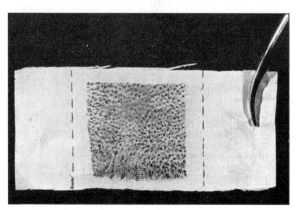

Left: Figures 3 and 4 from the classic Strauss-Pochi report cited above.

Figure 2: The cigarette papers, held in place by gauze squares, are secured by a three-inch wide rubber bandage. In this picture the lower border of the bandage has been reflected to show the underlying gauze.

Figure 3: After the three hour collection period, the central lipid containing area is cut is cut for extraction and gravimetric determination. For photographic purposes *only*, the lipid has been stained with osmic acid vapors, and the dotted lines have been drawn to demonstrate where the paper is cut with scissors.

Rees B. Rees, California born dermatologist affectionately known as "Gus" to friends and colleagues, received his M.D. from the University of California at San Francisco (UCSF) and his dermatologic training at the same school. He became chairman of the UCSF dermatology department in 1954. Recipient of almost every honor the specialty has to offer, he is retired now, and lives in Santa Rosa, CA.

Clinical expertise, a zest for clinical investigation, and a natural aptitude for teaching and organizational activities are united in Rees B. Rees. From the beginning, he was determined to elevate his department to the level of excellence he noted in the eastern schools. To accomplish this he convinced the university powers to create paid research positions and successfully recruited William Epstein and later Howard Maibach to fill them. The result was that UCSF has evolved into a dermatologic investigational center second to none, while managing to retain the reputation for clinical excellence it had always enjoyed. Clinical investigation and therapeutic innovation are Rees' real loves. The best known of his many contributions is his pioneering work with methotrexate in the treatment of psoriasis, noted below.

The list of administrative and teaching jobs Rees has been called upon to perform by grateful colleagues is endless. Among the "toughest," he admits, was his tour of duty on the American Board of Dermatology. He was in charge of the written examination for a number of years.

Rees is above all a people-person. When the *Journal of the American Academy of Dermatology* requested an account of his life for its "Contemporaries" feature in 1984, he complied and modestly listed his many contributions to the specialty, but he transformed the bulk of the article into a catalogue of the strong points and accomplishments of his enormous circle of friends and colleagues. It was an elegant literary performance and characteristic of the man.

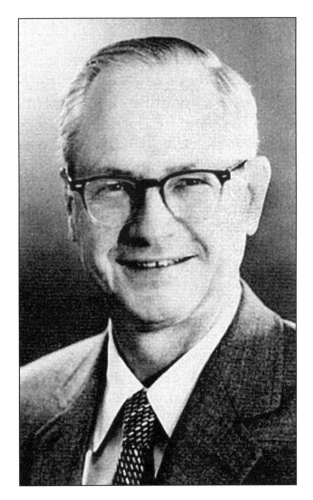

Rees B. Rees

Rees RB. Methotrexate vs. aminopterin for psoriasis. Arch Dermatol 1961;83:970-2

In 1984, Rees gave this account of his introduction to the antifolics: "I had previously become interested in the use of aminopterin for psoriasis when I heard Herbert Rattner's presentation of "What's new, and what's true of what's new" at the Academy meeting in 1951, when he presented work done by Richard Gubner, an internist from Brooklyn who was trying to find an alternative to the then-scarce cortisone for rheumatoid arthritis. One of his patients also had generalized psoriasis, which cleared miraculously. Many colleagues over the years assisted me in studying aminopterin, and subsequently methotrexate, for psoriasis. Dr. Gubner and I were subsequently awarded the Taub International Memorial Award for research in psoriasis."

In Rees' first publication on methotrexate (cited to the left) he compared it to its close relative aminopterin with respect to efficacy and safety and concluded that aminopterin is more effective, but also more toxic. He presented his findings at the 1960 Academy meeting in Chicago, where they were received with great interest. Soon after his presentation, aminopterin was removed from the market because of manufacturing difficulties, leaving methotrexate king of the antifolic hill. It took some time for the medication to be fully accepted, but it has taken its place now as a valuable component in the rotational therapy commonly employed in the management of psoriasis.

172

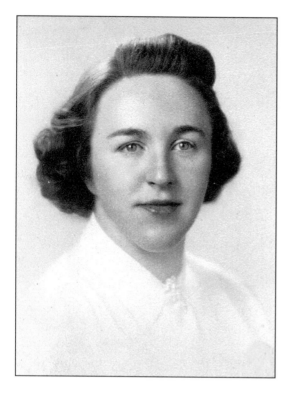

Margaret Ann Storkan (1919-1999)

Below: the famous SS Hope, hospital ship of Dr. Willam B. Walsh's Project Hope. From 1960 to 1974 this vessel carried physicians and other medical personnel to countries in the Third World where they helped their counterparts on the local scene enhance their clinical and laboratory skills and improve health care delivery systems.

Margaret Ann Storkan, American dermatologist of boundless energy, who combined professional excellence with social conscience and a willingness to serve, was a graduate of Creighton Medical School. She received her dermatologic training at the University of Southern California (USC) and the University of Minnesota. She was a clinical professor of dermatology at USC.

Her private office in Redondo Beach, a stone's throw from the Pacific Ocean, was an extremely busy place during her active years, and yet she managed somehow to put her practice on hold for two months at a time to sail with the famous SS Hope on its humanitarian medical missions to poorer countries. From 1962 to 1972, Storkan served seven hitches on the Hope, mostly on missions to South America. As the only dermatologist aboard it fell entirely on her shoulders to acquaint the local physicians at the ports of call with the latest diagnostic and therapeutic advances in cutaneous medicine in the First World and adapt them to the limitations of the Third. It was not an easy task.

Storkan also found the time for more than a decade to run USC's large and busy leprosy clinic, located then in San Pedro, California.

When examples of crass commercialism in the medical world leap out at us from TV screens and newspaper pages we are reminded that we need more physicians cast in the mold of Margaret Storkan.

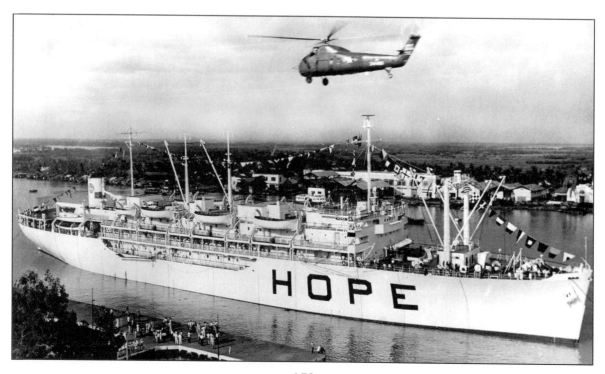

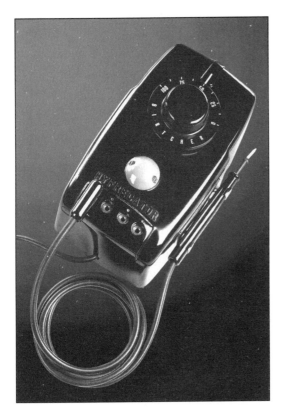

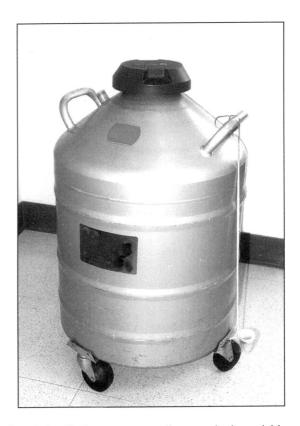

In 1937 Cecil Bircher of Los Angeles, California introduced the Hyfrecator, a small, rugged, dependable, inexpensive desiccation-fulguration unit that soon captured the lion's share of the market. The 1963 Model 709, shown above to the left, was easily the most popular instrument of its kind, sold by the thousands all over the world. Steady improvements in subsequent models by the ConMed Corporation have assured its continuing popularity.

Dry ice, introduced by William Allen Pusey early in the 20th century, remained the most popular form of dermatologic cryotherapy in North America until displaced by liquid nitrogen when the latter became readily available in the 1950s. Shown below, left, is the Kidde apparatus kit, a fixture in many offices at the time, used to produce small cylindrical pencils of dry ice from carbon dioxide cartridges. It is a collector's item now. Above and to the right is a large liquid nitrogen storage tank along with the long-handled dipper employed to remove suitably sized aliquots for immediate use or to fill the popular hand held spray can delivery system, an example of which is shown below, right. Both appeared in clinics and offices in the 1950s and 60s, and units of both types are still in use.

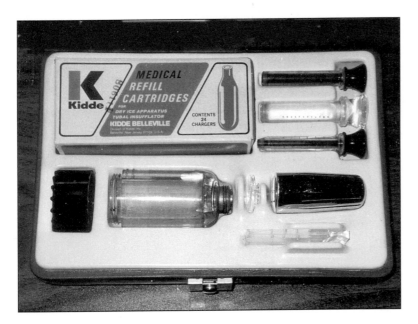

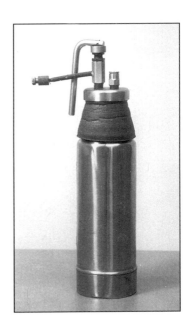

RECENT TIMES

Leon Goldman obtained his M.D. from the University of Cincinnati and his dermatologic training at the Cincinnati General Hospital; he also studied with Bruno Bloch at the University of Zürich. In 1933 he returned to Cincinnati to teach at his alma mater and became chairman of the department of dermatology in 1947.

A complete dermatologist, with an open mind and a wide range of interests, Goldman was a first class clinician. He was, among other things, a syphilologist of surpassing skill, when mastery of that subject was essential to success in the academic world of dermatology. He maintained throughout his life an irrepressible, youthful enthusiasm for everything new that came to his attention, including the field of interest for which he is best remembered, the laser and its potential uses in medicine.

The first operating laser was developed in 1960 by the Californian, Theodore Harold Maiman, and the device fascinated Goldman. He was certain it must have medical applications that cried out for investigation, and for Goldman, then in his late forties, it was as though he had discovered a whole new career. His initial laser publications, noted below, were tentative "toe in the water" reports, but they alerted dermatologists and others to the powerful new presence; henceforth Goldman became America's number one laser enthusiast. He was the first to treat skin cancer with the device, and he set up and was the first director of the course on the "biomedical laser" given by the American Society for Laser Medicine and Surgery. In 1985, he was given the Schawlow award by the Laser Institute of America for his contributions to the field.

Goldman was also devoted to the study of dermatologic history. He made valuable contributions to the study of skin diseases in ancient civilizations, and his reports on skin conditions depicted in the realistic paintings of the old masters are instructive and delightful reads.

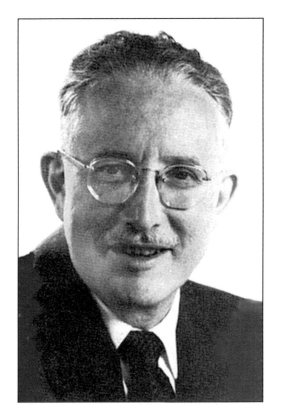

Leon Goldman (1905-1997)

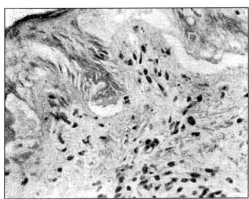

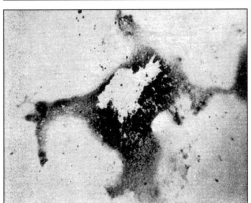

Goldman L, Blaney DJ, Kindel DJ Jr., Franke EK. Effect of the laser beam on the skin. J Invest Dermatol 1963;40:121-2

Goldman L, Blaney DJ, Kindel DJ Jr., Richfield D, Franke EK. Pathology of the effect of the laser beam on the skin. Nature 1963;197: 912-14

Conclusions from the classic Goldman laser report (J Invest Dermatol, 1963):
"From preliminary studies, eye lesions of pigmented rabbits and skin lesions of pigmented areas of rabbits and man may be produced by the coherent beam of a ruby laser of only light power intensity. Dark color of the skin increases absorption of the laser beam. Eye protection of operating personnel is necessary."

Left: Figures 2 and 3 from the classic Goldman laser report (Nature, 1963).
Upper: Colored skin after exposure to laser, showing marked epidermal change (H and E stain).
Lower: Cytological preparation from pigmented basal cell carcinoma. Tissue fragment of red cells and tumor masses on slide exposed to laser, then stained with May-Grünwald Giemsa. White area represents area of impact.

176

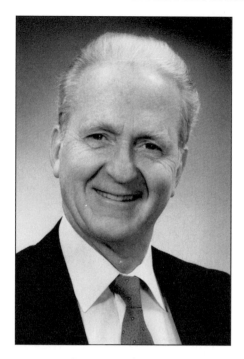

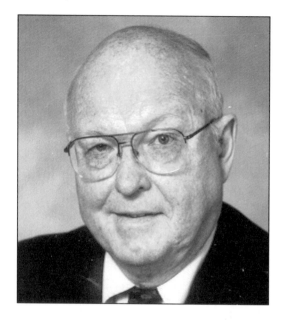

Robert E. Jordon

Ernst H. Beutner

Beutner EH, Jordon RE. Demonstration of skin antibodies in sera of pemphigus vulgaris patients by indirect immunoflourescent staining. Proc Soc Exp Biol Med 1964;117:505-10.

Below: Figure 1 from the Beutner–Jordon paper of 1964. I.I.F. stain of normal human skin with serum (1:10 dilution) of a pemphigus vulgaris patient (All.). The corium lies above the picture. I.I.F. staining in intercellular spaces occurs predominantly in prickle cell layer.

"This report," the authors stated, "sets forth our initial observations on the immunofluorescent demonstrations of antibodies to an intercellular substance of stratified squamous epithelium in the sera of some patients diagnosed as having pemphigus vulgaris and on the apparent in vivo reactions of these antibodies with the patient's own skin." The impact was immediate; this publication and subsequent ones by the same authors locating "basement zone" antibodies in bullous pemphigoid soon took their place among the most cited dermatological reports ever. They ignited an explosion in research on the bullous diseases that resulted in a short period of time in more insights into the pathogenesis of these entities than had been accumulated in all the years that had gone before.

Both authors were associated at the time with the State University of New York at Buffalo, School of Medicine, Buffalo, NY, and both have continued throughout their careers to make valuable contributions to immunologic research. Beutner, now an emeritus professor at the Buffalo school, runs a highly successful diagnostic laboratory. Jordon is now professor and chairman of the department dermatology of the University of Texas Medical School at Houston. His textbook on dermatologic immunology is current and widely read.

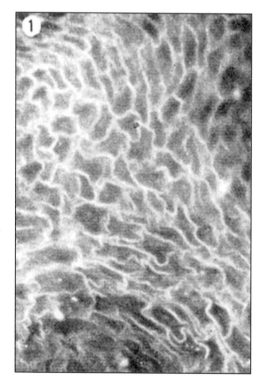

177

STEPHANIA JABLONSKA AND RUDI CORMANE, EUROPEAN PIONEERS IN DERMATOLOGIC IMMUNOLOGY

Stephania Jablonska, eminent Polish research dermatologist and Professor of Dermatology at the University of Warsaw, concerned herself early in her career with intensive investigations on the nature and cause of epidermodysplasia verruciformis. She and her colleagues demonstrated the oncogenic role of the human papilloma virus in the production of the carcinomata often associated with that condition. Since 1966 she has been involved in numerous studies on the immunopathology of the bullous skin diseases. In collaboration with Tadeusz Chorzelski she described the childhood disease linear IgA bullous dermatoses. When the time came in 1975 to move the newly perfected immunofluorescence techniques out of the laboratory and into the clinical world of dermatology, Jablonska captained the team that described the utilization of these techniques in the diagnosis of lupus erythematosus and the bullous diseases in a key role paper published simultaneously in four languages and five different journals.

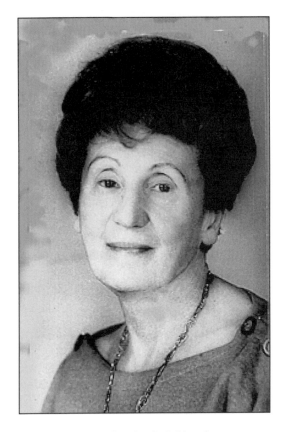

Stephania Jablonska

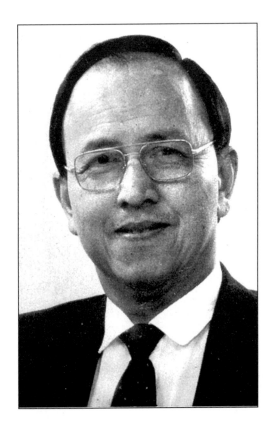

Rudi H. Cormane (1925-1987)

Rudi H. Cormane was born in Indonesia in 1925. He spent World War II imprisoned in a Japanese internment camp, and after the war emigrated to Holland. He received his medical degree from the University of Leiden, surviving an attack of poliomyelitis during his sophomore year that left him with a permanent partial paralysis of the lower extremities. He received his dermatologic training at Utrecht, joined the faculty there, and quickly made a name for himself in both basic and clinical research. His principle interests lay in immunology, immune-mediated skin diseases, and photochemotherapy. Co-author of a successful textbook on microbiology and immunology, he was among the very first in Europe to master, improve, and teach the new techniques associated with those fields, particularly immunofluorescence.

Cormane was a warm, friendly, cultured, and deeply religious man. He died at the age of 62 of a massive coronary attack while dining at home with friends.

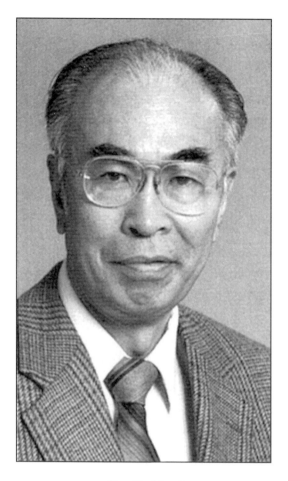

Ken Hashimoto

Born in Japan, Ken Hashimoto received his M.D. from Niigata University Medical School and his dermatologic training at the University of Maryland and the Massachusetts General Hospital. He joined the faculty of Tufts University School of Medicine, where he worked for the next 10 years, often collaborating with Walter Lever. He was for many years Professor and Chairman of the Department of Dermatology, Wayne State University School of Medicine, the first and only Japanese national ever to head and American dermatological department.

Hashimoto is a master of the electron microscope and a highly skilled histochemist. Both these forms of expertise were put to use in the well executed study noted below, in which Hashimoto and his coworkers explored the pathogenesis of the lethal metabolic disease angiokeratoma corporis diffusum (Anderson-Fabry's disease). He has applied his skills to many other subjects, to the study of cutaneous embryology, Kaposi's sarcoma, and particularly to the appendage tumors of the skin. His 1968 monograph on these neoplasms, coauthored by Lever, is a classic. Two previously undescribed diseases are associated with his name – congenital self-healing reticulocytoma (1973) and transient bullous dermolysis of the newborn (1985).

Hashimoto has also been most helpful in allaying the culture shock experienced by the many Japanese dermatology students who have come to North America over the years for postgraduate training.

Retired now, Hashimoto divides his time between the United States and Japan. Gardening, photography, and fishing occupy his time.

Hashimoto K, Gross BG, Lever WF. Angiokeratoma corporis diffusun (Fabry). J Invest Dermatol 1965;44:119-128

Right: Figure 6 from Hashimoto's classic paper on the pathogenesis of Anderson-Fabry's disease: *Large residual body*. This "residual body" was found in an endothelial cell lining a fairly large dermal vessel. Regularly arranged thick, wire-like structures are present. Lipid is deposited on some of them. Vesicles in varying sizes are scattered between the wire-like structures. The entire body is enclosed by a thin membrane. Several young lysosomes (L) in the "phagosome" stage are seen containing small deposits of lipid and small vesicles. The cytoplasm of this cell is markedly fibrous. ER: endoplasmic reticulum. M: mitochondria. Pi: pinocytotic vesicles. VL: vascular lumen.

Hashimoto concluded from his study that in Anderson-Fabry's disease "enormously engorged lysosomes are formed on the basis of a genetic deficiency of lysosomal enzymes essential for the digestion of phospholipoproteins."

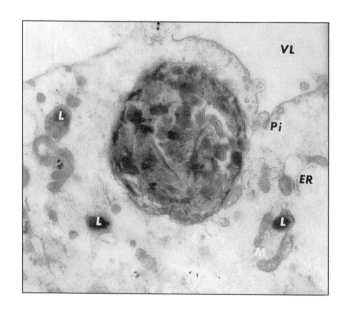

William E. Pace, Canadian dermatologist who first recognized the anti-acne properties of benzoyl peroxide, received his MD from the University of Western Ontario in 1941. He served in the Royal Canadian Air Force Medical Service in World War II, and after the war took his dermatologic training at the Montreal General Hospital and at the University of Michigan. In 1952, he returned to his hometown, London Ontario, where he opened an office and conducted an extremely busy practice for many years.

During his educational years, Pace had taken a special interest in biochemistry and mastered the technical tools that facilitated his work with benzoyl peroxide. He modestly describes his therapeutic discovery as "serendipitous." Perhaps it was, but it takes both an inquiring mind and uncommon drive to pursue such a project to the end, attributes clearly evident in Pace, and appreciated now by his colleagues everywhere.

Pace was also the first to use topical benzoyl peroxide in the successful treatment of decubitus ulcers.

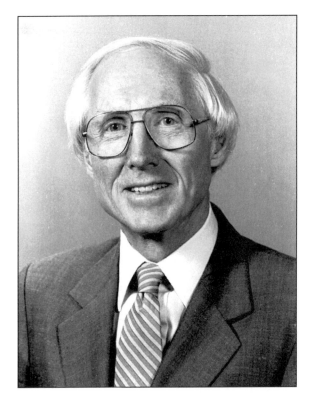

William E. Pace

Pace WE. A benzoyl peroxide sulfur cream for acne vulgaris. Canad Med Assoc J 1965;93:252-4

Above: The first appearance in print of Pace's work with benzoyl peroxide.

Below: the structural formula for benzoyl peroxide, the chief ingredient of numerous anti-acne topicals marketed in North America under the registered trade names, Brevoxyl, Benzac, Benzagel, Clearasil, Desquam-X, Fostex, and many more

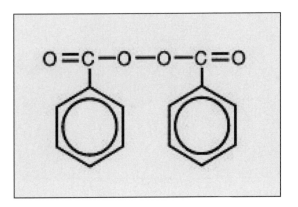

Pace noted in the 1950s that Squibb's antiseptic Quinolor Compound Ointment helped acne vulgaris, although its color limited patient acceptance. When the product was discontinued, he investigated its contents, found it contained 10% benzoyl peroxide (BP), a colorless bleach, and wondered whether the anti-acne properties of Quinilor might reside in that ingredient. With the help of a pharmacist, he began to formulate BP ointments of his own, and because of the instability of the substance and its explosive potential, mixed his early batches in the parking lot outside his clinic. To his delight, he found his new creations worked just as well as the Quinilor. He presented his findings in a paper read at a 1963 meeting of the Canadian Dermatological Association, where it raised eyebrows and generated a great deal of skepticism. But Pace persisted, and after he published the key paper cited to the left, the product took off. BP preparations, now available over the counter as well as by prescription, continue to be the most widely used anti-acne topicals on the market.

"Benzoyl peroxide was a lucky find," Pace told the Dermatology Times of Canada in 1993. "There was no brilliance involved in it at all, absolutely none. The discovery was all very serendipitous. I had years of absolute joy. I was monkeying with this, and I was the only person in the world who was."

Arthur Robert Birt, Canadian dermatologist with a sharp eye for the clinically new, was born in Winnipeg, Manitoba and received his M.D. from the University of Manitoba in 1930. After a few years in general practice he became interested in dermatology and entered the office of Dr. Andrew Davidson, Winnipeg's leading dermatologist, as a preceptee. Davidson's reputation as a superior teacher on a one-to-one basis was well deserved, and four years later Birt emerged from his preceptorship thoroughly trained in all aspects of the specialty. He opened his own office in Winnipeg, where maintained a busy practice until his retirement in 1989. He taught at the University of Manitoba, and was appointed chief of the section of dermatology at that institution in 1964.

Birt's diagnostic acumen and eye for the clinically new resulted in two classic papers. In 1968 he published the first of his landmark reports on the hereditary polymorphic light eruption of the Inuit and North and South American Indians (HPLE), noted below. In 1977, with G.R. Hogg and W. J. Dube, he described and named the rare syndrome, hereditary multiple folliculomas with trichodiscomas and acrochordons. The latter is often mercifully shortened to "Birt-Hogg-Dube disease."

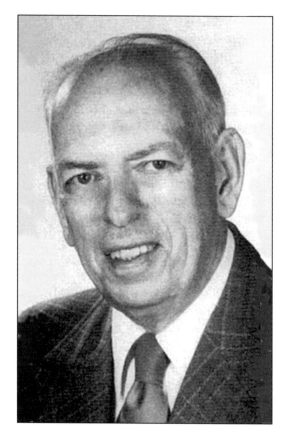

Arthur Robert Birt (1906-1995)

Below: Figure from Birt's classic paper on HPLE. Indian brothers, 6 and 8 years old, with eczematous eruptions on the face and papular, prurigo-like lesions on the arms.

Birt AR. Photodermatitis in Indians of Manitoba. Canad Med Assoc J 1968;98:392-7

Although photodermatitis had been noticed in native Americans as early as 1923 and was described later in several reports, it was Birt's classic 1968 paper, cited above, that brought the condition forcibly to the attention of the dermatologic world and established it as hereditary entity, transmitted as an autosomal dominant and different from other forms of photodermatitis. He later named the disease hereditary polymorphic light eruption (HPLE). Subsequent studies by Birt and others showed that the condition is not confined to North American Indians, but is also seen among the Inuit peoples, and indigenous Indians of Central America and parts of South America. Birt identified 175 examples in Manitoba alone. Eczematous lesions of the face, crusted papular lesions on extremities, and recurrent cheilitis are the usual findings.

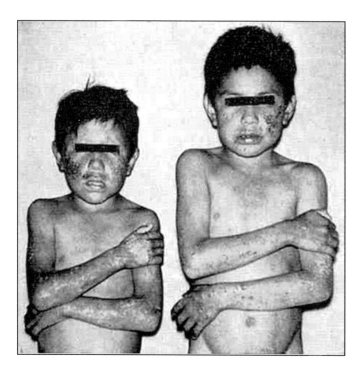

181

You have to be nimble and well read to keep up with Walter Shelley, long time professor of dermatology at the University of Pennsylvania and now Emeritus Professor of Dermatology at the Medical College of Ohio at Toledo. The most versatile of American dermatologists, he slides easily from the traditional to the cutting edge and back again. Clinical research, bench research, disease description, therapeutic and diagnostic innovations, yarns and stories – all are well within his purview.

Shelley's interest in the sweat gland early in his career resulted in the publication of a remarkable series of investigations on its function, abnormalities, and on therapeutic approaches to sweat gland problems. It was in these studies that he first made his mark in dermatology, but he went on to make outstanding contributions to our knowledge of itching, cutaneous innervation, cutaneous cytology (coined the term keratinocyte), the mysterious basophil, contact dermatitis, diseases of the hair and nails, cutaneous bacteriology, and much more - ten books and hundreds of papers filled also with observations and truisms that are integrated now into the workaday knowledge of every practicing dermatologist. In this respect he resembles that great dermatologic hero of the past, Paul Gerson Unna, who was also equally at home at the laboratory bench and in the clinic and, like Shelley, had a sharp eye for the homely and eminently practical tricks and tips that make life easier for the dermatologist on the firing line.

Shelley has been joined in much of his work in recent years by his wife, Dorinda, a talented dermatologist in her own right.

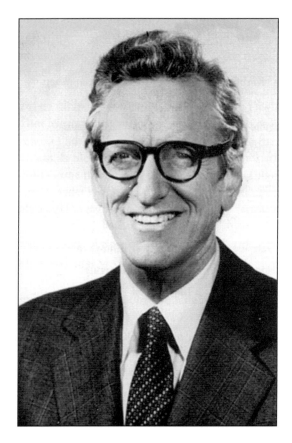

Walter B. Shelley

Shelley WB, Rawnsley HM. Aquagenic urticaria. JAMA 1964;189:895-98

"We discovered a totally new disease, aquagenic urticaria, with little more than a history and a wet towel to confirm it," Shelley wrote in a recent plea to younger colleagues to use their eyes and ears and not rely solely on the elaborate trappings of modern medical science. He was referring to the entity described in the publication cited above. The report describes two young women who developed cholinergic urticaria from contact with water - swimming, bathing, sweating, etc. The eruption had nothing to do with temperature or any identifiable factor other than surface contact with the water itself. Shown to the left is Figure 1 from the Shelley report: follicular hives on the back produced by 10 minutes' immersion in water at 92 F.

We chose to highlight this report because it illustrates Shelley's remarkable ability to spot the unusual blip on the radar screen of daily practice, follow it up, and show the rest of us what we are missing.

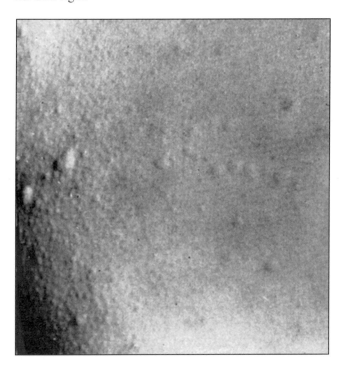

Albert Montgomery Kligman, Professor of Dermatology at the University of Pennsylvania, has for many years been center stage as American dermatology's one-of-a-kind man of ideas and also one its stormiest petrels. His contributions to the specialty are many and significant.

Trained as a botanist before entering medicine, he was naturally drawn to the mycotic skin diseases and early in his career discovered the PAS stain for visualizing fungi. With this tool and his botanical expertise, he clarified the pathogenesis of the dermatophyte infections, particularly tinea capitis. Contact dermatitis was next in line. He developed more reliable methods for identifying contact sensitizers (the Maximization test) and for the proper assessment of primary irritation, phototoxicity, and photoallergy.

In the 1960s, Kligman zeroed in on acne vulgaris, examining all aspects of that disease with the gimlet eye and calculated irreverence characteristic of the Kligman approach to dermatologic investigative activity. The landmark 1969 demonstration of the value of topically applied vitamin A acid in the treatment of acne vulgaris by Kligman, E.F. Fulton Jr., and Gerd Plewig is cited and noted below.

In recent years Kligman has concerned himself with the physiology of cutaneous aging. Topically applied retinoic acid plays an important role in that research as well.

Many research minded dermatologists of note cut their investigational teeth in Kligman's laboratory facilities.

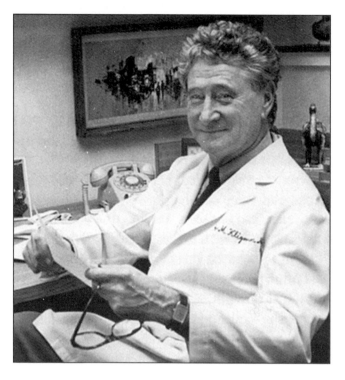

Albert Montgomery Kligman

Kligman A, Fulton EF Jr., Plewig G. Topical vitamin A acid in acne vulgaris. Arch Dermatol 1969;99:469-76

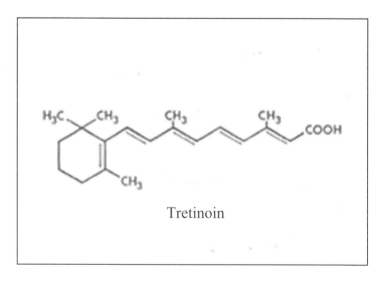

Tretinoin

The carefully controlled study of a large number of cases, cited above, established the effectiveness of topically applied vitamin A acid (retinoic acid, tretinoin) in the treatment of acne vulgaris. It also furnished evidence that the mechanism of action involved inhibition of comedone formation. Marketed later as Retin-A, tretinoin preparations eventually became the gold standard for topical acne therapy.

It has since been shown that topically applied tretinoin increases and alters collagen synthesis to reduce photo-aging wrinkling and roughness of skin and also redistributes melanin in sun-induced hyperpigmentation to produce lighter, more even skin tones.

The structural formula of tretinoin is shown to the left.

A refugee from Nazi Germany, Inga Silberg Sinakin emigrated as a child with her parents to the United States in 1938. She received her dermatologic training under Rudolph Baer at New York University and specialized training in electron microscopy at Wayne State University in Detroit under Yutaka Mishima. Silberberg-Sinakin put her new skills to work in 1966 in an electron microscope investigation of the percutaneous absorption of mercury. In the course of this study she noted that apposition of lymphocyte-like cells to Langerhans cells (LCs) occurred in individuals sensitive to mercury, but not in non-sensitive individuals. The conclusions she drew from this and other observations that LCs were actively involved in contact dermatitis were not accepted at first by the dermatologic world. Several years of frustration and rejection followed, during which she received the unwavering support of her mentor Rudolph Baer and her husband Herbert Sinakin. By 1979, corroborative evidence had put an end to the doubts, and Inga Silberberg-Sinakin received the credit she deserves for an immunologic discovery of the first magnitude.

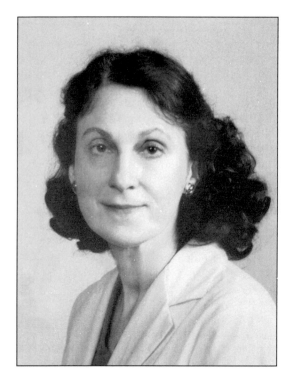

Inga Silberberg-Sinakin

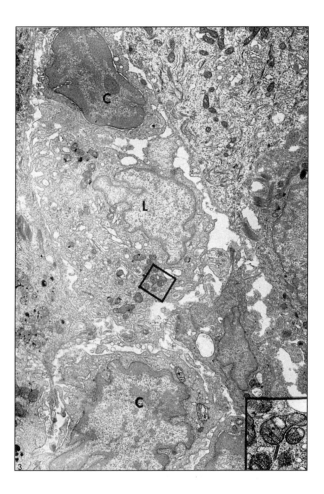

Silberberg I. Ultrastructural studies of the Langerhans cells in contact sensitive and primary irritant reactions to mercuric chloride. Clinical Research 1971;19:715.

The abstract cited above, and the definitive papers that followed, demonstrated the active participation of Langerhans cells in contact sensitivity reactions and not in primary irritation. Once accepted, they set off a wave of investigations on antigen presentation that continues to this day. Only a few decades ago the Langerhans cell was looked upon as some sort of effete melanocyte residing in the epidermis with nothing to do. In catching it in action Silberberg-Sinakin also reinforced the theory that whatever exists as structure in a living organism will sooner or later be shown to have function.

Left: Figure 3 from the definitive 1973 paper by Silberberg-Sinakin showing two mononuclear cells (C) juxtaposed to a Langerhans cell (L). The area demarcated by lines contains Langerhans granules and is seen at higher magnification in the inset.

Founders of the History of
Dermatology Society – June 23,
1973, Essex House, New York, NY

Lawrence C. Parish
Gerald N. Wachs
Saul Blau
Samuel B. Frank
Leon Goldman
Margaret Ann Storkan

Below: Marion B. Sulzberger, speaking at the first formal meeting of the History of Dermatology Society (then called "Club"), held in the Wrigley Building Restaurant, Chicago, December 4, 1973. Sulzberger described his experiences during his dermatologic training with Bruno Bloch in Switzerland in the 1920s and 30s. Some 40 people attended and were delighted with the whole affair. Parish had invited Samuel J. Zakon, the doyen of dermatologic historians in America at the time, to join Sulzberger on the podium. Zakon declined. "When the nightingale sings," he said with a smile, "all the other birds keep quiet." The list of dermatologists who have spoken at the annual meetings since includes many of the most illustrious among us, and they have never failed to amuse, surprise, or edify.

For some time Lawrence Charles Parish, Philadelphia dermatologist and medical historical buff, had dreamed of organizing a club where he and similarly afflicted individuals could get together and share their recent discoveries. The idea crystallized at an American Medical Association meeting in New York in 1973, when he organized a lunch meeting at the Essex House for the small group of like-minded enthusiasts listed in the box to the left and found that they shared his dream. By the time the dishes were cleared away, the group had founded a society and laid out plans for a formal meeting to be held later that year. Historical presentations were to be followed in the evening by a fine dinner and a distinguished guest speaker. Thoroughly energized, Parish set the wheels spinning. He convinced Marion B. Sulzberger to speak at the first formal dinner, contacted everyone he knew to be interested in dermatologic history, sent announcements to members who had signed up for a historical seminar he was to give at the Academy that year, shamelessly exploited the fame of the guest speaker, flaunted the delectable meal to be served - in short, behaved in the manner essential to the successful creation of a viable new enterprise. He was ably assisted in this work by Gerald N. Wachs, long time secretary and treasurer of the organization. Three decades later the society is still going strong, and Parish still spins the wheels when necessary.

The menu of the repast served at the first formal meeting of the society is shown below.

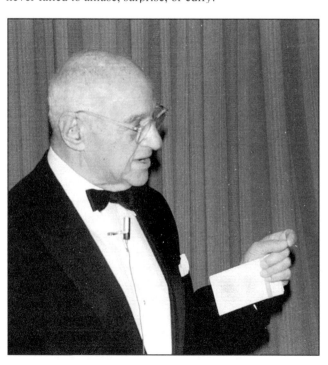

Menu

Consommé, Célestine
...with crêpes fines herbes

* * * *

Salade, Maison Wrigley
...kentucky bibb; hearts of palm and artichoke;
cherry tomato; vinaigrette

* * * *

Roast boneless Strip Sirloin
...Sauce Béarnaise
Potatoes Gaufrettes
Fresh Broccoli, polonaise

* * * *

Coupe, Romanoff
...vanilla; fresh strawberries in kirsch;
pulp of raspberries; chantilly

La Cave

Bourgogne Pinot Noir, André Simon, 1966

John A. Parrish, internist and dermatologist, received his dermatologic training under Thomas Fitzpatrick at Harvard and later succeeded his teacher as chairman of the dermatology department at that school. Like Fitzpatrick he has developed a life-long interest in photobiology. The pair, in collaboration with Lewis Tanenbaum and Madhukar Pathak, developed the novel and highly successful "PUVA" treatment for psoriasis described below. Klaus Wolff of Vienna also participated actively in this work.

Parrish's interests have also expanded into other fields with impressive results. As chairman and director of several large research foundations, he has been engaged in the study of the basic effects of laser radiation on tissue, introduced the procedure known as laser lithotripsy in the treatment of kidney stones, and pioneered in the selective laser treatment of cutaneous vascular lesions, including port wine stains.

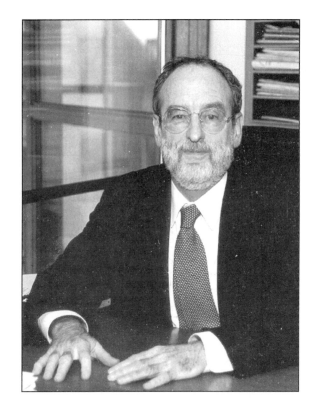

John A. Parrish

Parrish JA, Fitzpatrick TB, Tanenbaum L, Pathak MA. Photochemotherapy of psoriasis with oral methoxsalen and longwave ultraviolet light. New Engl J Med 1974;291:1207-11

Patients' psoriatic lesions were exposed to ultraviolet light emanating from a bed of 48 fluorescent bulbs, newly developed by GTE Sylvania, which emitted a continuous spectrum of high intensity radiation between 320 and 390 nm. Radiation below 320 nm was filtered out by a Mylar plastic sheet. The 8-methoxypsoralen was given by mouth. Sixteen patients were treated; all cleared completely. Conventional ultraviolet light (UVB) was used as a control. Differences in the response were obvious.

This paper generated enormous interest in the dermatologic world. When the results were confirmed by larger controlled studies the procedure, which came to be known as PUVA, took its place as an integral part of anti-psoriatic therapy worldwide.

Right: Figure 2 from the Parrish et al report: Psoriasis, before and after 16 treatments with methoxsalen followed by long wave ultraviolet light.

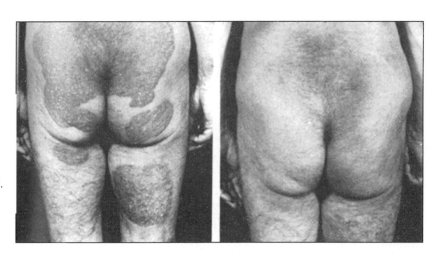

186

Within weeks of publication of the landmark paper of John Parrish et al. on the use of PUVA in the treatment of psoriasis, Klaus Wolff of Vienna set up a treatment center at his university and constructed a practical PUVA "couch." With this design as a starting point the highly respected German firm, H. Waldmann, GmbH + Co. of Schwenningen perfected and marketed in 1974 the PUVA treatment couch shown to the right. Equipped with 320-390 nm emitting tubes, it was the first PUVA machine on the market and was sold successfully in many different countries. Innovative technology such as built-in dosimetry systems and measurement sensors placed Waldmann in the upper eschelons of leadership in the field. Other firms have since developed and marketed excellent machines as well.

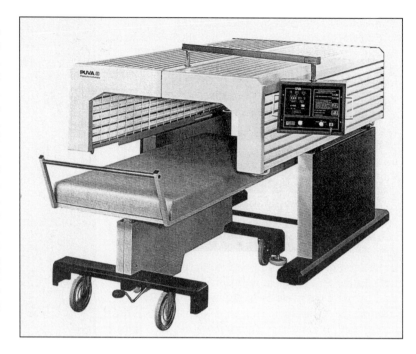

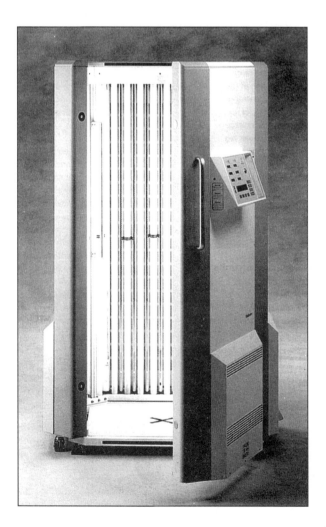

Early "couch" designs soon gave way to the more efficient cabinet or "light box" models in which the standing patient could be treated fore, aft, and laterally at the same time. A modern Waldmann design of this type is shown to the left. Many other specialized configurations have been developed by companies worldwide for partial body radiation or for the treatment of selected areas. One such device for the treatment of the hands is shown below.

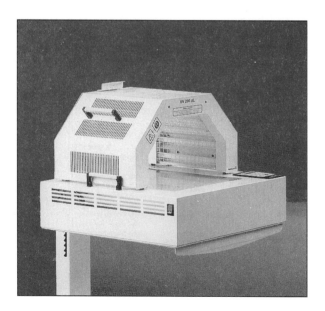

Eugene J. Van Scott, prominent American research dermatologist, received his M.D. from the University of Chicago and his dermatologic training at Chicago and at the University of Pennsylvania.. In 1961 he established and headed the Dermatology Branch at the National Cancer Institute. He later joined the faulty of Temple University School of Medicine in Philadelphia and in 1990 accepted a professorship in the Department of Dermatology at Hahneman University.

Early in his career, Van Scott succeeded in identifying the changes in scalp hair roots that followed exposure to ionizing radiation and the use of chemotherapeutic drugs. Soon after, he made valuable contributions to our knowledge of the kinetics of cell division in scalp hair roots and in normal and psoriatic skin. Of great interest and utility was his demonstration of the effectiveness of whole body application of nitrogen mustard in the production of long lasting remissions in mycosis fungoides. Also of great importance is his 1974 discovery (with Ruey J. Yu) of the remarkable response of ichthyosiform dermatoses to topical applications of the alpha hydroxy acids, as noted below. He later showed that these acids were capable of reversing the cutaneous signs of aging as well.

Retired now from the academic scene, Van Scott continues to engage in self-generated clinical research.

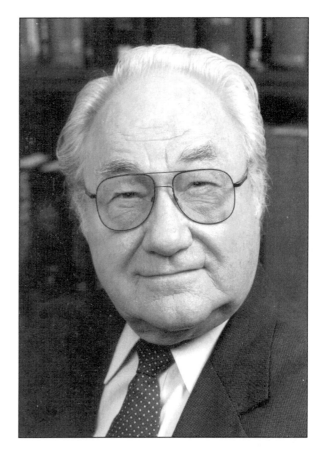

Eugene J. Van Scott

Van Scott EJ, Yu RJ. Control of keratinization with α-hydroxy acids and related compounds. Arch Dermatol

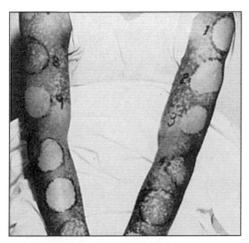

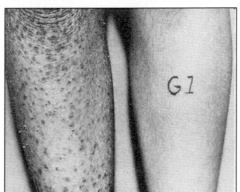

Left: Figures 1 and 2 from Van Scott's classic report of the effects of the alpha hydroxy acids on keratinization.

Figure 1 (top): Test sites on arms of patient with lamellar ichthyosis after four days of thrice daily topical applications of 10% test preparations. Abrupt appearance of normal appearing skin is apparent.

Figure 2 (bottom): Patient with lamellar ichthyosis. Right leg untreated. Left leg treated for three weeks with twice daily applications of 5% glycolic acid.

Fourteen patients with several types of ichtjyosiform dermatoses were treated with topical applications 12 different alpha hydroxy acids and related compounds. Both clinical and histologic responses were noted. The authors concluded that these materials appear to influence the process of keratinization per se, but do not seem to be keratolytic.

188

Jean-Hilaire Saurat, multi-talented French dermatologist working now in Switzerland, received his M.D. in Paris and his dermatologic training at l'Hôpital Saint Louis. From 1969 to 1981, he taught and was engaged in research in experimental pathology at the dermatology unit of the Hôpital Necker Enfants Malades in Paris. In 1981, he accepted the chairmanship of the Western Switzerland Department of Dermatology, headquartered in Geneva.

Recognition came early to Saurat for his work in the 1970s on cutaneous manifestations associated with graft versus host disease (GVHD). The sometimes fatal down side of allogeneic bone marrow transplantions, GVHD occurs most commonly in patients whose donors are unrelated or imperfectly matched, and in its acute form manifests itself early as an erythematous, scaling eruption of hands and feet. In the landmark publications cited and noted below, Saurat and his co-workers identified for the first time an important GVHD eruption characterized by lesions of skin and mucous membranes identical both clinically and histologically with the lesions of idiopathic lichen planus. The lichen planus-like eruption of GVHD may be a sign that more severe manifestations will follow. The hopes that Saurat's discovery would lead to clarifification of the pathogenesis of idiopathic lichen planus have not yet been fulfilled.

In recent years Saurat has been deeply involved in the investigation of the effects of the retinoids on human skin and in studies on the pathogenesis and treatment of toxic epidermal necrolysis.

An accomplished yachtsman, Saurat sails the waters of Lake Geneva and the Mediterranean. He also skis, plays tennis well, and enjoys a good book.

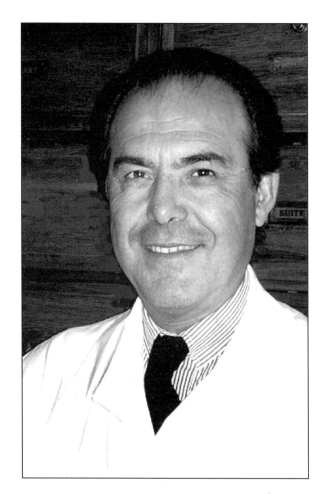

Jean-Hilaire Saurat

Saurat JH, Gluckman E, Bussel A, Didierjean L, Puissant A. The lichen planus-like eruption after bone marrow transplantation. Br J Dermatol

Saurat JH, Gluckman E. Lichen planus-like eruption following bone marrow transplantation: a manifestation of graft-versus-host disease. Clin Exper Dermatol 1977;2:335--44

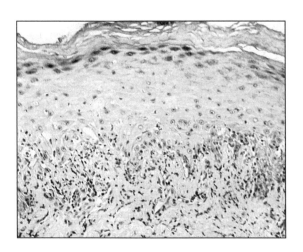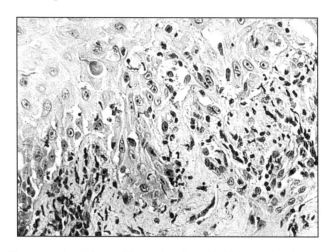

Figures 2 and 3 from the 1975 landmark report of Saurat and colleagues, cited above. Figure 2 – Case II 46 days after the graft (H&E x 100). Figure 3 – Higher magnification of the dermal-epidermal zone (H&E x 250)

John A. Kenney Jr., renowned African-American dermatologist, received his M.D. from Howard University College of Medicine and began his dermatologic training under Herman Beerman at the University of Pennsylvania Graduate School of Medicine. He completed his training with Arthur Curtis at the University of Michigan, set up a private practice in Cleveland, and taught at Western Reserve University in that city. In 1961 he joined the faculty at Howard, and later became chairman of the dermatology department. He retired as chief in 1980, having served with great distinction throughout his academic career.

Kenney's many publications deal for the most part with the special aspects of skin diseases as they appear in black patients. He is an expert in the management of the diseases of pigmentation.

From the beginning Kenney's aim was to train more black physicians in dermatology. In organizing and expanding his department at Howard and insisting at all times on the highest standards of excellence, he provided the ideal setting in which this goal could be achieved. A significant percentage of board certified black dermatologists in North America received their training under the keen and watchful eye of Dr. Kenney.

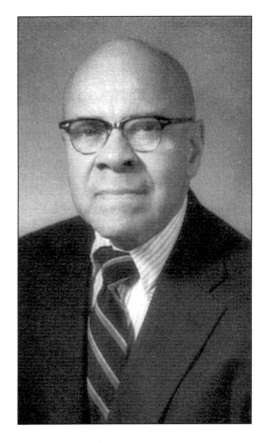

John A. Kenney Jr.

The department of dermatology at Howard began with Henry Honeyman Hazen (1879-1951), a much published Johns Hopkins graduate who made important contributions to the study of black skin dermatology, a subject that has since become traditional at the school. He was succeeded as chief by Charles Wendell Freeman. Freeman convinced John Kenney to leave his busy practice in Cleveland in 1961 to join him at Howard. Kenney took over as chief in 1965 and set up a complete residency training program and a dermatologic research laboratory. At the center of the program is the Howard University Hospital, shown below.

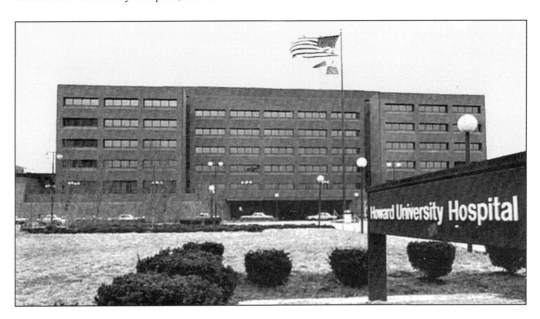

J. Graham Smith Jr., "Skee," as his friends call him, received his dermatologic training at Duke and the University of Miami. He became chief of dermatology at the Medical College of Georgia in 1967, and served later as chief at the University of South Alabama. Basic research occupied much of his time early in his career. He made important contributions to our knowledge of the effects of sun on elastic tissue at the molecular level and studied other damaging effects of solar radiation as well.

Smith has special organizational and planning talents that were soon discovered by colleagues and put to work in dermatologic venues of every description. There is scarcely any leadership position in the specialty he has not held, and in all of them he has acquitted himself with distinction. His role as the founding editor of the *Journal of the American Academy of Dermatology* (JAAD) is described below.

For the past eight years he has been editor in chief of the *Southern Medical Journal.*

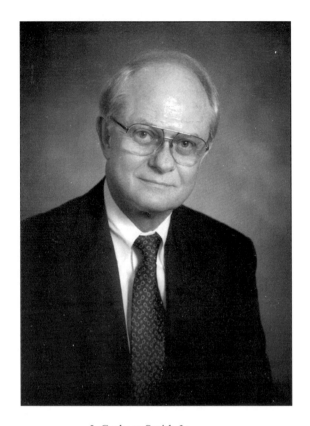

J. Graham Smith Jr.

JOURNAL of the AMERICAN ACADEMY OF DERMATOLOGY

Editors
J. Graham Smith, Jr., M.D. *Editor*
Donald C. Abele, M.D. *Associate Editor*

Assistant Editors
Robert A. Briggaman, M.D.   John H. Epstein, M.D.   Edgar B. Smith, M.D.
Richard L. Dobson, M.D.   John S. Strauss, M.D.

Editorial Board
Philip C. Anderson, M.D.   Leonard C. Harber, M.D.   George F. Odland, M.D.
David R. Bickers, M.D.   G. Thomas Jansen, M.D.   Richard B. Odom, M.D.
D. Martin Carter, M.D.   Stephen I. Katz, M.D.   William F. Schorr, M.D.
Philip M. Catalano, M.D.   Edward A. Krull, M.D.   Peyton E. Weary, M.D.
George W. Hambrick, Jr., M.D. Walter G. Larsen, M.D.   Dennis A. Weigand, M.D.

Volume 1, July-December, 1979

OFFICIAL PUBLICATION OF THE AMERICAN ACADEMY OF DERMATOLOGY

The C. V. Mosby Company, St. Louis, publisher

Published monthly

579

In 1978, the American Academy of Dermatology, then in its 40th year of existence and by far the largest body of its kind in the world, decided it was time it had a journal of its own. Harry Arnold Jr., Rees B. Rees, and John M. Shaw were the movers and shakers at the time. A committee chaired by John S. Strauss was appointed to select an editor. J. Graham Smith, whose executive ability and thorough knowledge of the Academy were combined with both clinical and basic research skills, seemed an ideal candidate. Smith, however, was convinced there were already too many journals devoted to the specialty. He declined at first and accepted only after a certain amount of judicious arm twisting and assurances of the full support of the Academy in all matters of importance. The early years were stormy, but under Smith's management the JAAD became the most successful journal of its kind. Smith's initial five-year commitment extended to ten, and he retired in 1988, after what was by universal agreement a job well done.

The masthead of the first issue of the JAAD is shown to the left.

Howard I. Maibach, indefatigable American research dermatologist, received his M.D. from Tulane University and his dermatologic training at the University of Pennsylvania. In 1961, he joined the faculty of the University of California at San Francisco, where he is now Professor of Dermatology and Chief of the Occupational Dermatology Clinic. Early in his career, he set for himself a research agenda, the main targets of which were contact dermatitis, cutaneous bacteriology, wound care, medical entomology, and percutaneous absorption. On a rotational basis he has managed to make meaningful contributions to each component over the years. All aspects of epicutaneous patch testing and insights into the mechanisms of sensitization have been a part of his work on contact dermatitis. New slants on the staphylococcus and *Candida albicans* have characterized his microbiologic investigations. In the 1960s, he and his colleagues took on the mosquito in a series of investigations that provided new insights into the feeding habits these potentially dangerous pests. He was also able to identify factors that attract and repel mosquitoes, quantitate individual susceptibility, and evaluate the effectiveness of various insect repellents. His work on wound healing anticipated the recent acceptance of occlusive dressings as the therapeutic gold standard. His percutaneous absorption investigations, noted below, have demonstrated convincingly that the value of dermatologic research extends well beyond the confines of the specialty.

A devoted family man, Maibach is also a hiking enthusiast and a connoisseur of art.

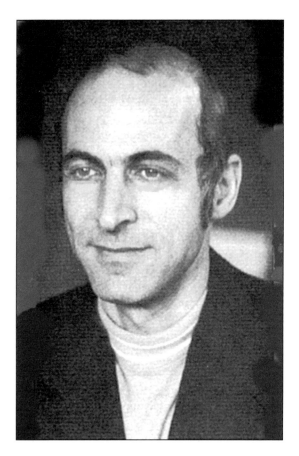

Howard I. Maibach

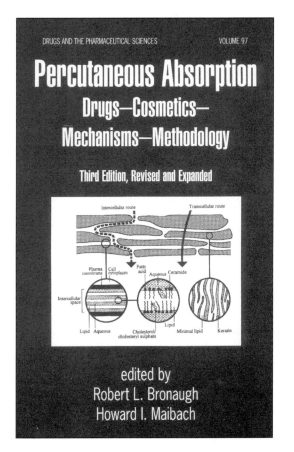

Maibach's interest in percutaneous absorption dates back to the 1960's when he participated in studies on the penetration of topical steroid preparations. Since that time, he has made many valuable contributions to the literature in the field, culminating in 1983 in a seminal work of great importance. With Robert L. Bronaugh of the U.S. Food and Drug Administration, he co-edited and contributed generously to the multi-authored textbook "Percutaneous absorption." The title page of the third edition (1999) is shown to the left. Interest in skin permeation has increased exponentially everywhere as it has become abundantly clear that an understanding of the process is essential to success and security in practical matters as well as theoretical. Skin penetration can be desirable, as in the case of drug delivery systems, or undesirable, as in exposure to potentially toxic agents in substances that may come into contact with the skin. The Bronaugh-Maibach work is therefore essential reading for personnel in the research, legal, and marketing departments of pharmaceutical, cosmetic, and pesticide manufacturers, and a host of other industries.

Maibach's abiding interest and contributions to the field have done a great deal to place dermatology where common sense and expertise indicate it ought to be – deeply involved in everything related to the penetration of substances into and through the skin.

A. Bernard Ackerman, internationally acclaimed dermatopathologist, much-read author, medical publisher, and outspoken idealist, received his M.D. from Columbia and his dermatologic training at Columbia, the Universty of Pennsylvania, and Harvard. He was for many years Professor of Dermatology and Pathology at New York University, and from 1993 to 1999 served in a similar capacity at Jefferson in Philadelphia. In 1999 he returned to New York, where he is associated with Cornell and is the Director of the Ackerman Academy of Dermatopathology.

Ackerman is the founder of two well-known journals, *Dermatopathology: Practical and Conceptual*, and *The American Jounal of Dermatopathology*. He is the author of some 35 books and innumerable scientific reports covering, among other things, the entire gamut of dermatopathology. All are written in a style characterized by unflinching honesty and a willingness to take a stand on the most controversial issues facing the dermatology of today. The best known of his publications, the "Histologic Diagnosis of Inflammatory Skin Diseases," is noted below. Ackerman is also justly proud of his new medical publishing house, Ardor Scribendi, dedicated to the production of "books that have ballast and are beautiful, too."

A dynamic lecturer, Ackerman participates regularly in courses, colloquia, and symposia. He leavens heavy material with asides, bon mots, and unexpected turns of phrase, and is at his pedagogical best at the helm of his 27-headed microscope. He has also emerged as the number one defender of both medical dermatology and dermatopatholgy, disciplines he believes to be headed for extinction if the specialty fails to institute reforms and exert itself vigorously to prevent it.

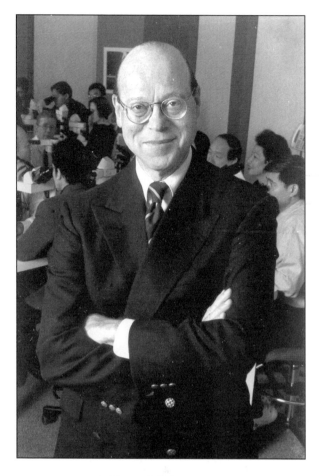

A. Bernard Ackerman

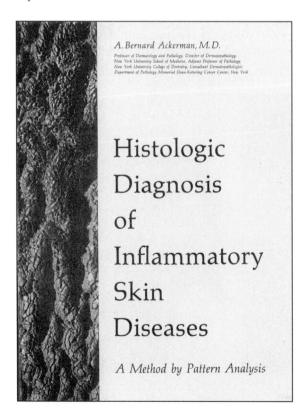

In 1978 Ackerman chose to enter the thorny thicket of inflammatory skin diseases with the intention of laying out the histopathology of these dermatoses in such a way that even the clinically illiterate could arrive at a diagnosis close to the mark. The result was the "Histologic diagnosis of inflammatory skin diseases," the title page of which is shown to the left. His approach was novel. He described the nine major histopathologic patterns peculiar to inflammatory skin diseases, most of which can be identified with the scanning objective of the microscope. Closer observation reveals subsets to these patterns, and often sub-subsets that can be followed in algorithmic fashion until a definitive diagnosis can be made.

Clearly Ackerman correctly perceived both the need for a work of this type and the appeal and utility of his new approach; the book is standard equipment in dermatology departments everywhere. It is often called "the gold book" by the residents, both for its worth and the color of its cover. A second edition appeared in 1997.

Ackerman is an admirer of Heinrich Auspitz and shares with the nineteenth century Viennese master the ability to transform static two-dimensional tissue sections into three-dimensional cellular theater, conveying to students the essential message that lesional changes are works in progress. It is an uncommon gift.

Gary L. Peck, dermatologist and retinoid expert, was graduated M.D. from the University of Michigan School of Medicine in 1962 and received his dermatologic training at the University of Chicago hospitals. From the beginning his preference was for dermatologic research, and in 1969 he joined the faculty of the National Cancer Institute at the NIH.

Peck's early work included investigations of the topical effects of vitamin A acid in psoriasis. In 1975 an opportunity presented itself to study the effects of the recently developed 13 cis-retinoic acid administered orally to patients suffering from several severe and recalcitrant dermatoses. He obtained surprisingly good results in the treatment of Darier's disease, lamellar ichthyosis, and pityriasis rubra pilaris, and noted in some of these patients a facial dermatitis side effect that reminded him of the reactions to topical all-trans retinoic acid observed in his earlier studies. With this in mind, he and his research team chose to treat cystic acne vulgaris (acne conglobata) with the 13 cis form by mouth and were delighted to observe that in a high percentage of cases the medication produced remissions that were long lasting or even permanent. Publication of the landmark paper on the subject noted below was greeted with great enthusiasm by dermatologists everywhere. Nothing other than X-ray (all but unacceptable by the 1970s) really worked in the treatment of cystic acne, and 13 cis-retinoic acid, marketed later as Accutane, soon took its place as the gold standard for the treatment of that condition.

Now associated with the Washington (DC) Hospital Center and the Washington Cancer Institute, Peck maintains a private practice in Bethesda, MD.

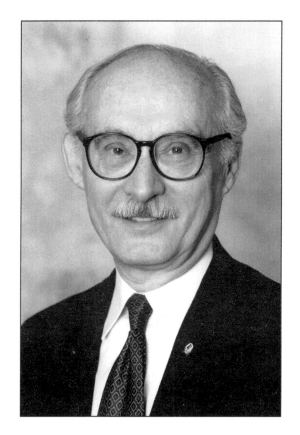

Gary L. Peck

Peck GL, Olsen TG, Yoder FW, Strauss JS, Downing DT, Mangala P, Butkus D, Arnaud-Battandier J. Prolonged remissions of cystic and conglobate acne with 13-cis-retinoic acid. N Engl J Med 1979:300:329-333.

Right: Figure from Peck's landmark paper cited above: Severe cystic acne vulgaris, before and after treatment with 13 cis-retinoic acid by mouth.

Fourteen cases, 8 men and 6 women, were treated. The average age was 24 years. The dose was 2 mg/kg/day, by mouth for 4 months. Thirteen cleared completely, one improved 75%. Side effects were discussed in detail; teratogenic effects were anticipated, and contraceptives were advised for female patients.

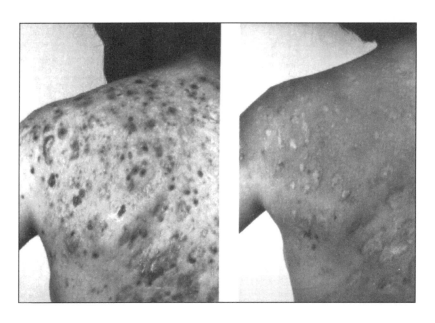

Raul Fleischmajer, much-honored Argentinian-American research dermatologist, received his M.D. from the University of Buenos Aires and his dermatologic training at Bellvue Hospital and New York University. He held a post-doctoral fellowship in biochemistry at New York University from 1960 to 1963, and in 1979 was appointed Professor and Chairman of the Department of Dermatology at the Mount Sinai School of Medicine in New York.

For the past twenty years, Fleischmajer has presided over laboratory facilities at Mt. Sinai engaged in important collagen research, particularly in the study of collagen fibrillogenesis. Among his many contributions are the identification of the amino propeptides of type I and Type III collagens in human skin and the elucidation of collagen fibril formation in embryogenesis. He also pioneered in the study of the cellular infiltrates in scleroderma. Recently, he has turned his attention to investigations on the role of integrin receptors in the formation of the epidermo-dermal junction and on alterations in the basement membrane associated with psoriasis.

Away from the laboratory, Fleischmajer is a history buff and is well versed in all aspects of music. He is also a jogger – at a very slow pace. He calls himself a "slogger."

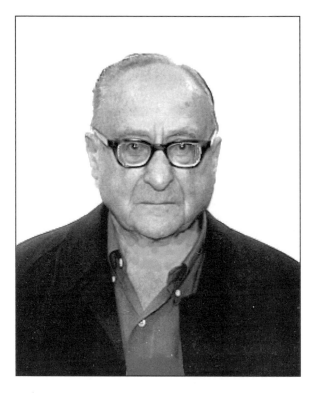

Raul Fleischmajer

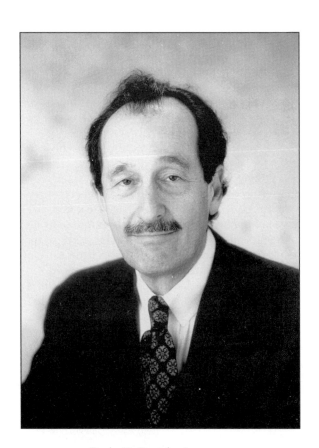

Ervin H. Epstein, Jr.

Son of a highly respected dermatologist, Ervin H. Epstein Jr. received his M.D. from the University of California at San Francisco, and his dermatologic training at the Massachusetts General Hospital, the National Cancer Institute, and New York University. In 1972, he joined the faculty of his San Francisco alma mater, where he continues his research and teaching activities.

Early in his career, Epstein concerned himself with basic collagen research and was among the very first to identify Collagen type III and confirm its presence in human skin. In the 1980s, he began to study of the deficiency of the enzyme steroid sulfatase in recessive x-linked ichthyosis. He realized that it might be possible to clone the DNA encoding this enzyme and identify the mutations responsible. In the pursuit of this goal he was led into the new, exciting, and rapidly expanding field of DNA research in general. His work evolved gradually from the initial approach of isolating genes by making antibodies to isolated proteins to the use of family linkage studies to identify the genes involved. With this approach he and colleagues J.M. Bonifas and A L. Rothman were able in 1991 to establish that epidermolysis bullosa simplex is linked to the keratin gene loci on chromosomes 12 and 17.

As important as the specifics of Epstein's genetic work are his enthusiastic presentations before many forums, calling the attention of dermatologists to the astonishing advances in the understanding of DNA-based diseases.

Jouni J. Uitto, Finnish-American research dermatologist and collagen expert, received his M.D., along with a Ph.D in medical biochemistry, from the University of Helsinki. He trained in dermatology at the Washington University School of medicine in Saint Louis, and since 1986 has been a professor of dermatology, cutaneous biology and biochemistry, and molecular pharmacology at Jefferson Medical College in Philadelphia.

Uitto's career, from the beginning to the present, has been closely associated with investigations on the structure and diseases of the extracellular matrix, the molecular biology and biochemistry of collagen and elastin, and particularly the molecular genetics of the cutaneous basement membrane zone. Our knowledge of epidermolysis bullosa, pseudoxanthoma elasicum, cutaneous photoaging, pachyonycia congenital, bullous pemphigoid, paraneoplastic pemphigus, and the Netherton syndrome has been greatly increased as a result of his assiduous research.

In addition to his innumerable contributions at the basic level, Uitto has been, through both written and spoken word, a potent force in acquainting dermatologists everywhere to the impressive progress being made in the field.

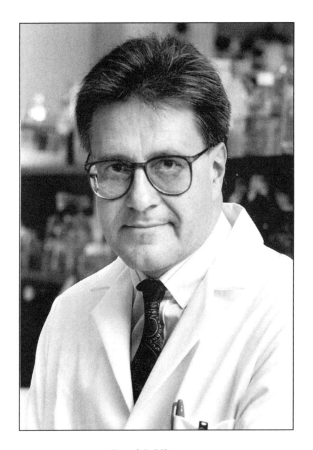

Jouni J. Uitto

Dr. Larry E. Millikan, internationally oriented New Orleans dermatologist, received his M.D. from Monmouth College, University of Missouti and his dermatologic training at the University of Michigan. He has been chairman of the dermatology department at Tulane University since 1981.

Millikan is an acknowledged expert on medical education. He has mastered the art of uniting successfully in his department the potentially divisive factions of modern American dermatology – patient care, clinical research, bench research, and dermatologic surgery. His personal contributions lie in the identification of animal models in melanoma research, in immuno-dermatology, and in the rigorous evaluation of dermatologic medications.

Millikan's influence in dermatologic teaching extends well beyond the borders of the United States. At Tulane, dermatologists from Mexico, Venezuela, Greece, Saudi Arabia, Jordan, and many other countries have trained alongside their American counterparts. The International Society of Dermatology and the International Academy of Cosmetic Dermatology have also benefited greatly from his participationn and counsel.

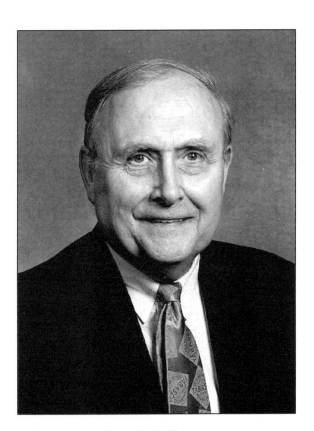

Larry E. Millikan

196

Stephen I. Katz, preeminent and much-honored American research dermatologist, received his M.D. from Tulane University Medical School, and trained in dermatology at the University of Miami. In 1974 he earned a PhD in immunology at the University of London. He has been Chief of the Dermatology Branch at the National Institutes of Health since 1980, and currently serves as Director of the Institute of Arthritis, Musculoskeletal, and Skin Diseases.

From the beginning Katz has been concerned with the skin immune system, focusing particularly on the use of contact dermatitis as a model through which to gain insights into immunologic, inflammatory, infectious, and neoplastic diseases of the skin. He was among the earliest to demonstrate that in addition to producing structural proteins, keratinocytes produce a variety of cytokines, interleukin-1 being the first to be discovered. The functions of these cytokines in the regulation of immune response is under intense scrutiny in his laboratory. Katz has also made valuable contributions to our knowledge of the pemphigus and pemphigoid antigens that serve as targets for autoimmune response.

In his directorial position, Katz is responsible for funding a broad spectrum of dermatologic research activities, from basic science investigations to studies more clinical in nature. He is most proud of his success in converting a large number of dermatologists into bonafide, productive immunodermatologists. Twenty-five of his trainees now chair dermatology departments in North America, Europe, and Japan.

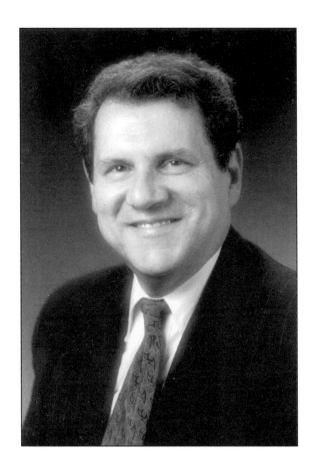

Stephen I. Katz

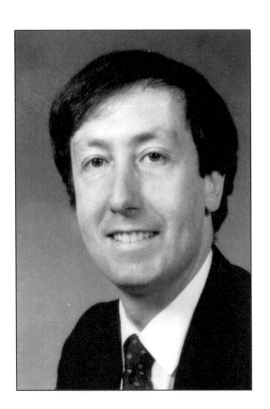

Daniel N. Sauder

Daniel N. Sauder, busy Canadian research dermatologist and cytokine expert, received his M.D. from McMaster University, Ontario, and his dermatologic training at at the U.S. National Institutes of Health and the Cleveland Clinic. In 1990 he was appointed chief of the Division of Dermatology at the University of Toronto, and was associated now with the Sunnybrook Health Science Centre. He is now chairman of the department of dermatology at Johns Hopkins in Baltimore.

Like Stephen Katz, with whom he often collaborated, Sauder personifies the "new model" dermatologist from the 1970s, destined for research from the beginning. Even his earliest reports deal for the most part with basic aspects of skin diseases, immunoregulation, cellular kinetics, and the like. In a landmark 1982 report, he furnished convincing evidence that keratinocytes are capable of synthesizing cytokines, and in particular interleukin-1. In further investigations he demonstrated that Langerhans cells also produce interleulin-1 and that this cytokine is a chemotactic factor for human keratinocytes. Sauder was the first to show that cyclosporine inhibits keratinocyte cytokines as a part of its mechanism of action.

Sauder has also been deeply involved in the evaluation of dermatologic treatment modalities, itraconazole, cyclosporine, immiquimod, calcipotriol , and many more. In 1996, he found time in his busy schedule to found a new publication, the *Journal of Cutaneous Medicine and Surgery*, and served as editor-in-chief during its early years.

David T. Woodley, American research dermatologist and bullous disease authority, received his M.D. from the University of Missouri and his dermatologic training at the University of North Carolina. He spent two years in France as a Research Fellow at the Université de Paris and from 1980 to 1983, served as an Expert Investigator at the National Institutes of Health in Bethesda. In 1992, he became chairman of the dermatology department at Northwestern University in Chicago, and in 1999 joined the faculty of the Keck School of Medicine, University of Southern California.

From the beginning Woodley concentrated his research on the immunology and pathogenesis of the bullous diseases. He participated actively in the exciting investigational events of the 1970s and 80s in which these entities, traditionally shoehorned into the two categories pemphigus and dermatitis herpetiformis, were shown in fact to number nine or more. Among his many contributions were his demonstration that the antigen of bullous pemphigoid is synthesized in vitro by human epidermal cells, and the landmark reports on the identification and characterization of the antigen of epidermolysis bullosa acquisita, noted below. In recent times, Woodley has also involved himself deeply in studies relevant to wound healing, with particular emphasis on the biomechanics of keratinocyte migration.

Away from the laboratory and clinic, Woodley enjoys tennis, bicycling, and basketball with his sons.

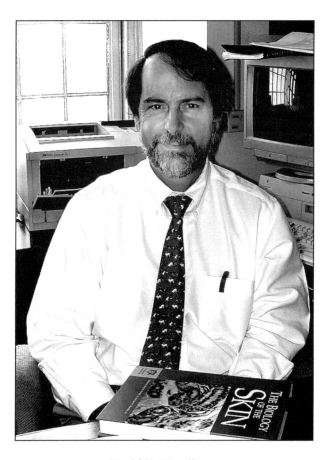

David T. Woodley

Below: Figure 4. Indirect immunofluorescent staining with serum from patient with epidermolysis bullosa acquisita of normal human skin in which epidermis has been separated from the dermis by the induction of a suction blister (x230).

The epidermolysis bullosa acquisita antigen, which is localized to the dermal-epidermal junction of intact skin, remains with the dermis (D) when the skin is separated (arrow). E denotes epidermis and B blister space.

Woodley DT, Briggaman RA, O'Keefe EJ, Inman AO, Queen LL, Gammon WR. Identification of the skin basement membrane autoantigen in epidermolysis bullosa acquisata. New Eng J Med 1984;310:1007-13

For many years the acquired, chronic, scarring, bullous disease known as epidermolysis bullosa acquisita (EBA) remained a questionable entity, suspected by many to be no more than an odd variant of bullous pemphigoid. In the landmark report by Woodley and co-workers cited above, the team investigated nine typical cases in which they identified and characterized a major protein of the basement membrane that served as the target of the autoantibodies in the disease. Figure 4 from this report is shown to the left. Woodley and his group were able later to show that EBA antigen is a connective tissue molecule distinct from laminin, fibronectin, elastin, and collagens I, IV, and V. It is type VII collagen, which is not targeted in any other bullous diseaese. That, QED, established EBA once and for all as an entity properly *sui generis.*

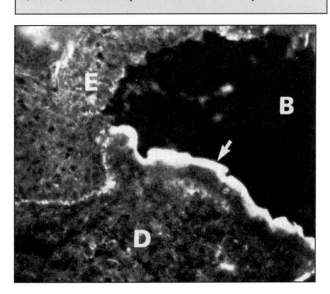

William H. Eaglstein, American dermatologist and wound healing expert, received his M.D. from the University of Missouri and his dermatologic training at the University of Miami. He served as chaiman of the dermatology department at Pittsburgh, and in 1986 became chaiman of the department at Miami.

Eaglstein is responsible to a great extent for the acceptance of wound healing as a legitimate area of interest to dermatology. As early as 1978, he was working to develop new methods for assessing the healing of epidermal injuries, and he pioneered in the clinical development and introduction of occlusive dressing therapy for the healing of cutaneous wounds. Particularly influential in this regard was the 1985 landmark report on biosynthetic dressings noted below. More recently, he has worked with composite skin substitutes, tissue engineered skin, and was the first to introduce these materials in the management of human surgical wounds.

Eaglstein has also made a pair observations of importance to the practicing dermatologist in his everyday work. He demonstrated that systemic steroids do not lead to the dissemination of zoster, and showed that removing tissue for biopsy from the edge of an ulcer does not result in enlargement of the lesion. On the more basic level, he clarified the mechanism of action of fluorouracil in the destruction of actinic keratoses and showed that the prostaglandin inhibitor, indomethacin, blocks the early stages of ultraviolet light induced inflammation.

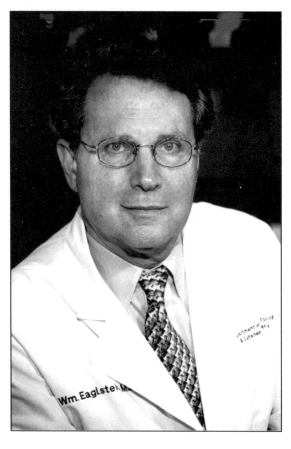

William H. Eaglstein

Eaglstein WH. Experiences with biosynthetic dressings. J Am Acad Dermatol 1985;12:434-40

Although some of the advantages of occlusive dressings and " moist wound healing" had been recognized by G.D. Winter, Howard Maibach, and others in the 1970s, fear of an increased incidence of infection, largely unjustified, retarded the commercial development of dressings designed to occlude. All that changed in the 1980s, when a number of new products appeared, marketed under the registered trade names Op-site, Tegaderm, Bioclusive, Vigilon, and Duoderm. In the widely discussed 1985 report cited above, Eaglstein called attention to the advantages and disadvantages of the new dressings, as indicated in the table from his paper, shown to the left. The "pros" outweighed the "cons," and the dermatologic world for the most part changed its approach to wound management from dry to wet.

Table IV. Advantages and disadvantages of occlusive dressings

Advantages	Disadvantages
Rapid healing	Accumulation of pus
Reduced pain	Hematoma or seroma
Fewer dressing changes	Silent infections
Exclusion of microorganisms	Folliculitis
Better cosmetic results	Need for healthy borders
	Trauma to adjacent skin
	Adherence to new tissue
	? Allergy
	Fear of infection
	Retarding of gain in tensile strength

Jeffrey A. Klein, California dermatologist and the originator of the revolutionary "tumescent" technique for liposuction, received his M.D. from the University of California at San Francisco and his dermatologic training at the University of California at Irvine (UCI). He is an associate clinical professor of the dermatology at UCI.

Liposuction was first developed in the 1970s by Arpad and Giorgio Fischer in Italy, and the early techniques were improved by Pierre Fournier and Illouz of Paris. The initial enthusiasm that greeted the work of these men and their immediate successors diminished when serious complications began to be reported. The procedure was given a new life when Klein developed his tumescent technique and described his innovations and impressive results in the classic 1987 report cited below. The Klein procedure included the injection of relatively large volumes of a dilute solution of lidocaine and epinephrine into the operative sites permitting the nearly bloodless removal of large quantities of fat without the need for general anesthesia. Smaller sized, blunt tipped cannulas, and post operative elastic support garments were also employed. The technique caught on immediately, and with improvements subsequently made by Klein and others has become standard. Klein has shared his knowledge in lectures, seminars, courses, and in hands-on instruction in his private office in San Juan Capistrano. Liposuction is now one of the most popular forms of dermatologic cosmetic or restorative surgery.

The figures shown below appeared in Klein's original report. Left: Lines drawn on the patient's abdomen prior to liposuction indicate the path along which the anesthetic solution is injected. Curved lines represent the contours of targeted fat compartments. Right: The Klein Needle allows deposition of vasoconstrictive/anesthetic solution exactly along the paths intended for the liposuction cannula. The IV line has a one-way check valve (cv) that prevents retrograde flow. After the needle is inserted into the subcutaneous fat and the flow regulator clamp (frc) is opened, the syringe is filled (or emptied) simply by pulling (or pushing) on the syringe plunger.

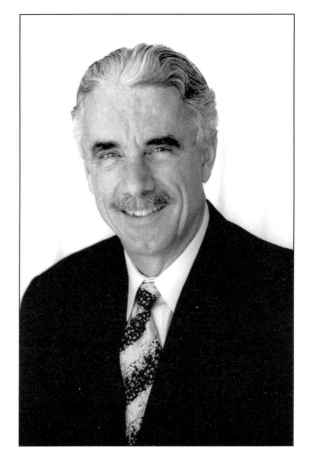

Jeffrey A. Klein

Klein JA. The tumescent technique for lipo-suction surgery. J Cosmet Surg 1987;4:263-7

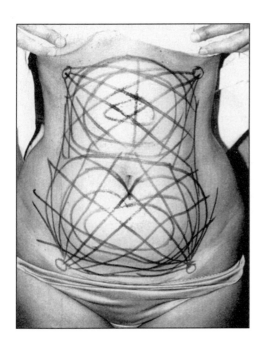

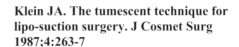
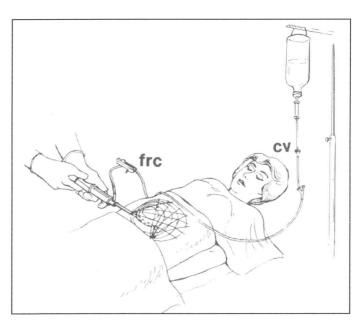

We have come a long way from the tentative ruby laser experiments of Leon Goldman in the early 1960s. The results of laser treatment of a significant number of dermatologic conditions have been so impressive that the presence of these instruments offices and clinics has become commonplace, and instruction in laser use is now an essential part of dermatologic training programs.

Destruction of melanocytic lesions began as early as the 1960s with normal mode ruby lasers and later argon lasers. Results have been improved with the development of Q-switched ruby, Nd:YAG, and alexandrite lasers. Since the 1980s, similar instruments have been used effectively in the treatment of tattoos. Lasers are chosen that emit wavelengths of light maximally absorbed by the different ink colors in the tattoo in accordance with the R.R. Anderson–John Parrish principle of selective thermolysis put forward in 1983.

Pulsed dye lasers have been used with great success in the treatment of port wine stains and other vascular lesions. Skin resurfacing to ameliorate the cosmetic damage associated with photoaging began in the 1980s, but caught fire in 1990s with development of Er:YAG and improved carbon dioxide lasers, which made the procedure much safer.

Recently, several new lasers and other light sources have been developed for the removal of unwanted hair. Results are encouraging.

The development of cleverly designed cooling devices to be used in conjunction with laser treatment to reduce the amount of unwanted thermal damage and associated discomfort has improved both results and patient acceptance.

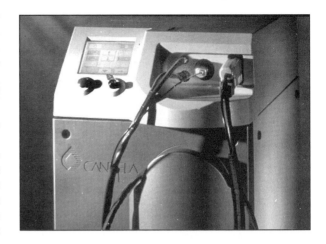

Modern pulsed dye laser (Candela Corporation, V-beam pulsed dye laser)

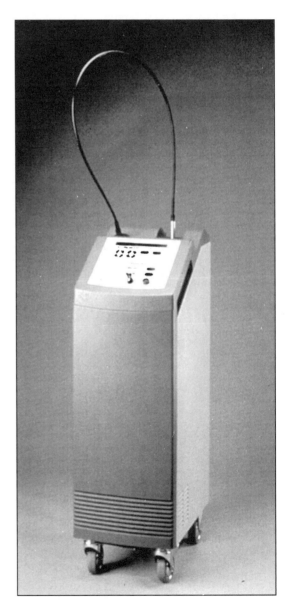

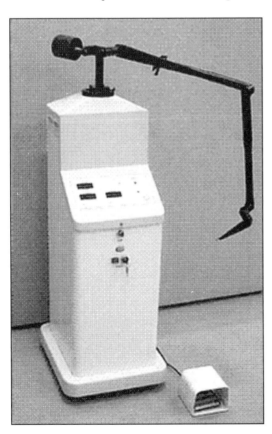

Modern carbon dioxide skin resurfacing laser (Tissue Medical Lasers Corporation, Tru-Pulse laser)

Modern alexandrite laser (Candela Corporation, ALEXlazr)

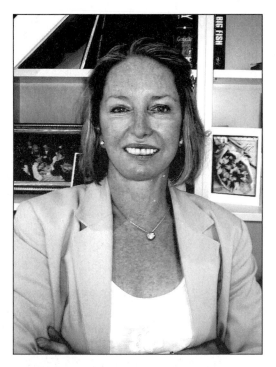

Jean Carruthers

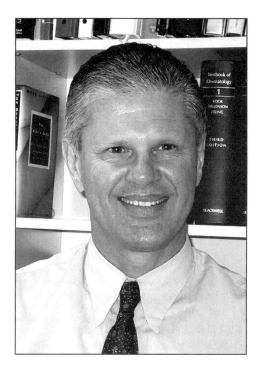

Alastair Carruthers

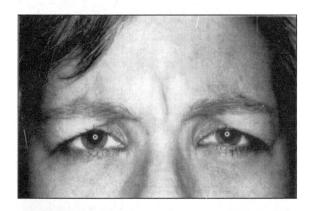

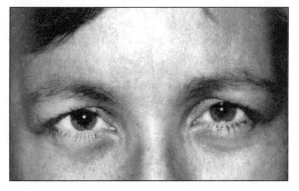

Before and after exotoxin injections, from the Carruthers' paper. Upper: intentional frown accentuates already prominent glabellar frown line. Lower: after exotoxin injection the line no longer appears, even when the patient attempts to produce it.

Carruthers JDA, Carruthers JA. Treatment of glabellar frown lines with C. botulinum-A exotoxin. J Dermatol Surg Oncol 1992;18:17-21

Jean Carruthers, ophthalmologist and cosmetic surgeon, collaborated with her husband, Alastair, a surgical dermatologist, in this persuasive study of local botulinum toxin injections in the treatment of glabellar frown lines. Both physicians are University of British Columbia (Canada) faculty members. The exotoxin had been employed earlier in the treatment of several ophthalmologic and neurologic conditions, but this report introduced it to the dermatologic world.

The medication is expensive and the results temporary, but the procedure is acceptably safe and is superior to any available alternative. It has become extremely popular with those individuals who are convinced that a permanently furrowed brow presents to the world a face at variance with a pleasant inner self. Acceptance and performance of the injections by dermatologists everywhere is still another sign of the inexorable trend of the specialty in North America away from exclusive concerns with disease and toward the inclusion of procedures designed to improve appearance.

The exotoxin, marketed as Botox ®, later proved to be useful in the management of hyperhidrosis.

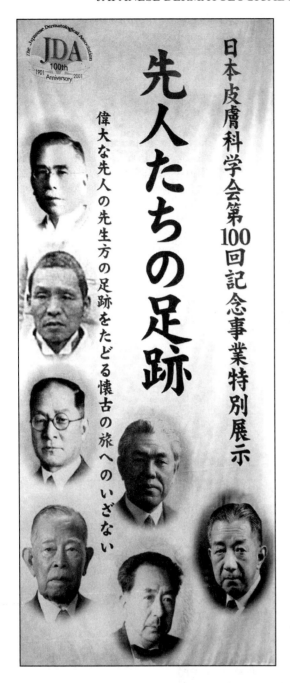

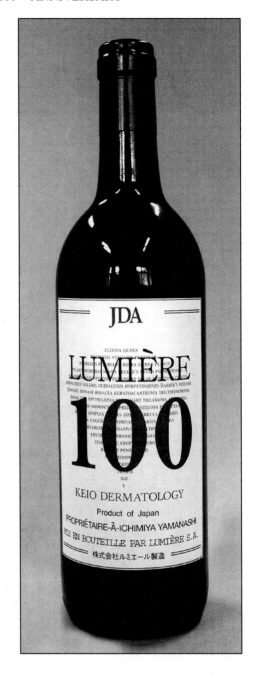

On 8 April 2001, 3200 participants, foreign and domestic, gathered at the Keio Plaza Hotel in Tokyo to celebrate the 100th anniversary of the founding of the Japanese Dermatological Association (JDA). Takeji Nishikawa, Professor of Dermatology at Keio University, presided over a three-day meeting that included scientific presentations along with celebratory activities. The society was founded a century earlier in Tokyo, with Keizo Dohi as its first president. There was at the time only one department of dermatology in Japan, and the founding members of the JDA numbered fifty. Membership today exceeds four thousand.

Among the memorabilia prepared for the present meeting are the two shown above, a banner featuring photographic portraits of the past presidents of the society, and a fine vintage, bottled specifically for the occasion. The names of the dermatologists featured on the banner are as follows - Left column, top to bottom: Keizo Dohi (1866-1931), Ushitaro Matsuura (1865-1937), Ikuzo Toyama (1877-1951), Seigo Minami (1893-1975). Middle column, top to bottom: Masao Ota (1885-1945), Minoru Ito (1894-1982). Right column: Kanehiko Kitamura (1899-1989). The text lines on the banner read R to L: "Japanese Dermatological Association 100th annual meeting memorial program, special exhibition." – "The Footprints of the founders of Japanese dermatology." – "An invitation to follow in the footsteps of the great founders of Japanese dermatology." Beneath the large "100" on the wine bottle label is printed a select list of dermatologic conditions – psoriasis, dermatitis herpetiformis , and the like - a clever and fitting touch to indicate the nature of the of the activities that brought the participants together.

The influential 1969 report presented to the National Institutes of Health by the Joint Committee on Planning for Dermatology recommended, among many other things, the establishment of a national biomedical communications network for the specialty. That recommendation resulted eventually in an informational leviathan that neither the committee chairman Rudolf Baer nor any of his colleagues could possibly have imagined. A task force, headed by Alfred Kopf and Darrell Rigel, was formed by the American Academy of Dermatology (AAD) and with the help of many volunteers spent the next decade assembling dermatologic databases of various kinds and searching out the best way to put dermatologists in touch with this information by electronic means. By 1986, a system had been developed that connected users' personal computers by phone to large computers maintained at the national headquarters of the AAD, and it was announced with pride in the landmark paper cited below. The hardware then in use is also shown below. Its monochromatic mini-monitor, five and a quarter inch floppy drive, and funky acoustical modem look a bit quaint now, but the combination successfully delivered quantities of information that would have taken many hours to dig out in the library, and it did so with what was for the time incredible speed. Dubbed the "Derm/Infonet," this impressive development served yet another purpose; it functioned as a training ground for a sizeable cadre of computer-literate dermatologists and helpers who were well prepared to take advantage of the next great advance in informational technology, the Internet.

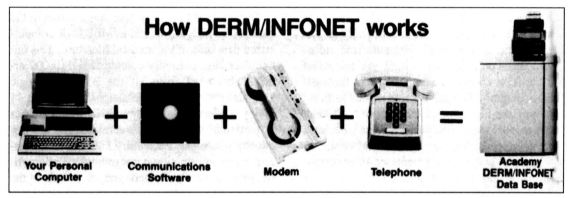

Kopf AW, Rigel DS, White R, Rosenthal L, Jordan WP, Carter DM, Everett MA, Moore J. Derm/Infonet: a concept becomes a reality. J Am Acad Dermatol 1988;18:1150-57

Ray TL, Collison DW. The American Academy of Dermatology on the World Wide Web. Dermatol Online J 1995;1:1-6

Although the Internet has its early roots in the 1960s, it remained to a great extent a tool for computer cognoscenti until the development in the 1990s of "hypertext" style programs that made it a great deal easier to use. In 1995, previously independent consumer networks such as America Online, Prodigy, and Compuserve linked themselves to the Internet, and the number of users shot up exponentially. In the same year a decision was made by the AAD to create a server-based World Wide Web site on the Internet for the benefit of the dermatologic community. To this end, the Academy appointed a task force, the members of which were Walter G. Larsen (chairperson), Daniel W. Collison, Scott M. Dinehart, Stephanie H. Pincus, Thomas L. Ray, and Lawrence E. Rosenthal. The frenetic and exhausting efforts that went into the creation of the Academy website are well described in the landmark paper by Ray and Collison cited above. Both authors were key players in the project.

The Academy of course was not the only dermatologic entity interested in the Internet, nor were Internet activities confined to the United States. Throughout the 1990s websites were set up worldwide by university dermatology departments, group practices, individual practitioners, and patient advocacy groups. Chat rooms appeared, giving voice to disgruntled patients, holistic and alternative medicine enthusiasts, hucksters, and desperate sufferers seeking help. By 1995, dermatologic informational difficulties had become exactly the opposite of those encountered in earlier times. The dearth of information on skin diseases in the 19th century had given way in the 20th to informational overload. The trend continues. It is an odd skin disease indeed that fails to appear on the monitor one way or another when summoned up by our efficient computer search engines. The danger in this embarrassment of riches lies in the fact that a significant portion of the information furnished is suspect, incomplete, outdated, or wrong; that constitutes a problem both for physicians looking for expert help and patients who with increasing frequency regard the Internet as a convenient route to a second opinion. It was the inaccuracy evident in many Internet postings that motivated the Academy to set up its own website in the first place, but the problem persists. *Caveat lector.*

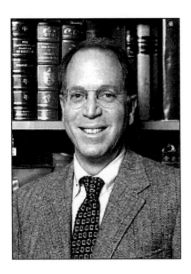

Jeffrey D. Bernhard
Worcester, Massachusetts

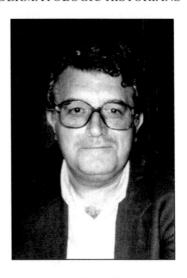

Joaquin Calap Calatayud
Cadiz, Spain

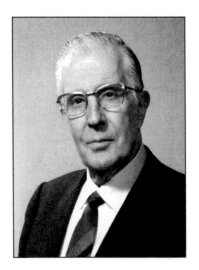

Aureliano Da Fonseca
Porto, Portugal

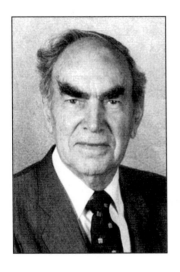

R. Roy Forsey
Montreal, Canada

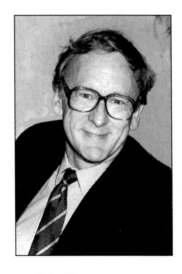

John Hunter
Edinburgh, Scotland

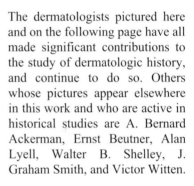

The dermatologists pictured here and on the following page have all made significant contributions to the study of dermatologic history, and continue to do so. Others whose pictures appear elsewhere in this work and who are active in historical studies are A. Bernard Ackerman, Ernst Beutner, Alan Lyell, Walter B. Shelley, J. Graham Smith, and Victor Witten.

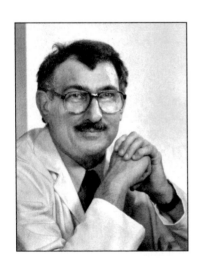

Robert Jackson
Ottawa, Canada

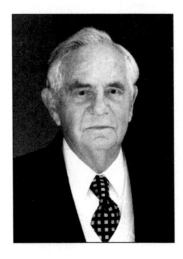

Willard L. Marmelzat
Los Angeles, California

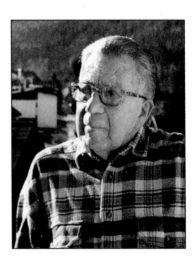

Emiliano Panconesi
Florence, Italy

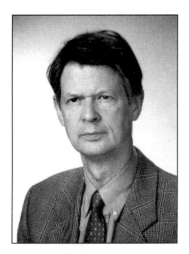

Albrecht Scholz
Dresden, Germany

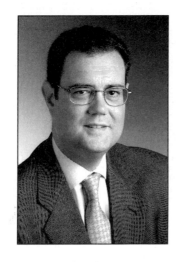

Xavier Sierra
Terrassa, Spain

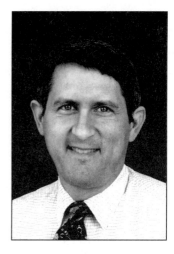

Robert J. Thomsen
Los Alamos, New Mexico

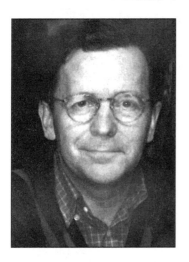

Gerard Tilles
Paris, France

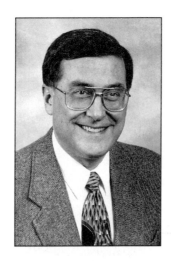

Mark C. Valentine
Everett, Washington

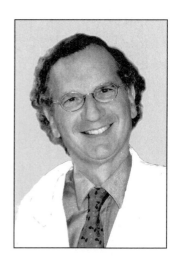

Daniel Wallach
Paris, France

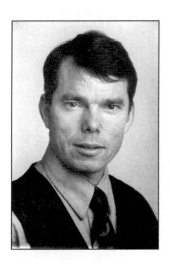

Wolfgang Weyers
Freiburg, Germany

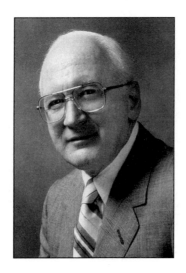

Joseph A. Witkowski
Philadelphia, Pennsylvania

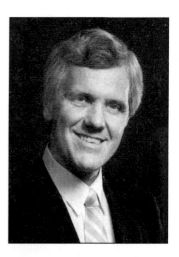

John E. Wolf Jr.
Houston, Texas

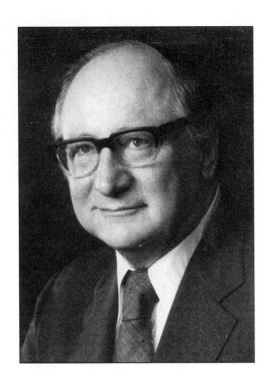

John Thorne Crissey

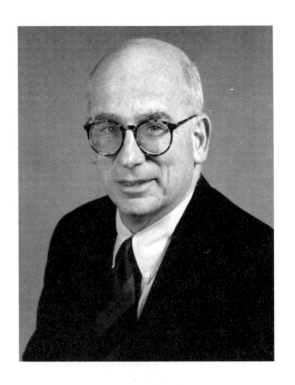

Lawrence Charles Parish

THE AUTHORS

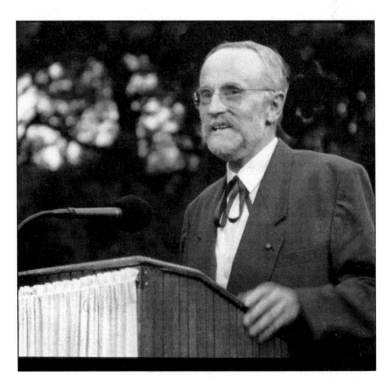

Karl Holubar

REFERENCES AND PICTURE SOURCES

EARLY OBSERVATIONS

Ancient Egyptian dermatology
    Picture source: Breasted JH. The Edwin Smith Surgical Papyrus, Chicago, University of Chicago Press, 1930, V. 1, p. 506.
    Ghalioungui P. Magic and Medical Science in Ancient Egypt, New York, Barnes and Noble, 1963
    Leake CD. The Old Egyptian Medical Papyri, Lawrence, Kansas, University of Kansas Press, 1952

Aristotle and lice
    Picture source: authors' collection
    Rayer P. Theoretical and practical treatise on the diseases of the skin, Philadelphia, Carey and Hart, 1845. p 395

Celsus and alopecia areata
    Picture source: authors' collection
    Collier GF. A translation of the eight books of Aul. Corn. Celsus on medicine, London, Simpkin and Marshall, second edition, 1831. p 222

Mercurialis and the first book on skin diseases
    Picture source: Mercurialis, authors' collection
    Mercurialis H. De morbis Cutaneis, Venice, Paulus and Antonium Meietos, 1572
    Sutton RL Jr. Sixteenth century physician and his methods, Mercurialis on diseases of the skin. Kansas City, The Lowell Press, 1986

Captain Smith and poison ivy
    Picture source: authors' collection
    Smith J. Journal excerpt, cited by McNair, JB, Rhus Dermatitis, Chicago, University of Chicago Press, 1923. p 1
    Unsigned article. Smith, John. The New Encyclopedia Britannica, Chicago, Encyclopedia Britannica Inc., 1974, 15th ed., Vol 10. p 895-6

Bernardino Ramazzini and percutaneous absorption
    Picture source: authors' collection
    Ramazzini B. Diseases of workers. Chicago, IL, Translation of Wilmer Cave Wright. University of Chicago Press, 1940, p xiii-xliv. p 45-6

EIGHTEENTH CENTURY "PROTODERMATOLOGISTS"

Daniel Turner
    Picture source: authors' collection
    Lane, J. E., Daniel Turner and the First Degree of Doctor of Medicine Conferred in the English Colonies of North America by Yale College in 1723. Ann Med Hist. 1919;2:367-80
    Wadd W. Nugae Chirurgicae, London, J. Nichols and Son, 1824, p. 154
    Turner D. De Morbis Cutaneis, 4th Ed., London, Walthoe, Wilkin, etc., 1731. p 312

Lyell A. Daniel Turner (1667-1740) LRCP London (1711) MD Honorary, Yale
(1723). Surgeon, physician and pioneer dermatologist: the man seen in the pages
of his book on the skin. Internat J Dermatol 1982;21:162-70

Lorry and his treatise

Picture source: authors' collection

Bayle and Thillaye. Biographie médicale, Amsterdam, B.M. Israel, 1967, V. 2. p
215-20

Huard P, Imbault-Huart MJ. Dictionary of scientific biography, New York,
Charles Scribners and Sons, 1973, V. 8. p 505-7

Rayer P. Theoretical and practical treatise on the diseases of the skin,
Philadelphia, Carey and Hart, 1845. p 17

Josef Plenck

Picture source: author's collection

Lane JE. Joseph Jacob Plenk [sic], Arch. Dermatol. Syphilol., 1933;28:193-214.

Graefer, R., cited by Neuberger, M., Das alte medizinische Wien in
Zeitgenössischen Schilderungen, Vienna, Moritz Perles, 1921. p 96.

EARLY NINETEENTH CENTURY DERMATOLOGY:
FOUNDING OF THE ENGLISH AND FRENCH SHOOLS

Robert Willan, founder of modern dermatology

Picture source: authors' collection

Booth CC, Robert Willan, M.D., F.R.S., F.S.A., Br. J. Dermatol. 1968;80:459-68

Hare PG. A Note on Robert Willan's Edinburgh Days. Br J Dermatol
1933;88:615-17

MacCormac H. At the Public Dispensary with Willan and Bateman, Br. J.
Dermatol 1933; 45:385-95

B. (Thomas Bateman), Biographical Memoir of the Late Dr. Willan, Edin Med
Surg J 1812;8:502-12

Crissey JT, Parish LCTwo hundred years of dermatology. J Am Acad Dermatol
1998;39:1002-1006

Thomas Bateman

Picture source: authors' collection

J. R. (J. Rumsey), Some account of the life and character of the late Thomas
Bateman, M.D., F.L.S., 2nd ed., London, Longman, Rees, Orme, etc., 1827.

Bateman T. A Practical Synopsis of Cutaneous Diseases, 3rd ed., London,
Longman, Hurst, Rees, etc., 1814

Baron Jean Louis Alibert

Picture sources: authors' collection; Desbordes painting, Prof. Daniel Wallach,
Paris

Alfaric AJL. Alibert, Fondateur de la Dermatologie en France. Paris, Baillière,
1917.

Brodier LJL. Alibert, Médecin de l'Hôpital Saint-Louis. Paris, A. Maloine et fils,
1923.

Huard P, Imbault-Huart MJ.l'École Dermatologique de Saint-Louis, Hist Sci Wd
1974;8:703-20

Siboutie P. Souvenirs d'un Médecin de Paris. Paris, Plon-Nourrit, 1910, 2nd ed. p 103-6.

Hardy A. Documents pour Servir à l'Histoire de l'Hôpital Saint-Louis au Commencement de çe Siècle. Ann Dermatol Syphilig 1885;6:629-38

Laurent Biett

Picture source: Institute for the History of Medicine, University of Vienna

Crissey JT, Parish LC. Dermatology and syphilology of the nineteenth century. New York, Praeger, 1981. p 47-8

Hardy A.. Documents pour Servir à l'Histoire de l'Hôpital Saint-Louis au Commencement de çe Siècle. Ann Dermatol Syphilig 1885;6:629-638

Tilles G, Wallach D. Robert Willan and the French Willanists. Brit J Dermatol 1999;140:1122-26

Renucci and the scabies mite

Picture source: Nékám L. Corpus Iconum Morborum Cutaneorum. Leipzig, Johann Ambrosius Barth, 1938

Crissey JT, Parish LC. Dermatology and syphilology of the nineteenth century. New York, Praeger, 1981. p 60-79

Luca Stulli and mal de meleda

Picture source: portrait, Dr. Stella Fatovic-Ferencic, Zagreb

Shelley WB, Crissey JT. Classics in Clinical Dermatology, Springfield, Ill., Charles Thomas, 1953. p 48-50

Johann Lukas Schoenlein and favus

Picture source: Institute for the History of Medicine, University of Vienna

Crissey JT, Parish LC. Dermatology and syphilology of the nineteenth century. New York, Praeger, 1981. p 97-8

THE FRENCH WILLANISTS

Pierre Rayer

Picture source: authors' collection

Beeson BB. Pierre François Rayer. Arch Dermatol Syphilol 1930;22:893-97

Rayer PF. Traité théorique et pratique des maladies de la peau. Paris, J.B. Baillière, 2nd ed., 1835, plate xxi

Gibert and pityriasis rosea

Picture source: authors' collection

Caffe (n.i.). Nécrologie (Camille-Melchior Gibert), J Conn Méd Prat Pharm, 1866;33:367-368

Beeson, BB. Camille Melchior Gibert. Arch Dermatol Syphilol 1934;30:101-03

Gibert, CM. A Practical Treatise on the Special Diseases of the Skin, 2nd ed., London, John Churchill, 1845. p 55

Alphée Cazenave

Picture source: authors' collection

Goodman H. Alphée Cazenave. Urol Cutan Rev 1947;51:301-3

Goodman H. Alphée Cazenave, Notable contributers to the knowledge of dermatology. New York, Medical Lay Press, 1953. p 187-90

Alphonse Devergie, eczema expert

Picture source: authors' collection.
Beeson BB. Alphonse Devergie. Arch Dermatol Syphilol 1939;21:1030-32
Crissey JT, Parish LC. Dermatology and syphilology of the nineteenth century.
New York, Praeger, 1981. p 334-5
Devergie A. Traité Pratique des Maladies de la Peau, 2nd ed., Paris, Masson,
1857. p 231
Devergie A. Traité Pratique des Maladies de la Peau Paris, Masson, 1854. p 237.

EARLY AMERICAN DERMATOLOGY

Henry Daggett Bulkley and his lectures
Picture sources: authors' collection
Bulkley HD. Clinical lectures on diseases of the skin. New York Med Times
1854;3:351-430

Noah Worcester and his pioneering treatise
Picture sources: authors' collection
Pusey WA. Noah Worcester, A.M., M.D., Pioneer Internist and Dermatologist in
the Middle West. Arch Dermatol Syphilol 1933;27:825-832
Marmelzat WL. Noah Worcester, M.D. - The Forgotten Pioneer. Ohio State Med
J 1948;44:282-84

MID-NINETEENTH CENTURY LEADERS

Karl Gustav Theodor Simon
Picture sources: authors' collection
Waldeck (n.i.). C.G.T. Simon. Allgem Med Centr Zeit 1857;26:446-8, 454-5
Simon GT. Ueber eine in den kranken und normalen Haarsacken des Menschen
lebende Milbe. Arch f Anat Physiol Wissenschf Med 1842, p 218-37.

Ferdinand Hebra and the Vienna school
Picture sources: authors' collection
Crissey JT, Parish LC. Dermatology and syphilology of the nineteenth century.
New York, Praeger, 1981. p 163-77
Lesky E. The Vienna Medical School of the 19th century, Baltimore, Johns
Hopkins University Press, 1976. p 128-40

Erasmus Wilson
Picture sources: authors' collection
Crissey JT, Parish LC. Dermatology and syphilology of the nineteenth century.
New York, Praeger, 1981. p 133-44
Wilson E. Leichen planus. J Cutan Med 1869;3:117-132

William Tilbury Fox
Picture sources: portrait, authors' collection; impetigo, Fox T, Atlas of skin
diseases. London: J. and A. Churchill, 1877
Unsigned obit. Brit Med J 1879;1:915
Fox WT. On impetigo contagiosa or porrigo. Brit Med J 1864;1:467

Ernest Bazin and the diatheses.
Picture source: authors' collection.

Beeson B. Ernest Bazin, a sketch of his life and his works. Arch Dermatol Syphilol 1929;20:866-72

Crissey JT, Parish LC. Dermatology and syphilology of the nineteenth century. New York, Praeger, 1981. p 150-62

Bazin E. Recherches sur la nature et le traitement des teignes. Paris, Poassielgue, Masson, 1853

Bazin E. Scrofulides érythémateuses, in Leçons théoriques et cliniques sur la scrofula. Paris, Adrien Delahaye, 2nd ed, 1861. p 146

Alfred Hardy and his photographic atlas

Picture source: portrait, authors' collection

Hardy A, de Montmâeja A, Clinique photographique des maladies de la peau. Paris, H. Lauwereyns, 1868.

Hallopeau H. Le Professeur Hardy. Ann Dermatol Syphilig 1893;4:113-15,

Beeson B. Alfred Hardy. Arch Dermatol Syphilol 1930;21:108-11

Fox GH. Reminiscences. New York, Medical Life, 1926. p 117.

LATE NINETEENTH CENTURY BRITISH DERMATOLOGY

"Brooke of Manchester"

Picture source: authors' collection

Graham-Little E. A Retrospect of Dermatology in Great Britain, in De Dermatologia et Dermatologis, edit. by L. Nékam, Budapest, International Congress Committee, 1936. p 140-50.

Henry Radcliffe-Crocker

Picture source: authors' collection

Unsigned obit., Henry Radcliffe Crocker, M.D., F.R.C.P., with add. by Butlin HT, Pernet G, Br Med J 1909;ii:729-32

Williams D, Taylor LT. Obituary:Henry Radcliffe Crocker, M.D., F.R.C.P. Brit Med J 1909;2:729-32

Graham-Little E., A Retrospect of Dermatology in Great Britain, in De Dermatologia et Dermatologis, edit. by L. Nékam, Budapest, International Congress Committee, 1936. p 140-50.

Thomas Colcott Fox

Picture source: authors' collection

Pringle J, Adamson H. Obituary, Thomas Colcott Fox. Br J Dermatol 1916;28:93

Graham-Little E. A Retrospect of Dermatology in Great Britain, in De Dermatologia et Dermatologis, edit. by L. Nékam, Budapest, International Congress Committee, 1936. p 140-50.

John James Pringle and adenoma sebaceum

Picture source: authors' collection

Morgan R, Wolfort F. The early history of tuberous sclerosis. Arch Dermatol 1979;115:1317-19

Graham-Little E. Obituary J.J. Pringle. Brit J Dermatol 1923;35:43

Malcolm Morris and the "BJD"

Picture source, author's collection.

Graham-Little E. Retrospect of Dermatology in Great Britain, in De Dermatologia et Dermatologis, edit. by Nékam L, Budapest, International Congress Committee, 1936. p 140-50.

Jonathan Hutchinson

Picture source: authors' collection

Klauder JV. Sir Jonathan Hutchinson. Med Life 1934;41:313-27

Wales AE. Sir Jonathan Hutchinson. Br J Vener Dis 1963;39:67-86

Graham-Little E., A Retrospect of Dermatology in Great Britain, in De Dermatologia et Dermatologis, edit. by L. Nékam, Budapest, International Congress Committee, 1936. p 140-50.

Hutchinson J. On the means of recognising the subjects of inherited syphilis in adult life. Med Times Gaz Sept. 11, 1858. p 264-65

LATE 19TH CENTURY AUSTRIAN DERMATOLOGY

Isidor Neumann

Picture source: authors' collection

Rille JH. Isidor v. Neumann, Deut Med Wchnschr 1906;52:2119-2120

Crissey JT, Parish LC. Dermatology and syphilology of the nineteenth century. New York, Praeger, 1981. p 252-54, 315

Neumann I. Beitrag zur Kenntnis des Pemphigus. Wiener Med Wchnschr 1876, p 409

Neumann I. Lymphgefässe der Haut. Vienna, Wilhelm Braumüller, 1873

Neumann I. Lehrbuch der Hautkrankheiten. Vienna, Wilhelm Braumüller, 2nd ed., 1870

Neumann I. Syphilis. Vienna, Alfred Hölder, 2 vol., 1896

Fox GH. Reminiscences. New York, Medical Life Press, 1926. p 106

Moriz Kaposi

Picture source: Institute for the History of Medicine, University of Vienna

Nobl G. Fünfzig Jahre Wiener Dermatologie, in Nékám L. De Dermatologia et Dermatologis, Budapest, International Congress of Dermatology, 1936, p 245-56

Crissey JT, Parish LC. Dermatology and syphilology of the nineteenth century. New York, Praeger, 1981. p 254-60

Filipp Pick, the Archiv, and the "DDG"

Picture source: authors' collection

Goodman H. Notable contributers to the knowledge of dermatology. New York, Medical Lay Press, 1953. p 244

Scholz A. Geschichte der Dermatologie in Deutschland. Berlin, Springer, 1999. p 60-1

Heinrich Auspitz

Picture source: Institute for the History of Medicine, University of Vienna

Bronson EB. The objects of dermatological classification, with especial reference to Auspitz's System. J Cutan Vener Dis 1884;2:161-168, 201-13

Crissey JT, Parish LC. Dermatology and syphilology of the nineteenth century. New York, Praeger, 1981. p 251-53, 315

Auspitz H. Ueber die Zellen-Infiltrationen der Lederhaut bei Lupus, Syphilis und Scrofulose. Med. Jahrb. Zeitschr. k.k. Gesell. Aerzte Wien 1864;20 (Part 2):208-242.

Auspitz H, Ueber das Verhältniss der Oberhaut zur Papillarschicht. Arch f Dermatol Syph 1870;2:24-57

Auspitz H, Unna PG. Die Anatomie der syphilitischen Initial-Sclerose. Viertelj Dermatol Syph 1876;9:161-200

Heinrich Koebner

Picture source: Institute for the History of Medicine, University of Vienna
Koebner H. Zur Aetiologie der Psoriasis. Viertelj Dermatol Syph 1876;8:559-61
Crissey JT, Parish LC. Dermatology and syphilology of the nineteenth century. New York, Praeger, 1981. p 232, 367-69

LATE 19TH CENTURY GERMAN DERMATOLOGY

Albert Neisser

Picture source: Institute for the History of Medicine, University of Vienna
Scholz A. Albert Neisser and his pupils, in Zur Geschichte der deutschen Dermatologie. Bremen, Joachim J. Herzberg, Mainz, Günter W. Korting, 1987. p 167-77
Jadassohn J. Albert Neisser. Arch f Dermatol Syph. 1916;123:xvii-lxiv
Fite GL, Wade HW. The contribution of Neisser to the establishment of the Hansen bacillus as the etiologic agent of leprosy and the so-called Hansen-Neisser controversy. Int J Leprosy 1955;23:418-28

Paul Gerson Unna

Picture source: Portraits, authors' collection; Dermatologikum, Prof. Albrecht Scholz, Berlin
Hollander A. Paul Gerson Unna of Hamburg (1850-1929), in Zur Geschichte der deutschen Dermatologie. Bremen, Joachim J. Herzberg, Mainz, Günter W. Korting, 1987. p 179-85
Crissey JT, Parish LC. Dermatology and syphilology of the nineteenth century. New York, Praeger, 1981. p 310-31

Talented trio

Picture source: authors' collection

LATE 19TH CENTURY FRENCH DERMATOLOGY

Charles Lailler and Emile Vidal

Picture source: authors' collection
Thibierge G. Notes sur les successeurs de Bazin a l'Hôpital St. Louis. Bull Soc Franc d'Hist Méd 1925;19:129-144
Crissey JT, Parish LC. Dermatology and syphilology of the nineteenth century. New York, Praeger, 1981. p 261-4
Beeson BB. Émile Vidal. Arch Dermatol Syphilol 1930;22:115-19
Brocq L. Émil Vidal. Ann Dermatol Syphilig 1893;4:805-13

Jules Baretta, moulage craftsman

214

Picture source: Musée de l'Hôpital St. Louis

Jeanselme E. Décès de M. Baretta. Bull Soc Franc Dermatol Syphilol 1923;17:218-220

Parish LC, Worden G, Witkowski JA, Scholz A, Parish DH. Wax models in dermatology. Trans & Studies Coll Phys Philadelphia Ser 5 1991;13:29-74.

Ernest Besnier

Picture source: authors's collection

Sabouraud R. Souvenirs de l'Hôpital St. Louis, in Nékám L. De Dermatologia et Dermatologis, Budapest, International Congress of Dermatology, 1936. p 323-26

Beeson BB. Ernest Besnier. Arch Dermatol Syphilol. 1929;20:95-9

Thibierge G. Ernest Besnier, Ann Dermatol Syphilig 1909;10:353-66

Besnier E, Thibierge G. Adrien Doyon. Ann Dermatol Syphilig 1907;7:577-83.

Besnier E, Doyon A. État actuel de l'enseignement dermatologique; Prominence de l'école de Vienne; Necessité d'une reforme en France. France Médicale 1881;28:742-769

Adrien Doyon and the Annales

Picture sources: portrait, authors' collection; journal page, Prof. Daniel Wallach, Paris

Besnier E, Thibierge G. Adrien Doyon. Ann Dermatol Syphilig 1907; 7:577-83

Wallach D. Ann Dermatol Syphil, 1868, 1:1. Ann Dermatol Venerol 1994;121:787-91

Jean-Louis Brocq and the fixed drug eruption

Picture source: authors' collection

Pautrier LM. Louis Brocq. Ann Dermatol Syphilig 1929;10:133-50

Jean Darier

Picture sources: portrait, authors's collectiom; Darier's disease plate, Darier J. De la psorospermose folliculaire végétante, Ann Dermatol syphilig 1889;10:397; Erythema annulare centrifugum figure, Darier J. De l'érythème annulaire centrifuge. Ann Dermatol syphilig 1916;6:57

Graham-Little E. Obituary, Jean Darier. Br J Dermatol 1938;50:384

LATE 19TH CENTURY AMERICAN DERMATOLOGY

Louis Duhring and Duhring's disease

Picture sources: portrait, authors' collection; dermatitis herpetiformis, Stelwagon HW. Treatise on diseases of the skin. Philadelphia, W. B. Saunders Co., 1907, fifth ed.

Parish LC. Louis A. Duhring, M.D., pathfinder for dermatology. Springfield,

Charles C. Thomas, 1967

Duhring L. Dermatitis herpetiformis. JAMA 1884;3:225-29

Morris Henry Henry and the first American dermatology journal

Picture source: authors' collection

Parish L C. Morris Henry Henry. Cutis 1966;2:260-261

Henry MH, in Specialists and Specialties in Medicine, New York, Wm. Wood, 1876.

Fox GH. Reminiscences, in De Dermatologia et Dermatologis, edit. by L. Nékam, Budapest, International Congress Committee, 1936. p 61-3

James Clarke White, America's first professor of dermatology

Picture source: author's collection

White JC. Sketches from my life. Cambridge, Massachusetts, Riverside Press, 1914

White JC. A case of keratoses (ichthyosis) follicularis. J Cutan Dis 1889;7:201-3

Lucius Duncan Bulkley

Picture source: authors' collection

Goodman H. Lucius Duncan Bulkley, Med. Life, 1928;35:399-403

Walsh JJ. History of Medicine in New York, New York, Nat. Americana Soc., 1919, V4. p 58-62

The "ADA"

Picture source: Transactions of the American Dermatological Association. New York, G.P. Putnam's Sons, 1878

Bechet PE. History of the American Dermatological Association in commemoration of its seventy-fifth anniversary, 1876-1951. New York, Froben Press, 1952. p 19-33

George Henry Fox

Picture source: author's collection

Fox GH. Reminiscences. New York, Medical Life Press, 1926

Fox, GH. Photographic illustrations of skin diseases. New York, E. B. Treat, 1880.

Foz GH. Photographic illustrations of cutaneous syphilis. New York, E. B. Treat, 1881.

"Brains" Piffard and the "JCVD"

Picture source: authors' collection

Fox GH. A memorial sketch of Dr. Henry Granger Piffard. J Cutan Dis 1911;29:82-7

Crissey JT, Parish LC. Dermatology and syphilology of the nineteenth century. New York, Praeger, 1981. p 290-2

Sigmund Pollitzer and acanthosis nigricans

Picture source: authors' collection

Wile UJ. Obituary, Sigmund Pollitzer. Arch Dermatol Syphilol 1938;37:499

Pollitzer S. Fifty-six years in medicine, in De Dermatologia et Dermatologis, edit. by L. Nékam, Budapest, International Congress Committee, 1936. p. 273-80

Curtis AC. Chronicle of the Society of Investigative Dermatology. J Invest Dermatol 1954;23:225-31

T. Casper Gilchrist and blastomycosis

Picture source: authors' collection

Unsigned obituary. Thomas Casper Gilchrist, M.D., 1862-1927. Arch Dermatol Syphilol 1928;17:392-4

Rippon JW. Medical mycology. Philadelphia, W.B. Saunders Company, 1988, 3rd ed. p 474

Pollitzer S. Fifty-six years in medicine, in De Dermatologia et Dermatologis, edit. by L. Nékam, Budapest, International Congress Committee, 1936 p 273-80

John Fordyce and his "affection"

Picture sources: portrait, authors' collection; disease plate, Fordyce JA. A peculiar affection of the mucous membrane of the lips and oral cavity. J Cutan Dis 1896;14:413-19

MacKee GM. Obituary, John Addison Fordyce. Arch Dermatol Syphilol 1925;12:268

LATE 19TH CENTURY ITALIAN DERMATOLOGY

Domenico Majocchi

Picture source: authors' collection.

Diasio F. Domenico Majocchi. Med Life 1932;39:597

Augusto Ducrey and his streptobacillus

Picture source: authors' collection

Ronchese F. Ducrey and His Streptobacillus. Cutis 1968;4:1400

Cappelli J. Obituary, Augusto Ducrey (abstract). Arch Dermatol Syphilol 1942;45:160

Schiavo AL, Ruocco V, Marino F, Ferraiolo S, Pinto F, Orlando G. Tommaso De Amicis, Augusto Ducrey, Lodovico Tommasi: three Neapolitan stars in the dermatovenerealogy firmament. Internat J Dermatol 1996;35:57-62.

Vittorio Mibelli, angiokeratoma, and porokeratosis.

Picture source: authors' collection

Ullman J. Obituary: Vittorio Mibelli. Archiv f Dermatol u Syph 1910;103:566-7

EARLY SCHOOLS IN OTHER COUNTRIES

Early Danish dermatology

Picture sources: authors' collection

Bonnevie P. Dermatology in Denmark. Internat J Dermatol 1983;22:193-200

Early Norwegian dermatology

Fyrand O. History of Norwegian dermato-venereology during the last two centuries. Internat J Dermatol 1983;22:593-7

Haarvaldsen J. Caesar Boeck. Dermatol Wchnschr 1917;65:763-5

Epstein WL. Commentary: what begot Boeck? Arch Dermatol 1982;118:721-2

Early Canadian dermatology

Picture sources: authors' collection

Unsigned obituary. Francis John Shepherd M.D. Arch Dermatol Syphilol 1929;19:679

Unsigned obituary. James Elliot Graham. J Cutan Dis 1899;17:407

Forsey RR. Historical vignettes of Canadian dermatology. Ville St-Laurent, QC, Canada, 1990. p 35, 62-4

Early Japanese dermatology

Picture sources: author's collection

Parish LC, Crissey JT. Japanese and American dermatology: Parallels and interactions. Japan J Dermatol 2001;111:688-95

Early Spanish dermatology: Olavide and his atlas

Picture source: authors' collection.

Sierra X. Olavide and the roots of Spanish dermatology. Internat J Dermatol 1997;36:870-74

Calatayud JC. The dermatological heritage in danger in Madrid:Rescue Olavide's moulages.Website of the Société Française d'Histoire de la Dermatologie 2001:1-4

Sierra X. Historia de la dermatologia. S.A.Spain, Menarini, 1994, p 275-6

Da Fonseca A. Dermatology in Europe, a historical approach. No city given, Schering-Plough Lda., 1997. p 320-3

NINETEENTH CENTURY TOOLS AND DEVICES

New items featured in the 1883-84 Journal of Cutaneous Diseases

Picture sources: J Cutan Dis. 1883; p 146 (syringe),p 154 (scabies tool), p 183 (epilation needle),p 398 (Auspitz instrument)

J Cutan Dis. 1883: p 126 (hollow comb)

Late 19th century dermatologic instruments

Picture sources: authors' collection

EARLY TWENTIETH CENTURY
DERMATOLOGISTS, EVENTS, AND DISCOVERIES

Alfred Blaschko, his lines, and his society

Picture source: authors' collection

Jackson R. The lines of Blaschko: A review and reconsideration. Brit J Dermatol 1976;95:349-60.

Weindling P, Slevogt U. Alfred Blaschko (1858-1922) and the problem of sexually transmitted disease in Imperial and Weimar Germany; a bibliography. Oxford: Wellcome Unit for the History of Medicine, 1992. p 27-117

Finsen and lupus vulgaris

Picture source: authors' collection

Finsen NR. Phototherapy. London, Edward Arnold, 1901, p70

Crissey JT, Parish LC. Dermatology and syphilology of the nineteenth century. New York, Praeger, 1981. p 210-14

Liquid air and liquid oxygen become available

Picture sources: Baker RS. Liquid air. McClure's Mag 1899;12:397-408

White AC, Liquid air, its application in medicine and surgery. Med. Rec 1899;56:109-112

Baker RS. Liquid air.McClure's Mag 1899;12:397-408

White AC, Possibilities of liquid air to the physician. JAMA 1901;36: 426-29

Whitehouse HH. Liquid air in dermatology; its indications and limitations JAMA 1907;49:371-77

Unsigned obit. Charles Tripler, N.Y. Times, June 23, 1906.

X-ray becomes available

Picture source: authors' collection

Brecher R, Brecher E. The rays, a history of radiology in the United States and Canada. Baltimore, Williams and Wilkens Company, 1969. p 1-10, 137-49

MacKee GM, Cipollaro A. X-rays and radium in the treatment of diseases of the skin. Philadelphia, Lea & Febiger, 1947. p 6

X-Ray equipment for sale

Picture source: authors' collection

William Allen Pusey and X-Ray

Picture source: authors' collection.

Crissey JT. Epitaph:William Allen Pusey. J Am Acad Dermatol 1984;11:702-08

Pusey WA. Report of cases treated with Roentgen rays. Chicago Med Record 1902;22:251-61, 269-304

Pusey WA, Caldwell EW. Practical application of Roentgen rays in therapeutics and diagnosis. Philadelphia, W.B. Saunders & Co., 1903

Walker W. History of the dermatological activities in the United States. Urol Cutan Rev 1919;23:645-50

Brown P. American martyrs to science through the Roentgen rays. London, Bailliere, Tindall, & Coc, 1936, p 175-76

Raymond Sabouraud

Picture source: authors' collection

Sabouraud R., Les Teignes, Paris, Masson, 1910. p 1-90

Sabouraud R., Contribution à l'Étude de la Trichophytie Humaine, Ann. Dermatol. Syphilig 1892;3rd s:1061-1087

McCarthy L. Raymond Sabouraud, M.D., mycologist, sacteriologist, and dermatologist. Arch. Dermatol. Syphilol 1938;37:843-846

Grigoraki L. Le Docteur Sabouraud. Mycopathologia, 1939-40;2:171-200 [contains complete list of Sabouraud's publications].

Civatte A. Raymond Sabouraud. Br J Dermatol 1938;50:206-208

Rippon JW. Medical mycology. Philadelphia, W.B. Saunders Company, 1988, 3rd ed. p 170-74

Crissey JT, Parish LC. Dermatology and syphilology of the nineteenth century. New York, Praeger, 1981. p 237-50

Radium, Becquerel, Ernest Besnier, and Henri Danlos

Picture source: authors' collection

Brecher R, Brecher E. The rays, a history of radiology in the United States and Canada. Baltimore, Williams and Wilkens Company, 1969. p 150-60, 279-89

Schaudinn, Hoffmann, and the spirochete

Picture source: Krusnayk drawing, Nékám L. De Dermatologia et Dermatologis, Budapest, International Congress of Dermatology, 1936. p 81

Schaudinn F, Hoffmann E. Vorlaüfiger Bericht ueber das Vorkommen von Spirocheten in syphilitschen Krankheitsprodukten und bei Papillomen. Arbeit Kaiserlichen Gesundheitsamte 1905;22:529-34

Schaudinn F, Hoffmann EA. Preliminary Note upon the Occurrence of Spirochaetes in Syphilitic Lesions and in Papillomata, in Selected Essays on Syphilis and Small-pox, London, New Sydenham Soc. (194), 1906, p 3-15

Winkler K. Dermatologie in Berlin–ein Rückblick, in Zur Geschichte der Deutschen Dermatologie, Berlin, Joachim J. Herzberg, 1987. p 17-40

Dennie CC. A history of syphilis. Springfield IL, Charles C. Thomas, 1962, p 94

Josef Jadassohn

Picture source: authors' collection

Eine eigentümliche Furchung, Erweiterung, und Verdickung der Haut am Hinterkopf. Verhandl Deutsch Dermat Gesell 1906;9:451

Sulzberger MB. Obituary, Josef Jadassohn. Arch Dermatol Syphilol 1936;33:1063-69

Bruno Bloch and dopa oxidase

Picture source: authors' collection

Bloch B. Chemische Untersuchungen ueber das spezifische pigmentbildende Ferment der Haut, die Dopaoxydase. Ztschr f physiol Chem 1916;98:226-54

Sulzberger MB. From there to here, my many lives. Skin & Allergy News for the Institute for Dermatologic Communications and Education, 1986. p 113-28

Ernst Kromayer

Picture source, Kromayer portrait: Dr Wolfgang Weyers, Freiburg, Germany

Winkler K. Dermatology in Berlin – a retrospective view, in Zur Geschichte der deutschen Dermatologie. Bremen, Joachim J. Herzberg, Mainz, Günter W. Korting, 1987. p 147-9

Scholz A. Geschichte der Dermatologie in Deutschland. Berlin, Springer, 1999. p 49-51

Felix Pinkus and lichen nitidus

Picture source: authors' collection

Michelson H. Obituary: Felix Pinkus. Arch Dermatol Syphilol 1948;58:92-94

Franjo Kogoj and the spongiform pustule.

Picture source: Institute for the History of Medicine, University of Vienna

Holubar K. Franjo Kogoj and the spongiform pustule. Am J Dermatopathol 1985;7:191-5

Ernest Graham-Little and Arthur Whitfield

Picture sources: authors' collection

MacLeod JMH. Obituary. Sir Ernest Graham-Little M.D., F.R.C.P., M.P. Arch Dermatol Syphilol 1951;63:672-4

Graham-Little E. A retrospect of dermatology in Great Britain, in Nékám L. De Dermatologia et Dermatologis, Budapest, International Congress of Dermatology, 1936. p 141-50

Unsigned Obituary. Arthur Whitfield M.D. (1868-1947). Arch Dermatol Syphilol 1947;56:394-6

Whitfield A. A note on some unusual cases of trichophytic infection. Lancet 1908;2:237-8

Henry W. Stelwagon and his textbook

Picture source: authors' collection

Hartzell MB. Memoir of Henry Weightman Stelwagon M.D., 1853-1919. Arch Dermatol Syphilol 1920;38:191-3

Stelwagon HW. Treatise on diseases of the skin. Philadelphia, W.B. Saunders & Co., 1902

John Templeton Bowen and Bowen's disease

Picture source: authors' collection;

White CJ. Obituary, John T. Bowen. J Cutan Dis 1941;43:386

Udo Wile and Lyle Kingery - warts and molluscum contagiosum

    Picture sources: authors' collection

    Bechet PE. History of the American Dermatological Association in commemoration of its seventy-fifth anniversary, 1876-1951. New York, Froben Press, 1952. p 173, 214

William H. Goeckerman and the Goeckerman treatment

    Picture source: authors' collection

    Obermayer ME. William H. Goeckerman M.D. U South Cal Med Bull 1954/55;7:28-29

Quartz mercury vapor lamps

    Picture source: Hall P. Ultra-violet rays in the treatment and cure of disease.St. Louis, Mosby Company, 1928, 3rd edition. p 84-101, 132

Louis Brunsting and pyoderma gangrenosum

    Picture source: authors' collection

    Perry HO. Louis A. Brunsting (1900-1980). J Am Acad Dermatol 1981;4:73-4A

The Canadian Dermatology Association

    Picture source: Dr. R. Roy Forsey, Montreal, Canada

    Forsey RR. Historical vignettes of Canadian dermatology. Ville St-Laurent, QC, Canada, 1990. p 84-114

    Bechet PE. History of the American Dermatological Association in commemoration of its seventy-fifth anniversary, 1876-1951. New York, Froben Press, 1952. p 262

    Goodman H. Notable contributers to the knowledge of dermatology. New York, Medical Lay Press, 1953. p 279, 295, 330

Barney Usher and William Garbe

    Picture source: authors' collection

    Forsey RR. Historical vignettes of Canadian dermatology. Ville St-Laurent, QC, Canada, 1990. p 32-4, 65-75

Henri Gougerot and Edouard Jeanselme

    Picture source: authors' collection

    Shelley WB, Crissey JT. Classics in Clinical Dermatology, Springfield, Ill., Charles Thomas, 1953. p 415-19

    Degos R. Henri Gougerot M.D. (1881-1955). Arch Dermatol 1955;71:782

    Da Fonseca A. Dermatology in Europe, a historical approach. No city given, Schering-Plough Lda., 1997, p 207-12

    De Beurmann L, Gougerot H. Les sporotrichoses. Paris, Felix Alcan, 1912

    Gougerot H, Brodier L. l'Hôpital St. Louis et la clinique d'Alfred Fournier. Paris, J. Peyronnet & Cie., 1932. p 121-7, 129-30

Twentieth Century Danes: Carl Rasch and Edvard Ehlers

    Picture source: authors' collection.

    Unsigned obituary: C.F. Rasch (1861-1938). Brit J Dermatol 1939;51:186-7

    Simon C. Edvard Ehlers. Ann Dermatol Syph 1937;8:458-9

Twentieth Century Danes: Holger Haxthausen and Svend Lomholt

    Picture source: authors' collection

    Bonnevie P. Dermatology in Denmark. Internat J Dermatol 1983;22:193-200

Haxthausen H. The pathogenesis of allergic eczema elucidated by transplantation experiments on identical twins. Acta Dermato-Venereologica 1942;23:438-57

Dowling GB. Obituary: Professor H.R. Haxthausen. Brit J Dermatol 1960;72:83-4

Fyrand O. History of Norwegian dermato-venereology during the last two centuries. Internat J Dermatol 1983;22:593-7

Hellerström S. Svend Lomholt, October 18, 1888-July 17, 1949. Acta Dermato-Venereologica 1950;30:91-4

Niels Danbolt and acrodermatitis enteropathica

Picture Source. authors' collection

K.W. Obituary: Niels Danbolt. Brit J Dermatol 1985;112:726

Danbolt N. Acrodermatitis enteropathica. Brit J Dermatol 1979;100:37-40

Louis Nékám and the 1935 International Congress

Picture source: Nékám L. De Dermatologia et Dermatologis, Budapest, International Congress of Dermatology, 1936

Nékám L. De Dermatologia et Dermatologis, Budapest, International Congress of Dermatology, 1936. p 185-209

Weyers W. Death of medicine in Nazi Germany. Philadelphia, Lippincott-Raven, 1998. p 127-33

The remarkable atlas

Picture source: Nékám L. Corpus Iconum Morborum Cutaneorum. Leipzig, Johann Ambrosius Barth, 1938

MID-TWENTIETH CENTURY
DERMATOLOGISTS, EVENTS, AND DISCOVERIES

Rose Hirschler, America's first woman dermatologist

Picture source: authors' collection

Witkowski J, Parish LC. Unpublished data, 2000, Philadelphia, PA

George Miller McKee and the "SID"

Picture source: authors' collection

McKee GM. Presidential address. J Invest Dermatol 1938;1:235-6

Wise F. Dr. George Miller McKee. J Invest Dermatol 1947;8:277-80

Curtis AC. Chronicle of the Society of Investigative Dermatology. J Invest Dermatol 1954;23:225-31

Naomi Kanof and the "JID"

Picture source: authors' collection

Wechsler HL. In memoriam: Naomi M. Kanof, MD, 1912-1988. Cutis 1989;43:89-90

Unsigned Announcement and Editorial. J Invest Dermatol 1938;1:1-7

The "AAD"

Picture sources: authors' collection

Parish LC. Founding of the Academy. J Amer Acad Dermatol 1988;18:Supp 786-92

Crissey JT. Epitaph: Earl D. Osborne, M.D. J Am Acad Dermatol. 1988;18 (Part 2);797-798

Frederic Mohs and microscopically controlled surgery

Picture source: authors' collection

Mohs FE. Chemosurgery: a microscopically controlled method of cancer excision. Arch Surg 1941;42:279-95

Robins P. A tribute to Dr. Mohs. J Dermatol Surg Oncol 1978;4:1

Mohs FE. Chemosurgery: microscopically controlled surgery for skin cancer – past, present, and future. J Dermatol Surg Oncol 1978;4:41-54

Brodland DG, Amonette R, Hanke WC, Robins P. History and evolution of Mohs micrographic surgery. Dermatol Surg 2000;26:303-7

Stephen Rothman and PABA

Picture source: authors' collection

Santoianni P. Stephen Rothman (1894-1963) Dermatologia Tropica 1963;2:193-4

Steigleder GK. Personal experiences with Stephen Rothman, M.D. J Am Acad Dermatol 1988;19:596-98

John Hinchman Stokes

Picture source: authors' collection

Beerman H, Lazarus GS. Tradition of excellence. Philadelphia, Herman Beerman and Gerald S. Lazarus Inc., 1986. p 41-58

Stokes JH, Beerman H, Ingraham NR Jr., Modern clinical syphilology. Philadelphia, W.B. Saunders Co., 3rd Ed., 1945

Achille Civatte

Picture source: authors' collection

Touraine A. Achille Civatte (1877-1956). Arch Dermatol 1957;75:783-5

Da Fonseca A. Dermatology in Europe, a historical approach. No city given, Schering-Plough Lda., 1997. p 216-7

Robert Degos

Picture source: authors' collection

Degos R. Malignant atrophic papulosis. Br J Dermatol 1979;100:21-35

Civatte J. Quelques aspects de la contribution de Robert Degos a la dermatologie. Website of the Société Française d'Histoire de la Dermatologie 1997:1-4

Da Fonseca A. Dermatology in Europe, a historical approach. No city given, Schering-Plough Lda., 1997, p 220-2

Abraham Buschke

Picture source: authors' collection

Curth W, Curth H. Abraham Buschke. Arch Dermatol Syphilol 1945;52:32

Gold JA, Nürnberger FG. A tribute to Abraham Buschke. J Am Acad Dermatol 1992;26:1019-22

Buschke A. Ueber eine durch Coccidien hervergerufene Krankheit des Menschen. Deutsche Med Wchnschr 1895;21:14

Busse O. Ueber parasitare zellinschlusse und ihre zuchtung. Zentralbl Bakterial 1894;16:175-180

Erich Urbach and necrobiosis lipoidica diabeticorum

Picture source: authors' collection.

Stokes JH. Obituary, Erich Urbach M.D. Arch Dermatol Syphilol 1947;55:545-47

Oscar Gans

Picture source: authors' collection

Weyers W. Death of medicine in Nazi Germany. Philadelphia, Lippincott-Raven, 1998, p 83-4

Braun-Falco O. Zum Gedenken an Oscar Gans (1888-1983) in Zur Geschichte der deutschen Dermatologie. Bremen, Joachim J. Herzberg, Mainz, Günter W. Korting, 1987. p 57-60, 159-162

Heinrich Gottron and Leopold Von Zumbusch

Picture source: Gottron, Prof. Albrecht Scholtz; von Zumbusch, authors' collection

Gottron H. Ausgedehnte, ziemlich symmetrisch angeordnete Papillomatosis cutis. Zentrlbl Haut- und Geschlects-kr 1932;40:445

Weyers W. Death of medicine in Nazi Germany. Philadelphia, Lippincott-Raven, 1998, p 201-2

Korting GW. Heinrich Adolf Gottron zum Gedenken in Zur Geschichte der deutschen Dermatologie. Bremen, Joachim J. Herzberg, Mainz, Günter W. Korting, 1987. p 61-4, 163-5

Alfred Marchionini and Der Hautarzt

Picture source: Marchionini portrait, British Journal of Dermatology, with permission; Hautarzt masthead, Springer-Verlag GmbH & Co. KG, with permission

Weyers W. Death of medicine in Nazi Germany. Philadelphia, Lippincott-Raven, 1998, p 88-91

Garretts M. Obituary, Professor Alfred Marchionini. Brit J Dermatol 1965;77:391-2

Otto Braun-Falco

Picture source: Portrait, Prof. Otto Braun-Falco, Munich; title page, Springer-Verlag GmbH & Co. KG, with permission

Braun-Falco O. Zum Gedenken an Oscar Gans (1888-1983) in Zur Geschichte der deutschen Dermatologie. Bremen, Joachim J. Herzberg, Mainz, Günter W. Korting, 1987. p 57-60, 159-162

Personal communication, 2001, Prof. Otto Braun-Falco to Dr. John T. Crissey

Klaus Wolff

Picture source: Portrait, Prof. Klaus Wolff, Vienna; figures, reprinted with permission from Nature, Vol 229, copyright 1971

Personal communication, 2001, Prof. Klaus Wolff to Dr. John T. Crissey

Thomas Fitzpatrick and human tyrosinase

Picture sources: portrait, Dr.Thomas Fitzpatrick; Weston, MA; Figures, reprinted from Science, 1950, with permission.

Personal communication, 2000, Dr. Thomas Fitzpatrick to Dr. John T. Crissey

Marion Sulzberger, Victor Witten, and the corticosteroids

Picture sources: authors' collection, Portrait, Dr. Victor H. Witten, Miami, FL; Figures, Journal of Investigative Dermatology, with permission

Sulzberger MB. From here to there, my many lives. Skin and Allergy News, 1986

Forman L. Marion B. Sulzberger. Brit J Dermatol 1984;111:367-9

Personal communication, 2000, Dr. Victor H. Witten to Dr. John T. Crissey

Unsigned article. Historical dermatology recordings donated to National Library of Medicine. Dermatology World 2000;10:15

Donald Pillsbury and Herman Beerman
> Picture source: authors' collection
> Beerman H, Lazarus GS. Tradition of excellence. Philadelphia, Herman Beerman
> and Gerald S. Lazarus Inc., 1986. p 58-67

Aaron Lerner and melatonin
> Picture source: Dr. Aaron B. Lerner, New Haven, CT
> Lerner AB. My 60 years in pigmentation. Pigment Cell Res 1999;12:131-144
> Personal communication, 2000, Dr. Aaron B. Lerner to Dr. John T. Crissey

Abner Kurtin and surgical planing (dermabrasion)
> Picture source: Portrait, Dr. Stephen Kurtin, New York, NY; Figure, AMA
> Archives of Dermatology, with permission
> Kurtin A. Corrective surgical planing of skin. Arch Dermatol 1953;68:389-97
> Kurtin SB. A look back at Abner Kurtin M.D. J Dermatol Surg Oncol
> 1987;13:603-3
> Burks JW. Wire brush surgery. Springfield, Charles C. Thomas, 1956. p 18-22
> Yarborough JM. Dermabrasion by wire brush. J Dermatol Surg Oncol
> 1987;13:610-15
> Personal communication, 2000, Dr. John M. Yarborough to Dr. John T. Crissey

Rudolf Baer.
> Picture source: Portrait, authors' collection; building, Dr Irwin M. Freedberg,
> New York, NY
> Unsigned Interview. Rudolf L. Baer, a clinician-investigator whose vision has
> shaped modern dermatology. Masters of Dermatology. 1984;1:1-21
> Freedberg IM, Kopf AW. A tribute to Rudolf L. Baer (1910-1997). J Am Acad
> Dermatol 1998;39:513-5
> Sulzberger MB. From here to there, my many lives. Skin and Allergy News,
> 1986. p 183-7

Walter F. Lever
> Picture source: Portrait, authors' collection; Figures, Medicine, with permission
> Lever WF. Contemporaries: Walter F. Lever, M.D. J Am Acad Dermatol
> 1984;10:321-5

Hermann Pinkus and alopecia mucinosa
> Picture source: Portrait, authors' collection; Figures, AMA Archives of
> Dermatology, with permission
> Lyell A. Obituary: Hermann Pinkus (1905-1985). Brit J Dermatol 1986;115:507-9
> Sulzberger MB. Homage to Pinkus: A genetic study. J Invest Dermatol
> 1975;65:418
> Birmingham DJ. Editorial: Hermann Pinkus. J Invest Dermatol 1975;65:419

Norman Orentreich and hair transplantation
> Picture source: Portrait, Dr. Norman Orentreich, New York, NY; Figures,
> Proceedings of the New York Academy of Sciences, with permission
> Orentreich N. Autografts in alopecias and other dermatological conditions. Ann
> NY Acad Sciences 1959;83:463-79
> Capiello V. Dr. Norman Orentreich, a true pioneering researcher on aging. LEF
> Magazine 1999;www.lef.org:1-4
> Unger WP. History of hair transplantation. Dermatol Surg 2000;26:181-89

Geoffrey B. Dowling and Archibald Gray
Picture source: authors' collection
Wallace H. Dr. G.B. Dowling. Brit J Dermatol 1976;95:677-81
Goldsmith WN. Sir Archibald Gray K.C.V.O., C,B.E., T.D., LL.D., M.D., F.R.C.P., F.R.C.S. Brit J Dermatol 1967;79:706-9

Alan Lyell and toxic epidermal necrolysis
Picture source: Portrait, Dr. Alan Lyell, Craigallion, Ayreshire, Scotland; Figure, British Journal of Dermatology, with permission
Holubar K. SSSS vs. TEN: Staphylococcal scalded skin syndrome versus toxic epidermal necrolysis. Acta Dermatolvenerel Croat. 2000;8:217-21
Lyell A. Toxic epidermal necrolysis (the scalded skin syndrome): A reappraisal. Brit J Dermatol 1979;100:69-73
Personal communication, 2001, Dr. Alan Lyell to Dr. John T. Crissey

Arthur Rook and the "Rook Book"
Picture source: Portrait, authors' collection; Figure, Blackwell Science, with permission
Wilkinson D. Arthur James Rook (1918-1991). J Am Acad Dermatol 1992;26:1024-6
Champion RH. Obituary: Arthur James Rook. Brit J Dermatol 1991;125:601-2
Personal communication, 2001, Dr. Darrell S. Wilkinson to Dr. John T. Crissey

Darrell S. Wilkinson and David I. Williams
Picture sources: Dr. Darrell S. Wilkinson, Amersham, England; authors' collection
Personal communication, 2001, Dr. Darrell S. Wilkinson to Dr. John T. Crissey
Wilkinson DS. Photodermatitis due to tetrachlorosalicylanilide. Brit J Dermatol 1961;73:213-9
Sneddon IB, Wilkinson DS. Subcorneal pustular dermatosis Brit J Dermatol 1956;68:385-90
Williams DI, Marten RH, Sarkany I. Oral treatment of ringworm with griseofulvin. Lancet 1958;2:1212-13
Williams DI. Contemporaries: De mortuis nil nisi bonum. J Am Acad Dermatol 1982;6:968-76
Sarkany I. Obituary: David Iorworth Williams FRCP. Brit J Dermatol 1995;133:328

Harvey Blank and griseofulvin
Picture source: Portrait, authors' collection; Figure, AMA Archives of Dermatology, with permission
Beerman H, Lazarus GS. Tradition of excellence. Philadelphia, Herman Beerman and Gerald S. Lazarus Inc., 1986. p 139-40
Blank H, Rake G. Viral and rickettsial diseases of the skin, eye, and mucous membranes of man, Boston, Little, Brown, 1955
Blank H, Roth FJ, Bruce WW, Engel MF, Smith JG, Zaias N. Treatment of dermatomycoses with orally administered griseofulvin. AMA Arch Dermatol 1959;78:259-66
Williams DI, Marten RH, Sarkany I. Oral treatment of ringworm with griseofulvin. Lancet 1958;2:1212-13

Clayton E. Wheeler, Jr.

Picture source: Portrait, Dr. Clayton E. Wheeler, Chapel Hill, NC. Figures, copyright 1959, the American Association of Immunologists, with permission Briggaman RA, Wheeler CE Jr. The epidermal-dermal junction. J Invest Dermatol 1973;65:71-84

Personal communication, 2001, Dr. Clayton E. Wheelet, Jr. to Dr. John T. Crissey

John S. Strauss

Picture source: Portrait, authors' collection; Figures, Journal of Investigative Dermatology, with permission

Personal communication, 2001, Dr. John S. Strauss to Dr. John T. Crissey

Rees B. Rees and methotrexate

Picture source: Dr. Rees B. Rees, Santasa, CA

Rees RB. Contemporaries: Rees B. Rees, M.D. J Am Acad Dermatol 1984;10:554-560

Margaret Ann Storkan and the SS Hope

Picture sources: portrait, Dr. Margaret Ann Storkan; SS Hope, Ms. Katie Bryson, Project Hope

Personal communication, 2000, Dr. Margaret Ann Storkan to Dr. John T. Crissey

Alumni Association, Project Hope. White Plains, NY, Bernard C. Harris Publishing Company, Inc.,1993. p xi-xiv

Mid-20th century office companions

Picture sources: Hyfrecator, Corey Strege, ConMed Corporation, Englewood, CO; Kidde set, Dr. Robert Jackson, Ottawa, Canada; Liquid nitrogen units, authors' collection

RECENT TIMES

Leon Goldman and the ruby laser

Picture source: Portrait, authors' collection; Figures, Nature, with permission

Lobitz WC Jr. A tribute with thanks to Leon Goldman M.D. J Am Acad Dermatol 1988;19:160-2

Ernst Beutner, Robert Jordon, and pemphigus vulgaris

Picture sources: Portraits, Drs. Ernst Beutner, Buffalo, NY and Robert Jordon, Houston, TX; Figure, Proceedings of the Society for Experimental Biology and Medicine, with permission

Beutner EH, Jordon RE. Demonstration of skin antibodies in sera of pemphigus vulgaris patients by indirect immunoflourescent staining. Proc Soc Exp Biol Med 1964;117:505-10

Stephania Jablonska and Rudi Cormane, European pioneers in dermatologic immunology

Picture sources: Portraits, Stephania Jablonska and the Institute for the History of Medicine, University of Vienna

Personal communication, 2000, Prof. Stephania Jablonska to Dr. John T. Crissey

Personal communication, 2001, Dr. Ernst Beutner to Dr. John T. Crissey

Ken Hashimoto

Picture source: Portrait, authors' collection; Figure, Journal of Investigative Dermatology, with permission

Personal communication, 2000, Ken Hashimoto to John T. Crissey

William Pace and benzoyl peroxide

Picture source: Portrait, Dr. Robert Jackson, Ottawa, Canada

Forsey RR.Historical vignettes of Canadian dermatology. Ville St-Laurent, QC, Canada, 1990. p 47-8

Johnston C. A conversation with William Pace, MD. Dermatology Times of Canada, Sept 1993, p 38

Arthur Robert Birt and HPLE

Picture source: Portrait, Dr. Robert Jackson, Ottawa, Canada; Figure, Canadian Medical Association Journal, with permission

Forsey RR. Historical vignettes of Canadian dermatology. Ville St-Laurent, QC, Canada, 1990. p 17-18

Everett MA et al. Arch Dermatol 1961;83:243-8

Birt AR, Davis RA. Hereditary polymorphic light eruption of American Indians. Internat J Dermatol 1975;14:105-11

Birt AR, Hogg G. The actinic cheilitis of hereritary polymorphic light eruption. Arch Dermatol 1979;115:699-702

Birt AR, Hogg GR, Dube WJ. Hereditary multiple fibrofolliculomas with trichodiscomas and acrochordons. Arch Dermatol 1977;113:1674-77

Walter B. Shelley and aquagenic urticaria

Picture source: Portrait, Dr. Walter B. Shelley, Grand Rapids, OH; Figure, copyrighted 1964, American Medical Association, with permission

Beerman H, Lazarus GS. Tradition of excellence. Philadelphia, Herman Beerman and Gerald S. Lazarus Inc., 1986. p 132-35

Shelley WB. A plea for clinical research. Arch Dermatol 2000;136:88-9

Albert Kligman and retinoic acid

Picture source: Portrait, Dr. Albert Kligman, Philadelphia, PA; Figures, AMA Archives of Dermatology, with permission

Beerman H, Lazarus GS. Tradition of excellence. Philadelphia, Herman Beerman and Gerald S. Lazarus Inc., 1986. p 67-70

Inga Silberberg-Sinakin and the Langerhans cell

Picture sources: portrait: Dr. Inga Silberberg-Sinakin, Vineland, NJ; Figure, Acta Dermato Venereologica, with permission

Personal communication, 2000, Dr. Inga Silberberg-Sinakin to Dr. John T. Crissey

History of Dermatology Society

Picture source: authors' collection

Archives of the History of Dermatology Society, in possession of Dr. Lawrence Parish, Philadelphia, PA

John Parrish, PUVA, and psoriasis

Picture source: Portrait, Dr. John A. Parrish, Boston, MA; Figures, copyright 1974, Massachusetts Medical Society, all rights reserved, with permission

Personal communication, 2000, Dr. John A. Parrish to Dr. John T. Crissey

PUVA and the light box

Picture source: Robert Zeller, Waldmann Medizintechnil, Villingen-Schwenningen, Germany

Eugene J. Van Scott and alpha hydroxy acids

Picture source: Portrait, Dr. Eugene J. Van Scott, Abington, PA; Figures, AMA Archives of Dermatology, with permission

Personal communication, 2001, Dr. Eugene J. Van Scott to Dr. John T. Crissey

Jean-Hilaire Saurat

Picture source: Portrait, Dr. Jean-Hilaire Saurat, Geneva, Switzerland; Figures, British Journal of Dermatology, with permission.

Personal communication, 2001, Dr. Jean-Hilaire Saurat to Dr. John T. Crissey

John A. Kenney Jr. and dermatology at Howard University

Picture source: authors' collection

Kenney JA. The department of dermatology of the Howard University College of Medicine. Cutis 1983;32:334,336,341

J. Graham Smith and the "JAAD"

Picture source: Portrait, Dr. J. Graham Smith Jr., Mobile, A; Figure, Journal of the American Academy of Dermatology, with permission

Smith JG Jr. The birth of the blues–2. J Am Acad Dermatol 1988;18: Supp 969-78

Howard I. Maibach

Picture source: Portrait, authors' collection; Figure, Marcel Dekker Inc., with permission

Personal communication, 2001, Dr. Howard Maibach to Dr. John T. Crissey

A. Bernard Ackerman and the gold book

Picture source: Portrait, Dr. A. Bernard Ackerman, New York, NY;

Personal communication, 2000, Dr. A. Bernard Ackerman to Dr. John T. Crissey

Gary L. Peck and 13 cis-retinoic acid

Picture source: Leslie E. Kossoff Photos, Bethesda, MD; Figures, copyright 1979, Massachusetts Medical Society, all rights reserved, with permission

Personal communication, 2000, Dr. Gary L. Peck to Dr. John T. Crissey

Raul Fleischmajer and Ervin H. Epstein Jr.

Picture sources: Dr. Raul Fleischmajer, New York, NY; Dr. Ervin Epstein Jr., San Francisco, CA

Personal communication, 2001, Dr. Raul Fleischmajer to Dr. John T. Crissey

Personal commubication, 2001, Dr. Ervin H. Epstein Jr. to Dr. John T. Crissey

Jouni J. Uitto and Larry E. Millikan

Picture sources: Portraits: Dr. Jouni J. Uitto; Dr. Larry E. Millikan

Personal communication, 2001, Dr. Jouni J. Uitto to Dr. John T. Crissey

Personal communication, 2001, Dr. Larry E. Millikan to Dr. John T. Crissey

Stephen I. Katz and Daniel N. Sauder

Picture sources: Dr. Stephen I. Katz, Bethesda, MD; Dr. Daniel N. Sauder, Toronto, Canada

Personal communication, 2000, Dr. Stephen I. Katz to Dr. John T. Crissey

Personal communication, 2000, Dr. Daniel N. Sauder to Dr. John T. Crissey

Sauder DN, Carter S, Katz SI, Oppenheim JJ. Epidermal cell production of thymocyte activating factor (ETAF). J Invest Dermatol 1882;79:34-9

David T. Woodley

Picture source: Authors' collection. Figures, copyright 1974, Massachusetts Medical Society, all rights reserved, with permission

Personal communication, 2001, Dr. David T. Woodley to Dr. John T. Crissey

William H. Eaglstein and wound healing

Picture source: portrait, Dr. William H. Eaglstein. Miami, FL

Personal communication, 2001, Dr. William H. Eaglstein to Dr. John T. Crissey

Eaglstein WH, Falanga V. Tissue engineering: an update. J Am Acad Dermatol 1998;39:1007-10

Jeffrey A. Klein and tumescent liposuction

Picture source: Dr. Jeffrey Klein, San Juan Capistrano, CA

Personal communication, 2001, Dr. Jeffrey A. Klein to Dr. John T. Crissey,

Flynn TC, Coleman WP III, Field LM, Klein JA, Hanke CW. History of liposuction. Dermatol Surg 2000;26:515-9

Lasers

Picture sources: AlexLAZR Q-switched alexandrite laser and V-beam pulsed dye laser, courtesy of Candela Corporation, Wayland, MA; Tru-Pulse laser, courtesy of Medical Lasers Corporation

Hruza GJ, guest editor. Seminar: Lasers. Seminars in Cutaneous Medicine and Surgery. 2000;19:205-92

Anderson RR, Parrish JA. Selective photothermolysis: Precise microsurgery by selective absorption of pulsed radiation. Science 1983;220:524-7

Drs. Carruthers, the furrowed brow, and C. botulinum-A exotoxin

Picture sources: Portraits, Dr. Jean Carruthers, Vancouver, BC, Canada; Figures 2 and 3, Journal of Dermatologic Surgery and Oncology, with permission

Personal Communication, 2000, Dr. Jean Carruthers to Dr. John T. Crissey

Japanese Dermatological Association, 100th Anniversary

Picture source: authors' collection

Holubar K, Saurat JH. The centenary of the Japanese dermatological association. Dermatology 2001;202:85-6

Infonet and Internet

Picture source: J Am Acad Dermatol

Dermatologic historians

Picture sources: all from the individuals themselves.

The Authors

Picture sources: all from the individuals themselves

INDEX